D1685424

Biopsy Pathology of
Bone and Bone Marrow

BIOPSY PATHOLOGY SERIES

General Editors

Professor Leonard S. Gottlieb, MD, MPH
Mallory Institute of Pathology,
Boston, USA

Professor A. Munro Neville, MD, PhD, MRC Path.
Ludwig Institute for Cancer Research,
Sutton, UK

Professor F. Walker, MD, PhD
Department of Pathology,
University of Aberdeen, Scotland

Biopsy Pathology of Bone and Bone Marrow

B. FRISCH MD

Associate Professor of Haematology,
Institute of Haematology, Ichilov Hospital,
Sackler School of Medicine,
University of Tel Aviv, Israel

S. M. LEWIS BSc MD FRCPath.

Reader in Haematology,
Royal Postgraduate Medical School,
University of London,
and Consultant Haematologist,
Hammersmith Hospital,
London, UK

R. BURKHARDT Prof. Dr Med.

Head, Department of Bone Marrow Diagnosis,
Medical Clinic Innenstadt,
and of Haematology Department,
Society for Radiation and Environmental Research,
Munich, FRG

R. BARTL Prof. Dr Med.

Professor of Internal Medicine,
Department of Bone Marrow Diagnosis,
Medical Clinic Innenstadt,
Munich, FRG

LONDON
CHAPMAN AND HALL

First published 1985
by Chapman and Hall Ltd
11 New Fetter Lane, London EC4P 4EE
© *1985 Frisch, Lewis, Burkhardt and Bartl*
Printed in Great Britain at the
University Press, Cambridge

ISBN 0 412 24920 0

British Library Cataloguing in Publication Data
Biopsy pathology of bone and bone marrow.——
  (Biopsy pathology series)
  1. Marrow——Biopsy   2. Marrow——Diseases——
  Diagnosis   3. Bones——Biopsy
  I. Title   II. Frisch, B.   III. Series
  616.4'10758   RB55.2

ISBN 0-412-24920-0

Contents

To Professor U. Seligsohn
in appreciation of his encouragement
B.F.

Preface

Morphology has been the basis of haematology from the very beginning of this clinical and scientific discipline. Bone marrow aspiration by means of needle puncture has provided material for recognizing abnormal haematopoietic cells and for diagnosing blood diseases for over 50 years since M. J. Arinkin described (in *Folia Haematologica,* **38,** 233, 1929) the method for needle aspiration of the bone marrow. Smears made from aspirated samples and stained by one of the Romanowsky staining combinations provide excellent cytomorphological detail. However, because the distribution of haematopoietic cells differs from one area to another in the marrow, aspiration does not always reflect true distribution of cells in the marrow; nor will an aspiration demonstrate the spatial relationships of haematopoietic cells and their precursors within the marrow framework; nor the extent of marrow involvement in lymphomas and other malignant diseases, nor the effect of intramedullary diseases on bone, and that of osseous condition on the marrow.

Marrow biopsy by surgical trephine is an older procedure than needle aspiration; the earliest published reports of this technique include those of Pianese in 1903 who obtained marrow from the epiphyses of the femur and Ghedini in 1908 who trephined the upper third of the tibia. Subsequent workers developed the technique of trephine biopsy from sternum and from iliac crest. This became established as a diagnostic procedure to supplement a bone marrow puncture in haematological diagnosis. But the ease of aspiration contrasted with the difficulty in obtaining adequate material for sectioning, and the laborious procedure for preparing sections was hardly justified by the end product. Whilst the technique was helped by improved needle and trephine design, sections of decalcified biopsies remained a poor substitute for aspirated material in studying cell morphology.

In the past decade major changes have taken place—new needles have been developed ensuring that the biopsy can be carried out with little discomfort to the patient and with little or no damage to the biopsied tissue. Finally, methods of plastic embedding, largely pioneered by one of us (RB) enable the preparation of semi-thin and undecalcified sections of bone marrow which can then be stained to reveal cytological features in detail equal to that obtained with smeared cells, but without the artefact of the smearing. This has opened up a new field for investigating the pathophysiology of the bone and the bone marrow.

Traditionally, interpretation of bone marrow aspirates has been the responsibility of the haematologist whilst interpretation of sections has been the responsibility of the histopathologist who is equally concerned with the histology of the adjacent bone; but bone and bone marrow are intertwined tissues and the expression of their interdependence in practically every disease affecting either one or the other, has only recently been recognized. In addition biopsy is becoming an important tool for exploring the pathogenesis of cancer metastases, angiogenic and endothelial cell factors, the stimulus of cytotoxicity and other fundamental aspects of cellular biology. For essential diagnostic purposes and for the studies mentioned above, bone biopsy has become a procedure of importance equally to the haematologist and the histopathologist as well as to the general physician.

There are a relatively large number of atlases on blood cell morphology which amply illustrate the haematopoietic cells of the bone marrow. Conversely, there have been few atlases or textbooks dealing exclusively with the histological morphology of bone and bone marrow biopsies; our intention was to provide a comprehensive textbook illustrating the features which are likely to be encountered in trephine biopsies in various conditions, and to supplement the descriptive text with an outline of the pathophysiology based on the morphological features.

The nature of the subject requires illustrations and we hope that we have provided these in sufficient abundance to serve a useful purpose. The monochrome figures have been supplemented by 16 colour plates. The cost of these have been partly offset by a generous grant from the Gesellschaft für Strahlen- und Umweltforschung mbH, München.

This has enabled the publishers to keep the price of the book lower than would otherwise have been possible; for this and for invaluable editorial help we are grateful to Dr Peter Altman and Chapman and Hall Ltd. The authors would also like to express their gratitude to all colleagues who referred patients or sent biopsies, to the technical staff of the laboratories in which the work was undertaken and the photographic units where the photomicrographs and sketches were prepared. This work was supported by the Gesellschaft für Strahlen- und Umweltforschung mbH, Munich.

B. Frisch, S. M. Lewis, R. Burkhardt, R. Bartl

1 Introduction

In recent years the indications for bone marrow biopsy (BMB) have broadened, so that they are now employed in the investigation of many disorders in haematology, internal medicine, oncology and osteology (Burkhardt, 1971; Byers, 1977; Krause, 1981; Gruber *et al.*, 1981; Westerman, 1981; Burkhardt *et al.*, 1982; Rowden *et al.*, 1982; Bartl *et al.*, 1982). The upsurge of interest was spurred by improvements in instrumentation for taking BMB (Burkhardt, 1971; Jamshidi and Swaim, 1971) as well as in processing the undecalcified cores into plastic embedding media, thus providing optimal histology for evaluation in the light microscope (TeVelde *et al.*, 1977; Brinn, 1979; Takamiya *et al.*, 1980; Burkhardt, 1981; Westen *et al.*, 1981; Beckstead *et al.*, 1981; Moosavi *et al.*, 1981; Block *et al.*, 1982; Frisch *et al.*, 1982).

There have been previous atlases and textbooks describing results with wax-embedded biopsies (e.g. Krause, 1981). But because of the advantages of plastic embedding (and also because this technique is rapidly being adopted in many centres), this book is based on the results of biopsies embedded without decalcification. Moreover this book deals strictly with diagnosis of bone marrow histology, with the emphasis on the findings in iliac crest biopsies, as these are clinically the most widely used.

A list of biopsy instruments, description of the techniques for taking them, a method for the rapid processing of the biopsy cores and the most commonly used staining methods are given in the Appendix.

In view of the large number of papers on BMB which have appeared in the literature in the last few years since the early publications of Burkhardt (1971), Duhamel (1974), Block (1976), and Rywlin (1976) only recent review articles will be cited as far as possible. In addition, this book relies heavily on observations made in the authors' laboratories on over 30 000 biopsies. Due to the limitation of space, and because this is intended principally to be a diagnostic text for bone marrow histopathology, some conditions in which a bone biopsy is unlikely to be performed, have been omitted.

1

1.1   Patients

Bone marrow biopsies may be taken from patients at all ages from birth onwards. Specially designed needles are available for babies and very young children. Informed consent is obtained from the patients after the procedure has been fully explained, or from either parents or guardians if the patients are under the legal age for consent.

1.2   Biopsy sites

The anterior and the posterior iliac crests are the preferred sites from which the biopsies are taken after local anaesthesia (see p. 281). This does not apply to biopsies taken under radiological guidance (Burkhalter *et al.*, 1983) or surgical biopsies obtained under general anaesthesia in the operating theatre, when the site depends on the diagnostic requirements and the surgeon's choice. There are differences in the amounts of trabecular bone and marrow in different regions of the ilium, but these have no practical significance (Whitehouse, 1977; Whitehouse *et al.*, 1971). Likewise, the proportions of bone, parenchyme and fat vary in the different parts of the skeleton containing the red haematopoietic marrow, but the basic constituents are the same (Wintrobe, 1981; Trubowitz and Davies, 1982). For example, the volume percentages of trabecular bone are less, and those of the marrow cavities are greater in sternum and vertebral bodies, than in the ilium, and they also have a higher paren-chyme to fat ratio, (a factor contributing to the popularity of the sternum as a site for aspiration).

1.2.1   *Contra-indications and complications*

Bone biopsies are (relatively) contra-indicated in patients with bleeding disorders; if absolutely necessary, the same precautionary measures must be taken as for other operations in such patients. Infections occur rarely, about once in a thousand biopsies (see also Appendix, p. 282).

1.3   Biopsy instruments

There are two main groups of instruments, namely electric drill and manual trephines, various types of which are on the market (see Appendix). The drill is used for vertical, and the wide-bore manual trephine for horizontal trans-ilial biopsies—both provide relatively wide cylinders (4 mm and 8 mm respectively), and are recommended when histo-morphometric measurements of cortical and trabecular bone are envisaged.

However, in most cases the 11 or 8 gauge trephines (2 or 3 mm width) are employed and the biopsies are taken from the superior spinous process of the posterior iliac crest. The length of these biopsies varies, but may reach 3–4 cm (details for the use of the different instruments are given in the Appendix). Representative sections of biopsies taken with the various needles are shown in Figs. 1.1 and 1.2.

In a retrospective series of 15 000 biopsies taken with the electric drill,

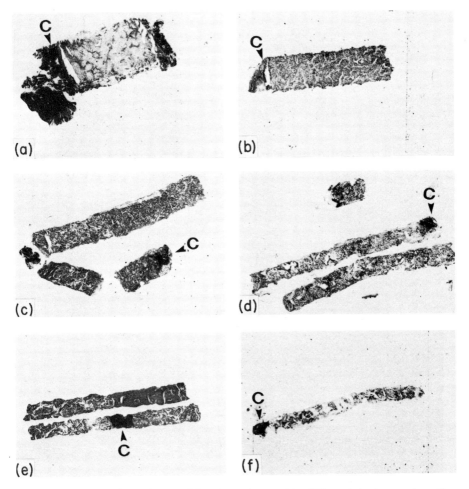

Fig. 1.1 Examples of bone biopsies taken with different instruments, all photographed at the same magnification. Actual sizes: (a) transilial 7 × 18 mm; (b) myelotomy drill 4 × 17 mm; (c) disposable regular bore 2 × 20, 2 × 22 mm; (d) Islam needle 2 × 22 mm; (e) Islam needle 2 × 25 mm; (f) Jamshidi, regular bore 1.5 × 21 mm. c = cortex.

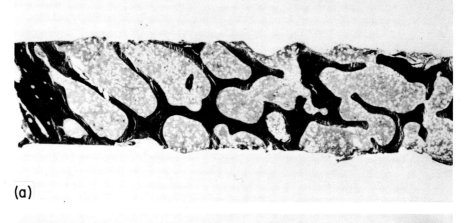

(a)

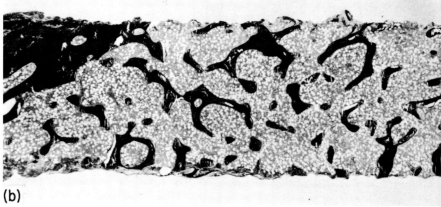

(b)

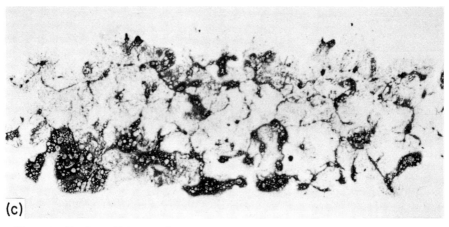

(c)

Fig. 1.2 Section of biopsy taken (a) with the Jamshidi needle. × 10, Gomori; (b) with the electric drill. × 10, Gomori; (c) biopsy imprint. × 10, Giemsa.

about 1% were inadequate; and about 10% of 18 000 taken with the Jamshidi needle. However, with the recent modifications and new models of the manual trephines, the results with both methods are comparable.

Scintigraphic investigation of the ilium after bone biopsies revealed no abnormalities when the biopsies had been taken with the manual trephines (Tyler and Powers, 1982). Previous studies on biopsies taken from the sternum, the thoracic and lumbar vertebrae and the iliac crest, have demonstrated that the iliac crest biopsy may be regarded as representative of the haematopoietic marrow, though there are quantitative differences in the amount of bone present (Whitehouse, 1977; Bartl *et al.*, 1982).

1.4   Indications

A long list of indications has now been established in haematology, internal medicine, oncology and osteology; it can be summarized as follows:

(1) In all cases in which aspiration of the bone marrow is considered as a diagnostic procedure there are advantages in taking a biopsy at the same time. The patient is psychologically prepared, the local anaesthetic will have been administered, and the mental and physical stress of another procedure later on will be avoided. Moreover, since aspiration and biopsy are complementary procedures, if the biopsy is omitted, the physician does not get the maximum information and therefore the patient does not have the full benefit of the investigation.

(2) In all conditions that might affect the bone, either primarily or secondarily.

(3) Clarification of numerous other disorders, such as infections, including toxo- and histoplasmosis (Jones and Goodwin, 1981), granulomatous conditions, amyloidosis, vascular disease, pyrexia of unknown origin, and the effects of metabolic disturbances (Kass, 1979; Krause, 1981; Frisch *et al.*, 1982).

(4) Whenever a dry tap or insufficient material is obtained on aspiration.

(5) In all patients with suspected or clinically established myelo- and lymphoproliferative disorders, other malignancies, myelodysplastic states, cytopenias, storage diseases and assessments of haematopoietic tissue for whatever reason (Burkhardt *et al.*, 1982; Bartl *et al.*, 1982; Frisch *et al.*, 1982).

(6) For monitoring of therapy or the evolution of the disease process, detection of residual foci of malignant cells; for assessment of the marrow

before and after autografts and transplants (Golembe *et al.*, 1979; Wittels, 1980; Chessels *et al.*, 1981).

1.5   Evaluation of iliac crest biopsies

Sections of biopsies illustrating the range of normal quantitative relationships between cortical and trabecular bone, haematopoietic and adipose tissue, and their topographic inter-relationships are shown in Fig. 1.2.

Most of the cortex of the anterior part of the iliac crest is porous (Whitehouse, 1977), about 25% void, and of varying thickness (Figs 1.3 and 1.4); moreover the thickness of the trabecular bone is also very variable. The same most probably also applies to the posterior part of the ilium. It is important to bear these considerations in mind especially when histomorphometric measurements and comparative studies are made and conclusions drawn from them.

Histomorphometric measurements are given in Table 1.1 and Fig. 1.5. Only sections without crushing or distortion artefacts and containing at least 5 but preferably more architecturally well-preserved marrow spaces should be used for qualitative and quantitative assessments (Fig. 1.6). When histomorphometric measurements are planned, a surface area of 60–80 mm^2 is required for reliable and representative measurements. This may be done with or without computerized evaluation of results and calculation of their correlations and statistical significance (Dixon and Brown, 1979).

1.5.1   Histomorphometry

This refers to the quantitative evaluation of any of the components or parameters of bone and marrow (Bordier *et al.*, 1964; Kerndrup *et al.*, 1980; Bartl *et al.*, 1982). Plastic embedded material is always used for histomorphometry, to avoid the shrinkage inherent in decalcification and paraffin embedding (Lane and Ralis, 1983).

There are several ways in which histomorphometry may be performed:

(1) Subjective assessment by naked eye of the structures and components of the biopsy section as observed in a number of fields in the light microscope (Hennig, 1975).

(2) Assessment by means of a graticule in the ocular (Merz and Schenk, 1970); for example, see Table 1.2.

(3) Semi-automatic or automatic measurements with or without computerized evaluation of the results, their correlations and their statistical significance (Malluche *et al.*, 1982a, b; Revell, 1983). Comparative studies have recently demonstrated the reliability of histomorphometric

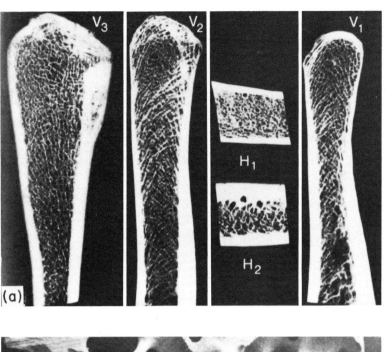

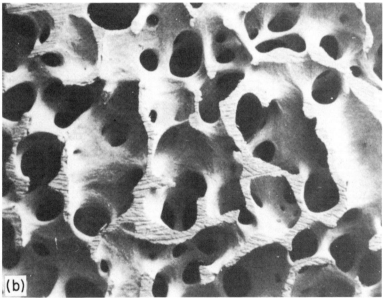

Fig. 1.3 (a) Vertical sections through the anterior part of the ilium from a 25 year old woman (accidental death) showing the variability in structure and thickness of the cortical bone; taken at different levels from along the ilium; (b) Scanning electron microscope view of representative cancellous bone structure of iliac crest. (Reproduced with permission from: W. J. Whitehouse. Cancellous bone in the anterior part of the iliac crest. *Calcif. Tissue Res.*, **26,** 67–76, 1977.)

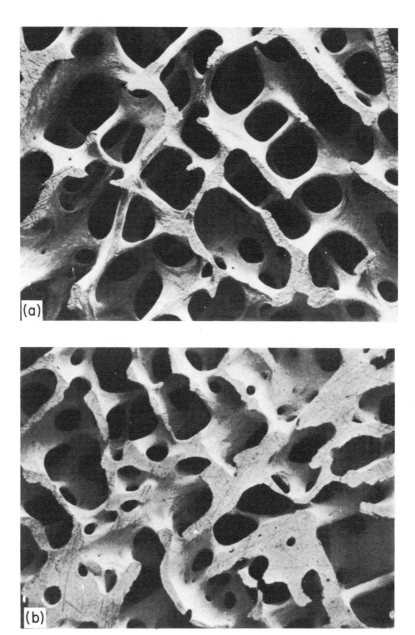

Fig. 1.4 Scanning electron microscope pictures of cancellous bone from Section V2 in Fig. 1.3, about 30 mm from the iliac crest, showing variability in cancellous bone structure. (a) usual range; (b) wide trabecular. (From W. J. Whitehouse. Cancellous bone in the anterior part of the iliac crest. *Calcif. Tissue Res.*, **26**, 67–76, 1977.)

Table 1.1 Histomorphometry of normal bone and bone marrow[1]

Variables	Mean value (SD)		Dimension
Haematopoietic tissue	40	(9)	Vol %
Fatty tissue	28	(8)	
Trabecular bone	26	(5)	
Osteoid	0.3	(0.2)	
Sinusoids	4.5	(2.1)	
H/F Index[2]	1.4		
G/E Index[3]	2.8		
Lymphocytes (diffuse)	20	(12)	/mm²
Mast cells	2	(1)	
Megakaryocytes	8	(4)	
Macrophages (containing iron)	16	(10)	
Plasma cells	21	(18)	
Lymphoid nodules	2		%
Arteries	3	(4)	/100mm²
Arterioles	26	(18)	
Capillaries	101	(61)	
Sinusoids	1700	(825)	
Osteoblastic Index (OB)[4]	5	(5)	%
Osteoclastic Index (OC)[5]	4	(3)	/100 mm

[1] These values are derived from 158 biopsies of normal healthy individuals.
[2] H/F Index = haematopoietic tissue (vol%)/fatty tissue (vol%).
[3] G/E Index = granulopoietic cells (n)/erythropoietic cells (n).
[4] OB = percentage of trabecular circumference covered by cuboidal osteoblasts.
[5] OC = number of osteoclasts per 100 mm trabecular circumference.

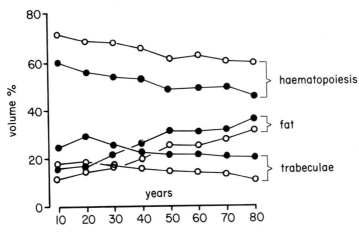

Fig. 1.5 Quantitative estimation of haematopoiesis, fat and trabecular bone in bone biopsies of 158 individuals without evidence of disease. Note steady decline in haematopoiesis and trabecular bone with increasing age.
● = iliac crest, o = lumbar vertebrae.

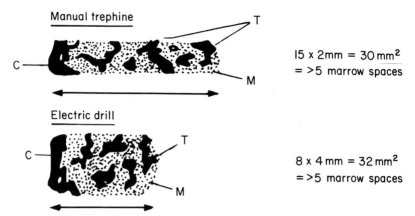

Manual trephine

15 x 2mm = 30 mm² = >5 marrow spaces

Electric drill

8 x 4 mm = 32 mm² = >5 marrow spaces

Fig. 1.6 Minimal biopsy size for diagnostic evaluation. C = cortical bone, T = trabecular bone, M = marrow. If the sub-cortical areas are occupied by fat cells as frequently happens in patients over 60 years, a correspondingly larger area is required.

Table 1.2 Histomorphometric correlations in various diseases

	Trab. bone vol%	Haematopoiesis vol%	Fat vol%	Osteoblast index	Osteoclast index
Normal 42(15–74)[+]	25[++] 20–32	54 40–63	21 8–31	4 1–8	5 0–9
Hyperparathyroid (HPT) 51(25–66)	23 14–33	42 18–46	27 18–86	18 6–81	20 16–109
Osteoporosis 45(26–78)	14 6–19	42 18–51	42 32–52	5 1–7	6 0–9
Paget's disease 63(48–81)	48 12–82	5 0–32	18 4–28	24 6–64	13 2–42
Polycythaemia vera 56(32–76)	21 15–28	62 34–85	12 0–18	7 0–11	2 0–5
CML 46(26–96)	20 10–29	75 62–90	2 0–16	5 1–8	2 0–4
Myelofibrosis/ osteomyclosclerosis 57(37–74)	32 21–69	33 12–41	14 4–28	5 2–16	5 1–8
Aplasia 49(34–81)	23 8–28	22 3–31	53 46–82	3 0–6	4 0–8
Multiple myeloma 61(33–84)	23 2–41	28 0–35	26 0–44	9 2–18	22 12–62

+ Age, mean (range in brackets).
++ All upper numbers are mean values; lower numbers show range.
Osteoblast Index = % of trabecular circumference covered by cuboidal osteoblasts.
Osteoclast Index = No. of osteoclasts per 100 mm trabecular circumference.
Measurements were made by means of an ocular graticule.

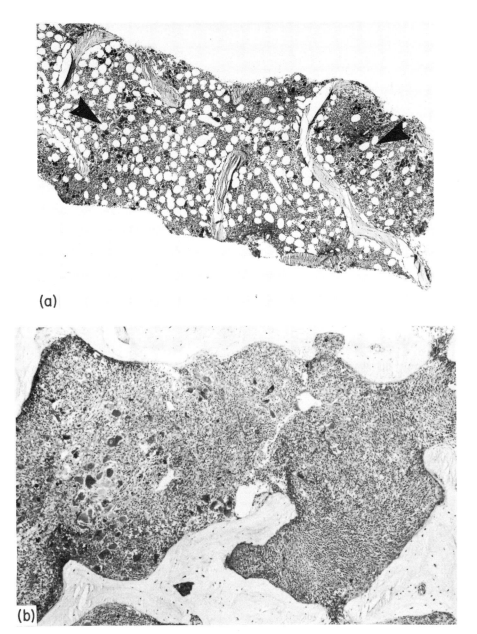

Fig. 1.7 Unequal distribution of cell lines in the marrow in myeloproliferative disease; (a) mature megakaryocytic myelosis, evident only in spaces indicated by arrows (right and left). × 60, Giemsa; (b) in chronic myeloid leukaemia. Left: marrow space both granulocytic and megakaryocytic; right: only granulocytic hyperplasia. × 100, Giemsa.

measurements of trabecular bone (Schwartz and Recker, 1981; de Vernejoul *et al.*, 1981).

(4) Functional studies by means of tetracycline labelling (Fallon and Teitelbaum, 1981).

1.5.2   *Pitfalls in histological diagnosis*

(1) Histological variation within the biopsy (Fig. 1.7).
(2) Subcortical hypoplasia.

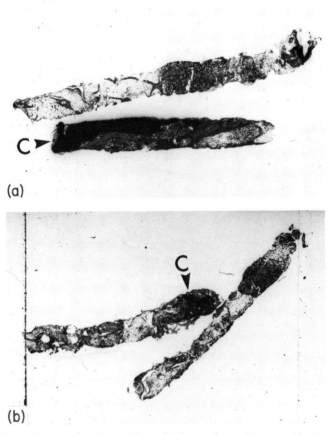

(a)

(b)

Fig. 1.8   Bone biopsy of patient with multiple myeloma diagnosed by this biopsy; actual biopsy size 2 × 15, 17, 18 and 22 mm. (a) and (b): two cores taken from adjacent spots on the anaesthetized area, each cut into two pieces and blocked separately; note hypercellular and aplastic areas. C = cortex. × 4.

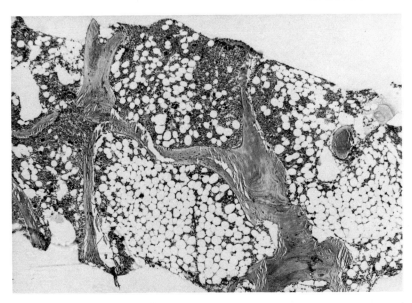

Fig. 1.9 Section of bone biopsy of 33 year old patient with thrombocytosis, after colectomy for carcinoma of the colon. Note variability in marrow cellularity, no increase in megakaryocytes. × 40, Giemsa.

(3) Alternating fatty and hyperplastic areas in deeper parts of the biopsy (Figs. 1.8, 1.9), and concentration of one cell type in single marrow spaces (Fig. 1.7).

(4) Presence of misleading artefacts. It should be remembered that artefacts are easily produced when taking bone biopsies—for example pieces of epidermis, skeletal muscle, cartilage or bone may be displaced into the biopsy, and it is important to recognize them for what they are. In addition, changes in the haematopoietic cells may be due to a variety of technical errors in processing. Some of these common artefacts are illustrated in Fig. 1.10.

Diagnostic evaluation. This is made in the first instance with respect to the histological and histopathological findings *per se* (Table 1.3); then, taking account of the patient's clinical status and the results of other diagnostic procedures, and thirdly together with the peripheral blood smear and the smears of the bone marrow aspirate and/or the imprints of the biopsy. In addition, where necessary, account is also taken of enzyme and marker studies, smears, imprints, or cryostat sections (Zucker-Franklin *et al.*, 1981).

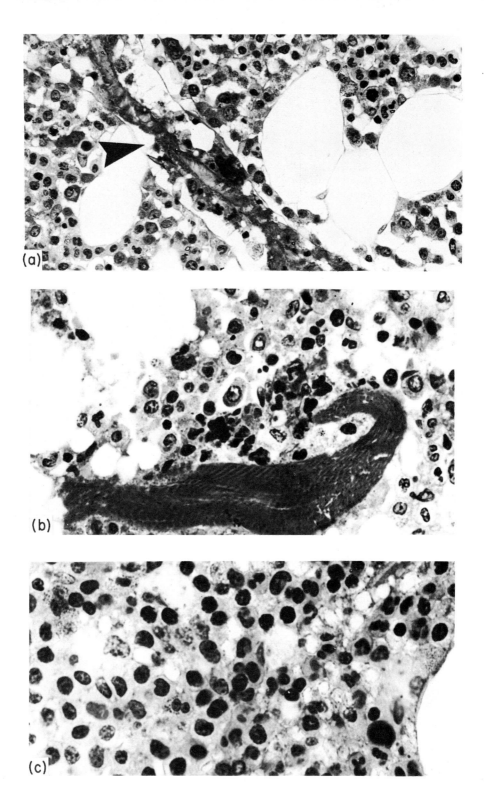

(a)

(b)

(c)

Table 1.3 Evaluation of bone marrow biopsy sections

1. Periosteal tissues and cortical bone
2. Trabecular bone marrow, overall architecture
3. Trabecular bone—normal range
   osteoporosis: osteolysis
   osteomalacia
   osteosclerosis—appositional, woven, both
4. Remodelling—reduced/increased
   osteoblasts—reduced/increased
   osteoclasts—reduced/increased
   osteocytes
5. Haematopoiesis/fat—normal range
                        other
   Erythropoiesis maturation
   Myelopoiesis maturation
   Megakaryocytes maturation
6. Stroma   fat   ferrum
             fibres   phagocytes
             vessels   lymphoid cells
                        plasma cells
                        mast cells
7. Artefacts
8. Malignant cells
9. Summary: Bone marrow findings in context
                     of all clinical and other tests
                     available; differential diagnosis
10. Diagnosis (when possible); remarks; recommendations

References

Bartl, R., Frisch, B., and Burkhardt, R. (1982), *Bone Marrow Biopsies Revisited. A New Dimension for Haematologic Malignancies*, Karger, Basel.

Beckstead, J. H., Halverson, P. S., Ries, C. A. and Bainton, D. F. (1981), Enzyme histochemistry and immunohistochemistry on biopsy specimens of pathologic human bone marrow. *Blood*, **57**, 1088–98.

Block, M. (1976), *Text Atlas of Hematology*, Lea and Febiger, Philadelphia.

Block, M. H., Trenner, L., Ruegg, P. and Karr, M. (1982), Glycol methacrylate embedding technique emphasizing cost containment, ultrarapid processing, and adaptability to a variety of staining techniques. *Lab. Med.*, **13**, 290–8.

Bordier, F., Matrait, H., Miravet, L. and Hioco, D. (1965), Mesure histologique de la masse et de la resorption des travees osseuses. *Pathol. Biol.*, **12**, 1238–43.

Brinn, N. T. (1979), Glycol methacrylate for routine, special stains, histochemistry, enzyme histochemistry and immunohistochemistry. A simplified cold method for surgical biopsy tissue. *J. Histochem.*, **3**, 125–30.

Fig. 1.10   Artefacts in bone marrow biopsies: (a) debris and bone within a sinus (arrow); (b) striated muscle fibres; (c) loss of nuclear detail due to inadequate fixation. × 400, Giemsa.

Burkhalter, J. L., Patel, B. R. and Harrison, R. B. (1983), Radionuclide bone scan as an aid in localizing lesion for bone biopsy. *Skeletal Radiol.*, **9**, 246–7.

Burkhardt, R. (1971), *Bone Marrow and Bone Tissue: Colour Atlas of Clinical Histopathology*, Springer-Verlag, Berlin.

Burkhardt, R. (1981), Bone marrow histology. In *Methods in Hematology. The Leukemic Cell* (ed. D. Catovsky), Churchill Livingstone, Edinburgh, pp. 49–86.

Burkhardt, R., Frisch, B. and Bartl, R. (1982), Bone biopsy in haematological disorders. *J. Clin. Path.*, **35**, 257–84.

Byers, P. D. (1977), The diagnostic value of bone biopsies. In *Metabolic Bone Disease, Vol. 1* (eds L. V. Avioli and S. M. Krane), Academic Press, New York, pp. 183–236.

Chessels, J. M. and Breatnach, F. (1981), Late marrow recurrences in childhood acute lymphoblastic leukemia. *Brit. med. J.*, **283**, 749–51.

Dixon, W. J. and Brown, M. B. (eds) (1979), *BMDP Biomedical Computer Programs*, University of California Press, Berkeley.

Duhamel, G. (1974), *Histopathologie Clinique de la Moelle Osseuse*, Masson et Cie, Paris.

Fallon, M. D. and Teitelbaum, S. L. (1981), A simple procedure for the rapid histologic diagnosis of metabolic bone disease. *Calcif. Tissue Int.*, **33**, 281–3.

Frisch, B., Bartl, R. and Burkhardt, R. (1982), Bone marrow biopsy in clinical medicine: An overview. *Haematologia*, **3**, 245–85.

Golembe, B., Ramsay, N. K., McKenna, R., Nesbit, M. E. and Krivit, W. (1979), Localised bone marrow relapse in acute lymphoblastic leukemia. *Med. Pediat. Oncol.*, **6**, 229–34.

Gruber, H. E., Staufer, M. E., Thompson, E. R. and Baylink, D. J. (1981), Diagnosis of bone disease by core biopsies. *Sem. Haemat.*, **18**, 258–78.

Hennig, A. (1975), Kritische Betrachtungen zur Volumen- und Oberflächenmessung in der Mikroskopie. *Zeiss Werkzeitschr*, **30**, 78–86.

Jamshidi, J. and Swaim, R. W. (1971), Bone marrow biopsy with unaltered architecture: a new biopsy device. *J. Lab. Clin. Med.*, **77**, 335–42.

Jones, R. C. and Goodwin, R. A. (1981), Histoplasmosis of bone. *Am. J. Med.*, **70**, 864–6.

Kass, L. (1979), *Bone Marrow Interpretation*, J. Lippincott, Philadelphia.

Kerndrup, G., Pallesen, G., Melsen, F. and Mosekilde, L. (1980), Histomorphometrical determination of bone marrow cellularity in iliac crest biopsies. *Scand. J. Haematol.*, **24**, 110–14.

Krause, J. R. (1981), *Bone Marrow Biopsy*, Churchill Livingstone, Edinburgh

Lane, J. and Ralis, Z. A. (1983), Changes in dimensions of large cancellous bone specimens during histological preparation as measured on slabs from human femoral heads. *Calcif. Tissue Int.*, **35**, 1–4.

Malluche, H. H., Meyer, W., Sherman, D. and Massry, S. G. (1982a) Quantitative bone histology in 84 normal American subjects. *Calcif. Tissue Int.*, **34**, 449–55.

Malluche, H., Sherman, D., Meyer, W. and Massry, S. G. (1982b), A new semiautomatic method for quantitative static and dynamic bone histology. *Calcif. Tissue Int.*, **34**, 439–48.

Merz, W. A. and Schenk, R. K. (1970), Quantitative structural analysis of human cancellous bone. *Acta Anatomica*, **75**, 54–66.

Moosavi, H., Lichtman, M. A., Donnelly, J. A. and Churukian, C. J. (1981), Plastic-embedded human marrow biopsy specimens. *Arch. Pathol. Lab. Med.*, **105**, 269–73.

Revell, P. A. (1983), Histomorphometry of bone. *J. clin. Path.*, **36**, 1323–31.

Rowden, G., Sacher, R. A. and More, N. S. (1982), Plastic embedded specimens for evaluation of bone marrow. In *Topical Reviews in Haematology*, Vol. II (ed. S. Roath), Wright, Bristol.

Rywlin, A. M. (1976), *Histopathology of the Bone Marrow*, Brown and Company, Boston.

Schwartz, M. P. and Recker, R. R. (1981), Clinical investigation: comparison of surface density and volume of human iliac trabecular bone measured directly and by applied stereology. *Calcif, Tissue Int.*, **33**, 561–5.

Takamiya, H., Batsford, S. and Vogt, A. (1980), An approach to postembedding staining of protein (immunoglobulin) antigen embedded in plastic: prerequisites and limitations. *J. Histochem. Cytochem.*, **28**, 1041–9.

Trubowitz, S. and Davies, S. (eds) (1982), *The Human Bone Marrow Anatomy, Physiology and Pathophysiology*, Vols I and II, CRC Press, Boca Raton, Florida.

Tyler, J. L. and Powers, T. A. (1982), Bone scanning after marrow biopsy. *J. nucl. Med.*, **23**, 1985–7.

TeVelde, J., Burkhardt, R., Kleiverda, K., Leenheers-Binnendijk, L. and Sommerfeld, W. (1977), Methyl-methacrylate as an embedding medium in histopathology. *Histopathology*, **1**, 319–30.

de Vernejoul, M. D., Kuntz, D., Miravet, L., Goutallier, D. and Ryckewaert, A. (1981), Bone histomorphometric reproducibility in normal patients.*Calcif. Tissue Int.*, **33**, 369–74.

Westen, H., Mück, K.-F. and Post, L. (1981), Enzyme histochemistry on bone marrow sections after embedding in methacrylate at low temperature. *Histochemistry*, **70**, 95–105.

Westerman, M. P. (1981), Bone marrow needle biopsy: an evaluation and critique. *Sem. Haematol.*, **18**, 293–300.

Whitehouse, W. J., Dyson, E. D. and Jackson, C. K. (1971), The scanning electron microscope in studies of trabecular bone from a human vertebral body. *J. Anat.*, **108**, 481–96.

Whitehouse, W. J. (1977), Cancellous bone in the anterior part of the iliac crest. *Calcif. Tissue Res.*, **23**, 67–76.

Wintrobe, M. M. (1981), *Clinical Hematology*, 8th edn., Lee and Febiger, Philadelphia.

Wittels, B. (1980), Bone marrow biopsy. Changes following chemotherapy for acute leukemia. *Am. J. Surg. Path.*, **4**, 135–42.

Zucker-Franklin, D., Greaves, M. F., Grossin, C. E. and Marmont, A. M. (1981), *Atlas of Blood Cells: Function and Pathology*, Lea and Febiger, Philadelphia.

2 Normal bone and bone marrow

2.1 Definition of terms

2.1.1 Osteons

The osteons are cylindrical structures (which may be branching) composed of concentric layers (or lamellae) of bone (Fig. 2.1b) disposed around a central (Haversian) canal within which are capillaries and venules. As the osteons are oriented in the long axis of the bones, they provide mechanical strength along the stress lines.

2.1.2 Cortical bone (cortex)

This is seen in BMB as a layer of compact bone of variable thickness (Fig. 2.1) to which the periosteum is attached on the outside and which is lined with a single layer of cells, the endosteum, on the inside (Figs 2.1a and 2.2a). Osseous remodelling, as indicated by the presence of osteoclasts in the scalloped niches (Howship's lacunae) and by a row of cuboidal osteoblasts on a layer of osteoid (Figs 2.2b, 2.3a) (unmineralized bone) or on the trabecular surface, is often present in the sub-cortical regions even when the cancellous bone is almost devoid of it. There is a delicate balance between bone formation and resorption in which highly complex regulatory mechanisms are involved (Rodan and Martin, 1981; Raisz and Kream, 1983).

Fig. 2.1 Sections of biopsies of posterior iliac crest to illustrate cortical bone structure: (a) layer of compact bone with lamellar arrangement (arrow) × 40, Giemsa; (b) compact bone showing Haversian systems (arrows). × 100, Giemsa; (c) cortex with few spaces. × 100, Giemsa; (d) cortical bone showing porosity. × 20, Gomori; C = cortex, P = periosteum, M = marrow.

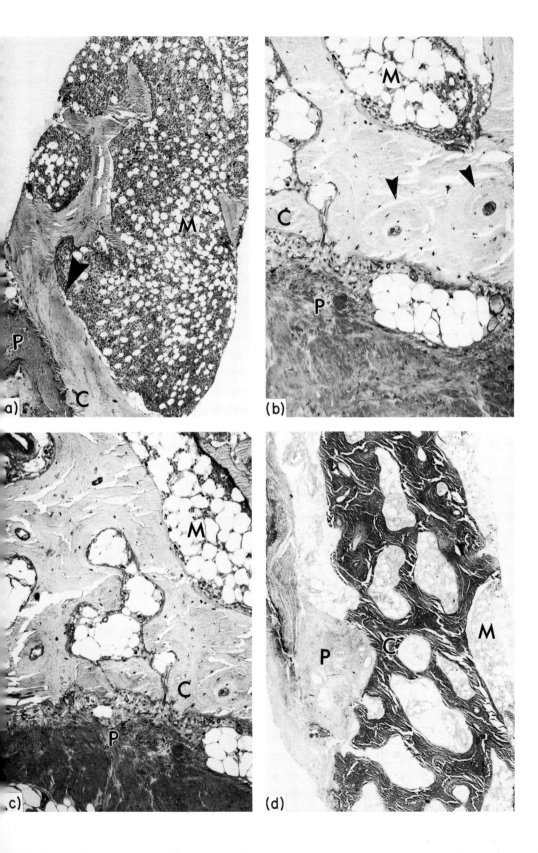

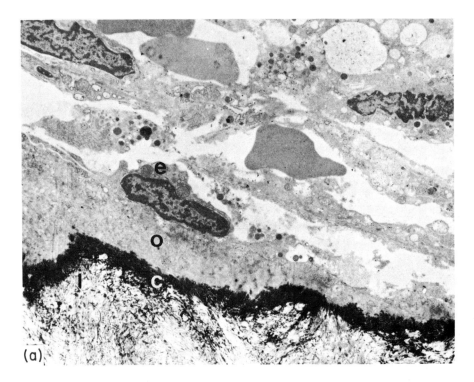

(a)

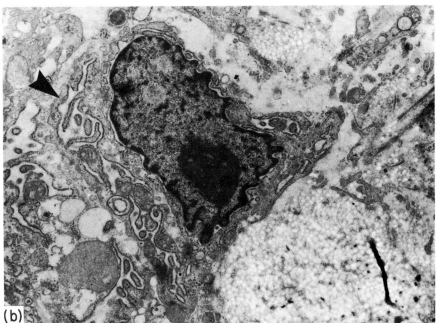

(b)

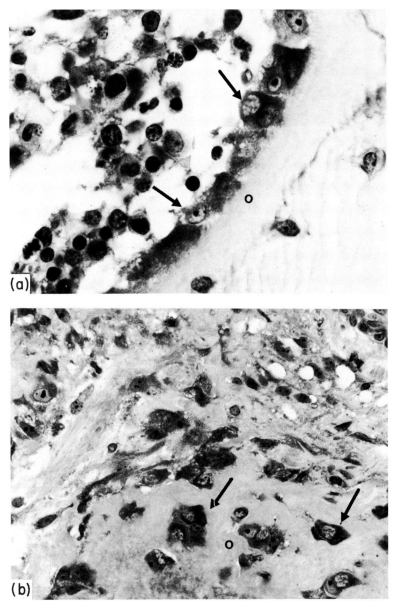

Fig. 2.3 (a) Appositional new bone formation: layer of osteoblasts (arrows) on trabecular surface; (b) osteoblastic bone formation, entrapment of osteoblasts (arrows) in the newly-formed osteoid (o) in their transition to osteocytes. × 800, Giemsa.

Fig. 2.2 (a) Electron micrograph showing trabecular bone surface with endosteal lining cells (e), layer of osteoid (o) and calcification front (c), lumen of sinus and endothelial cells, upper left and right. × 3700; (b) electron micrograph showing active osteoblast on trabecular bone surface; note dilated endoplasmic reticulum (arrow), and large nucleolus. × 6400.

2.1.3   Trabecular bone (cancellous bone, trabeculae, ossicles) (Plate Ia)

This refers to the honeycomb of bone (Figs 1.3 and 1.4) which partitions the space enclosed by the cortical bone and which is lined by the endosteum continuous with that of the cortices.

Osteopenia (or osteoporosis) signifies a reduced trabecular bone volume, mostly due to attenuation (rarefaction) with the consequent enlargement of the marrow cavities.

Osteosclerosis means thickening of the cancellous bone resulting in a decrease in size of the intertrabecular cavities (or marrow spaces).

2.1.4   Osteoblasts

These are cells that produce bone matrix. They arise, or develop, out of progenitor cells in the stroma 'mesenchyme' of the bone marrow, and also from the endosteal cells lining the surfaces of the cancellous bone; indeed, these are looked upon by some as a resting form of osteoblasts (Plate Id). When activated, they become cuboidal (Fig. 2.2b) and fibres and blood vessels in the vicinity appear more prominent. Occasionally (in the light microscope) there appears to be direct continuity as well as contiguity between the endosteal cells and the endothelial cells of the paratrabecular sinusoids. In this context it is worth noting that both the endosteal cells and the endothelial cells in their proximity have PAS-positive droplets in their cytoplasm while this is absent from the endothelial cells of the sinusoids further away. In areas of increased osseous remodelling, especially obvious in tangential cuts, the osteoblasts may form several layers. Osteoblasts lay down the bone matrix, osteoid, which later becomes mineralized to form lamellar bone (Frost, 1962). Following deposition of osteoid and its mineralization, the osteoblasts within that layer are enclosed and embedded in their own matrix and thus become osteocytes (Plate Ie) whose processes connect by means of the canaliculi with those of other osteocytes and with the osteoblasts on the surface of the bone (Figs 2.3–2.5). Thus, an osseous circulatory system is formed: this guarantees the sustenance of the osteocytes, exchange and transfer between bone and the intercellular (interstitial) fluid and the bloodstream. Moreover, it is thought that this is one mechanism by which the osteocytes participate in the homeostasis of minerals, and respond to stimuli, e.g. to initiate osteocytic osteolysis.

2.1.5   Osteoclasts

These are cells that resorb bone. They have 1–6 nuclei, and are found on the trabecular bone surface, in association with the endothelia of blood

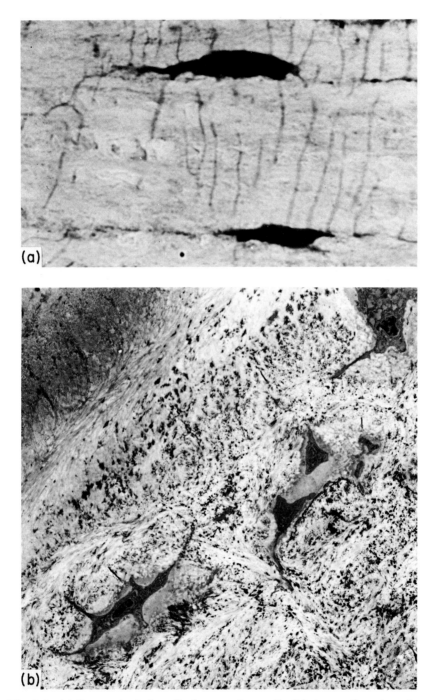

Fig. 2.4 (a) Osteocytes in lamellar bone; note canaliculi between the osteocytes. × 1200; (b) lamellar bone with osteocytes; note nuclei, cytoplasm and cytoplasmic processes in canaliculi; electron micrograph. × 2000.

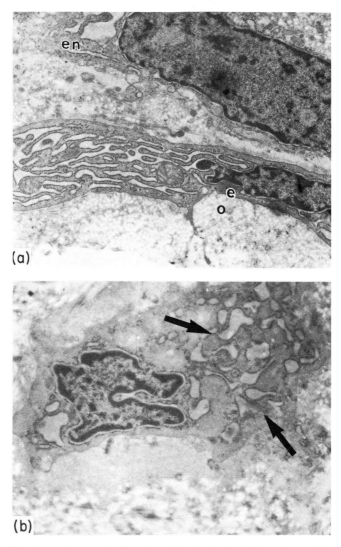

Fig. 2.5 Electron micrograph showing (a) endosteal cell (e) on layer of osteoid (o) with endothelial cell (en) above; note cisternae of endoplastic reticulum; (b) osteocyte in lacuna; note nucleus with only peripheral condensation of chromatin and dilated cisterna of endoplasmic reticulum (arrows). × 10 000.

Fig. 2.6 Electron micrographs: (a) part of osteoclast in Howship's lacuna; note nuclei and fragment of bone in cytoplasmic vacuole (arrow); bone at left and lower part of picture, ruffled membrane of osteoclast at right. × 10 000; (b) higher magnification of area indicated by arrow in (a); note folds of ruffled membrane at left, bone at right. × 40 000.

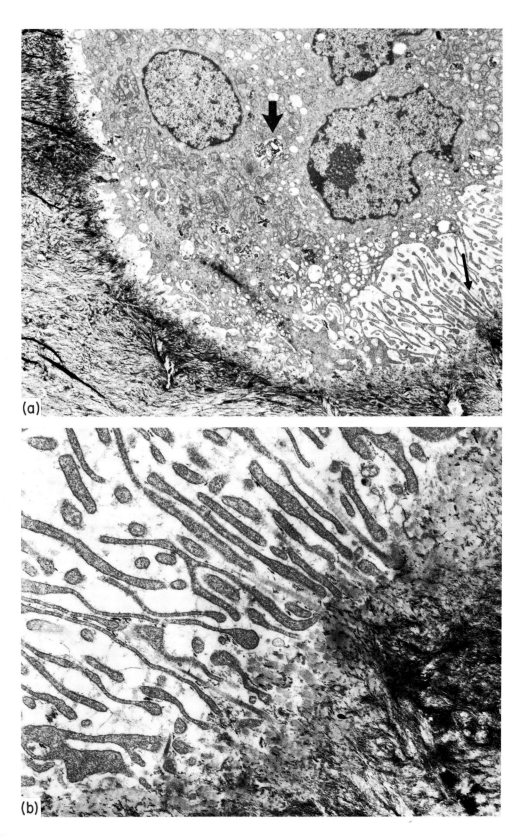

vessels; in the erosion cavities Howship's lacunae occur on both cortical and cancellous bone (Plate Ic; Fig. 2.6).

Osteoclasts may be observed interposed between adjacent endothelial and endosteal cells as well as between bone and endothelium on the trabecular and sub-cortical bone surfaces, especially on the resorbing surfaces (Chambers, 1980; Jonell, 1980).

In some disease states and after certain physiological stimuli there appears to be an association between the number of nuclei and activity; however, it is now believed that the relatively flat and uni-nucleated osteoclasts are also able to (and do) resorb bone. Osteoclastic resorption is accompanied by increase in blood vessels and blood flow (a classic example is Paget's disease). Recent experimental studies appear to have elucidated the origin of osteoclasts—they are now thought to develop from a precursor of the monocytic series, i.e. they belong to the haematopoietic cell lines (Owen, 1980; Loutit and Nisbet, 1982). However, from a morphological point of view, cells with the cytological characteristics of osteoclasts may be seen in areas of stimulated mesenchyme, as well as in close proximity to blood vessels and their endothelium. In these situations there appears to be a close association between the developing mesenchymal cells, the endothelial cells of the blood vessels, the endosteal cells, the osteoblasts and the osteoclasts. It should be noted that mitotic figures in cells that are identified unequivocally as osteoclasts are extremely rare and it is assumed that these multi-nucleated cells arise by means of coalescence; endomitosis may also contribute to osteoclast multinuclearity. Whether osteoclasts derive exclusively from the monocytic series, or also from local precursors or progenitors in the stimulated mesenchyme is not yet fully clarified. However, as noted earlier, physiological processes in the bone marrow are extremely rapid, may leave little or no trace and, therefore, extreme caution should be exercised in the interpretation of, and drawing conclusions from one-time snap-shot observations made on bone-marrow morphology.

2.2   Bone marrow

This term is generally used to refer to the tissue occupying the cavities between the trabecular bone. Normal marrow is either red, containing the

---

Fig. 2.7   (a) Bone biopsy section of 12 year old child, showing cellular bone marrow throughout the section; (b) bone biopsy of adult showing a normocellular bone marrow, which has more fat than that of the child; (c) bone biopsy section, elderly individual; overall cellularity is reduced especially in the sub-cortical regions (left); note also striking patchy reduction in trabecular bone (arrows). All × 25, Gomori.

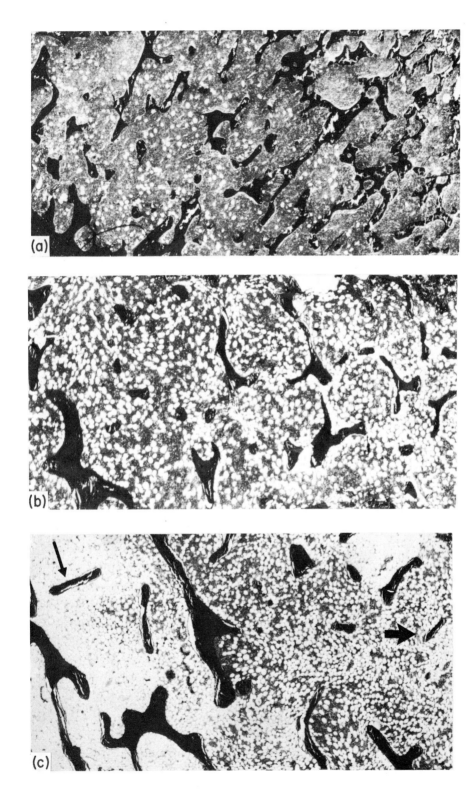

haematopoietic elements, or yellow, composed mainly of adipose tissue (fat cells) (Plate Ib). In the adult, red marrow is found in the skull, sternum, clavicles, scapulae, vertebrae, ribs, pelvic bones and the proximal ends of the long bones. The weight of the bone marrow is 1600–3700 g, approximately the same as the liver. The red marrow weighs about 1000 g. Why haematopoiesis in the adult organism is confined to these bones is not clear. Stem cells circulate in the peripheral blood and 'home' to the bone marrow. Under special circumstances other bones and organs—liver, spleen, lymph nodes—also support haematopoiesis. With advancing age, there is a reduction in the trabecular bone volume and the numbers of associated endosteal cells, osteocytes and para-trabecular sinusoids (Fig. 2.7). Haematopoietic tissue is also decreased, accompanied by an increase in fat cells, particularly in the sub-cortical regions (Fig. 2.7) (Mauch *et al.*, 1981; Williams *et al.*, 1981). However, there is a great individual variability in these age (and sex) related changes. They are not consistently observed, and they may be influenced by numerous other factors. In addition, other cells normally present in the bone marrow, such as lymphocytes, plasma cells and mast cells, may show increases in the bone marrows of older people (see below).

2.3   Marrow cellularity

This refers to both haematopoietic and fat cells and it indicates the relative amounts of these two components (Plate Ib). *Normocellular* implies marrow with approximately the proportions given in Table 1.1 and illustrated in Fig. 2.8. *Hypocellular* indicates a reduction in haematopoiesis and a corresponding increase in fat cells. *Hypercellular* is used when the fat is decreased and replaced by other elements. A concomitant reduction in haematopoietic tissue and trabecular bone is frequently observed.

These spatial differences represent potential pitfalls as mentioned earlier, especially the sub-cortical hypoplasia which frequently occurs in older individuals. Selective hypoplasia in the iliac crest has also been observed in certain conditions, (Ferrant *et al.*, 1980), such as auto-immune states, and it may be seen after radiotherapy to that region.

2.4   Topography

The haematopoietic tissue is distributed in the marrow spaces in the

---

Fig. 2.8   (a) Section illustrating normal bone marrow cellularity; note small blood vessels (arrow) with plasma cells, megakaryocytes, myelopoiesis and erythropoiesis. × 250, Giemsa; (b) higher magnification showing arteriole; note perivascular plasma cells. × 400, Giemsa.

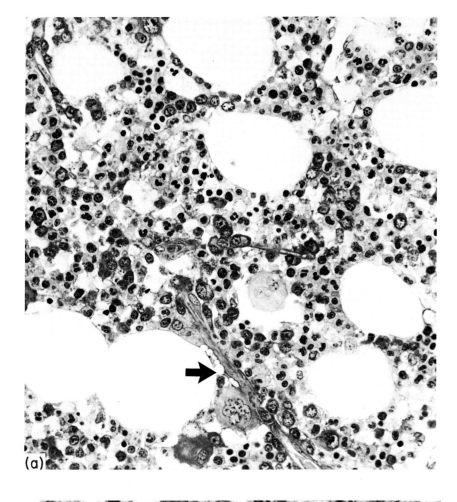

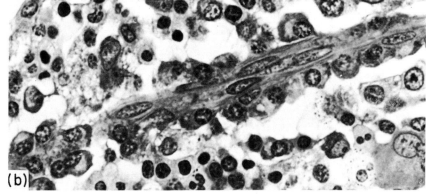

extravascular compartment, erythropoietic islands and megakaryocytes are associated with the marrow sinusoids in the central regions of the marrow cavities, early myeloid precursors lie close to the endosteal surfaces, and to the arterioles, while the more mature forms of the granulocytic series are also found in the central intertrabecular areas (Fig. 2.9). There are, however, normally considerable variations in the quantitative and qualitative distribution of the components of the bone marrow.

2.5   Cellular constituents of marrow

2.5.1   Haematopoiesis

This is the term applied to the process of production of the formed elements of the blood; it takes place in the extravascular compartments of the marrow within the intertrabecular cavities. The normal values in the peripheral blood are maintained by the haematopoietic tissues in the bone marrow. The stem cell compartment gives rise to the pluripotent cells for both myeloid and lymphoid cell lines, which in turn produce

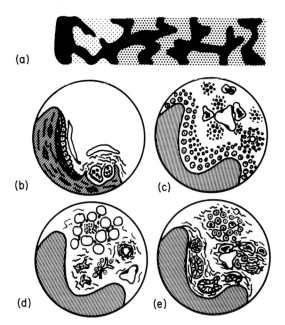

Fig. 2.9   (a) Representative bone marrow biopsy; note hypocellularity in subcortical region; (b) osteoblastic/osteoclastic remodelling; (c) histotopography of the three haematopoietic cell lines; (d) stromal elements of bone marrow; (e) patterns of tumour invasion.

progenitor cells of progressively restricted potential. In addition to erythrocytes, granulocytes, lymphocytes and platelets, the stem cells give rise to mast cells, macrophages and osteoclasts, but not to the bone marrow fibroblasts.

2.5.2 Erythrocytes

The nucleated precursors of the red cells are found in small and large clusters of cells exhibiting the range of maturational sequences from the earliest recognizable erythroblast to normoblast. A macrophage (reticular cell) with long cytoplasmic processes, and containing haemosiderin and possibly some cellular or nuclear debris is usually located in the vicinity of a medium to large cluster of 5 or more erythroid cells. However, the classical appearance of an erythropoietic island with a central macrophage (the erythron) is rarely seen in the light microscope in biopsy sections, possibly due to the plane of sectioning. Morphologically normal erythroid maturation (normoblastic) is observed in the clusters and usually there is a mixed population from early to late normoblasts ready to extrude their nuclei. The myeloid:erythroid ratio is 1.5:1 to 3:1 in BMB. A decreased ratio found in a normo- or hypocellular marrow indicates erythroid hyperplasia in the absence of decreases in the other elements. When one considers the astronomical numbers of erythrocytes produced per unit time (millions per mm^3 per second) it is astonishing that extruded nuclei and macrophages containing them are so rarely observed in normal bone marrow biopsies. This strongly indicates that the engulfment and/or lysis of normoblast nuclei must be remarkably efficient and fast.

2.5.3 Granulocytes

The granulocytic series consists of neutrophils, eosinophils, basophils. Myeloblast, promyelocyte, myelocyte, metamyelocyte, band and segmented forms are all identifiable in sections of the bone marrow. An increase in the myeloid:erythroid (M:E) ratio in a normocellular or hypocellular marrow, in the absence of a decrease in erythroid precursors, indicates granulocytic hyperplasia. There may be normal proportions of cells in the maturational stages, or a 'shift to the left', i.e. a preponderance of immature forms, or a 'shift to the right' with a greater number of mature polymorphonuclear leucocytes present. The paratrabecular and the periarteriolar regions constitute the granulocytic generation zones, but precursors are also scattered throughout the rest of the marrow. Neutrophilic (punctuate, brownish) granules and eosinophilic (slightly larger and yellowish-red) granules are readily distinguished, even in early myelocyte development. Basophils (having partially water soluble granules) are recognized infrequently though mature basophils are occasionally seen. They have fewer, larger and dark red granules.

Under normal circumstances, granulopoiesis is very effective, so that practically all the cells produced reach the circulation. The normal neutrophil:erythroid ratio in bone marrow sections is 1.5 ± 0.07 (Dancey et al., 1976).

2.5.4   Megakaryocytes

These are the largest cells normally present in the bone marrow (Figs 2.10–2.12). Their size ranges from 12 to 150 μm. The smaller ones may be difficult to identify at first, so that occasionally (particularly in haematopoietic neoplasias) enzymic or marker techniques are required. Three stages are recognized in megakaryocytes at maturation:

(1) The megakaryoblast, 15–20 μm, with an oval or kidney shaped nucleus and basophilic cytoplasm.*

(2) The pro-megakaryocyte, 20–80 μm, cytoplasm less basophilic, but with a zone of developing granules, especially perinuclear.*

(3) Mature megakaryocytes, with eosinophilic cytoplasm, and with variable granularity. The nucleus is coarsely cerebriform, multilobed, but not necessarily so. DNA synthesis proceeds as polyploidy goes through 8, 16, 32 or 64 n, while lobulation may continue after that, though there is no definite correlation between ploidy and lobulation of the nucleus and the extent of cytoplasmic differentiation. However, there is some link, as 95% of platelet-shedding megakaryocytes are 16–32 n as shown by Levine et al. (1982). Differentiation of the cytoplasm commences after DNA synthesis has ceased (in most cases) and three cytoplasmic zones are distinguished in the mature megakaryocyte: perinuclear, intermediate and marginal (Fig. 2.10). The first contains the synthetic apparatus, the second the developing demarcation membranes and the third, which is found only in non-platelet releasing megakaryocytes, contains filaments. In cases of extreme demand, large megakaryocyte fragments are released into the circulating blood—megaplatelets or megathrombocytes. Emperipolesis—the presence of other cells within megakaryocyte cytoplasm—may be found in megakaryocytes of any size, though it is

* These measurements are approximate and related to the method of preparation, i.e. whether smears or sections, paraffin or plastic embedding.

Fig. 2.10   Section of bone biopsy of patient with carcinoma of colon and thrombocytosis, to illustrate variability in megakaryocytes. (a) Note light and dark (peripheral) cytoplasmic staining. × 400, Giemsa; (b) and (c) bare megakaryocyte nuclei in sinusoids. × 1000, Giemsa.

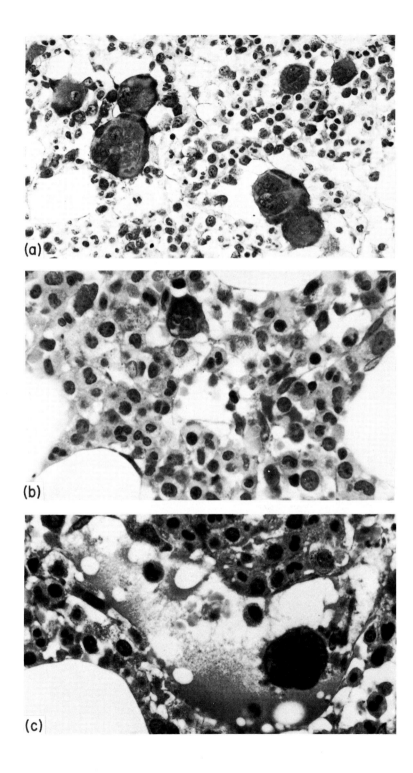

(a)

(b)

(c)

more frequently observed in the larger ones, and also when there are more megakaryocytes in the section, i.e. in hyperplasia of megakaryocytes. The cells within may be granulocytes, lymphocytes, erythroblasts, and erythrocytes (Fig. 2.11) and they are not apparently phagocytosed.

Examples of megakaryocytes of various sizes and nuclear configurations are shown in Figs 2.10–2.12. Megakaryocytes typically appear to abut on or project into the sinusoids, and the platelets are shed directly into their lumina. Whole megakaryocytes or portions of their cytoplasm

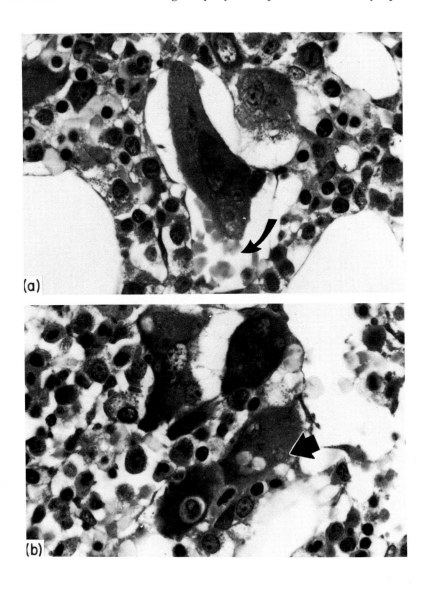

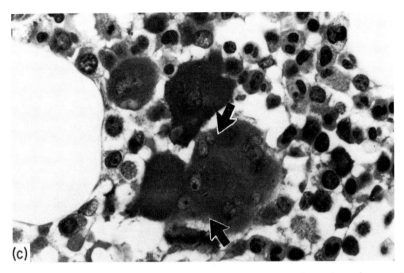

Fig. 2.11 Section of bone biopsy of patient with secondary thrombocytosis, showing range in megakaryocyte size and nuclear configuration. (a) Megakaryocyte in sinus; note erythrocytes (arrow); (b) emperipolesis; note erythrocytes (arrow) within megakaryocyte cytoplasm; (c) megakaryocyte with peripheral ring of small nuclei (arrows). × 1000, all Giemsa.

may also enter the sinuses and fragment in the vascular system (Crosby, 1977) (Fig. 2.10). Megakaryocytes frequently appear to be connected with or interposed between endothelial cells. In the light microscope and even more so in the electron microscope (Fig. 2.12) megakaryocytes have a variably granular cytoplasm, with clear and dense areas; occasional denuded megakaryocyte nuclei are also found in normal bone marrows. Emperipolesis is more frequently observed when their numbers are increased; its significance is unknown.

2.6   Cells of the mononuclear-phagocyte (reticulo-endothelial) system

Monocytes (though produced in the bone marrow) are not often encountered, even in optimal histological sections. Perhaps the problem is one of recognition as they are easily confused with granulocytic precursors; like the latter, they have oval to kidney shaped vesicular nuclei; and they have abundant eosinophilic cytoplasm with variable granulation (see van Furth *et al.,* 1979 for review).

Macrophages (reticular cells) are discussed separately from monocytes because there is still some uncertainty about their derivation in the bone marrow. Macrophages appear to be a heterogeneous population and there are several views as to their origin, which may be from the fixed

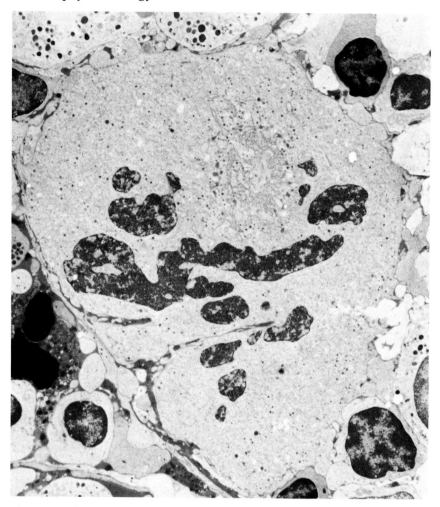

Fig. 2.12   Electron micrograph: megakaryocyte in bone marrow of patient with CLL; note condensed nuclear chromatin and very poorly granulated cytoplasm. × 2000.

reticular cells or their derivatives, from the granulocyte–monocyte precursors, or from mature monocytes. Macrophages may be very large, with nuclei which resemble those of histiocytes, and their abundant cytoplasm may contain granules, vacuoles, lipid, cellular and nuclear debris. Typical bone marrow macrophages (reticular cells) containing haemosiderin and/or cellular debris are shown in Fig. 2.13. These cells form part of the reticulo-endothelial system (RES) or the mononuclear phagocyte system, which is responsible for the breakdown of senescent

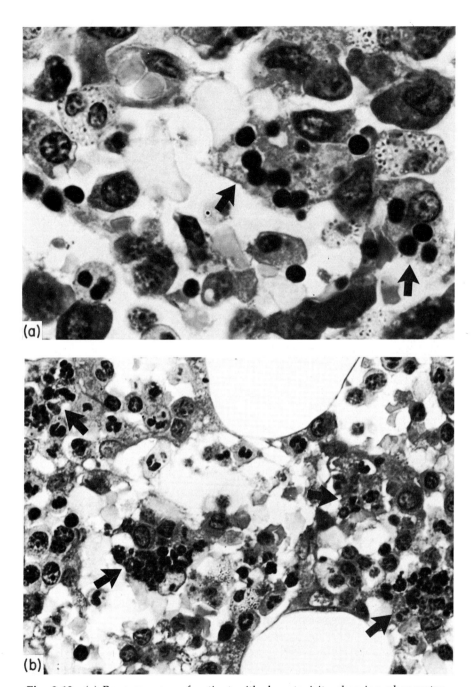

Fig. 2.13 (a) Bone marrow of patient with drug toxicity showing phagocytes (arrows) with engulfed erythroid precursors and eosinophils. × 1000, Giemsa; (b) bone marrow of patient after chemotherapy for malignancy; note numerous phagocytes with nuclear debris (arrows). × 400, Giemsa.

red cells and the storage of iron. Iron stain on bone marrow sections demonstrates overload, depletion and normal storage. There is generally a good correlation between serum ferritin levels, iron absorption, and marrow stores, except in cases of sideroblastic anaemia, haemosiderosis, some cases of neoplasia, infections and hepatic diseases (Krause and Stolc, 1980). Lipo-macrophages and foam cells (Plate IId) (as well as Gaucher cells as seen in the storage diseases) are thought also to develop out of reticular or adventitial cells (or even endothelial cells). Tissue histiocytes are derived partly by recruitment of monocytes and partly by mitotic division of local histiocytes. This term is used for cells which take up vital dyes and are capable of phagocytosis. Tissue histiocytes have oval or kidney shaped vesicular nuclei, with variable amounts of cytoplasm and inclusions. Histiocytes in different situations may have different properties.

Some sub-groups of histiocytes are recognized. Littoral cells are the sinus histiocytes which line the venous sinuses of the bone marrow (and other organs); they are spindle shaped with cytoplasmic processes. Epithelioid histiocytes have nuclei similar to those of histiocytes, and abundant eosinophilic and granular cytoplasm. Giant cells are thought to be derived from the histiocyte–monocyte series by endomitosis and/or by fusion or coalescence.

2.6.1   Lymphocytes

Some measure of lymphopoietic function (as in the embryo) is most probably retained by the adult bone marrow (Osmond et al., 1981). Whether or not, lymphoid cells belong to the normal marrow population, they are dispersed among the haematopoietic and fat cells, or aggregated to form lymphoid nodules (Fig. 2.14) whose incidence increases with age (Rywlin et al., 1974; Rywlin, 1976). They are found in 1% to over 40% of bone marrow biopsies with the higher incidence in the older age groups. The nodules or aggregates especially when small, are readily observed in sections stained for reticulin fibres, as they contain more fibres than their surroundings. Capillaries, reticular cells, a few plasma cells and mast cells may also be associated with these lymphoid nodules (Fig. 2.14).

Four configurations of lymphoid aggregates have been described: (a) nodules with germinal centres; (b) sharply demarcated nodules; (c) nodules with irregular borders; (d) small aggregates of lymphoid cells

---

Fig. 2.14   (a) Lymphoid follicle with germinal centre in iliac crest biopsy of 72 year old patient with femoral neck fracture and osteoporosis. × 400; (b) lymphoid cell aggregate, in normal biopsy. × 400; (c) parasinusoidal aggregate of lymphoid cells, × 450, in normal biopsy. Giemsa.

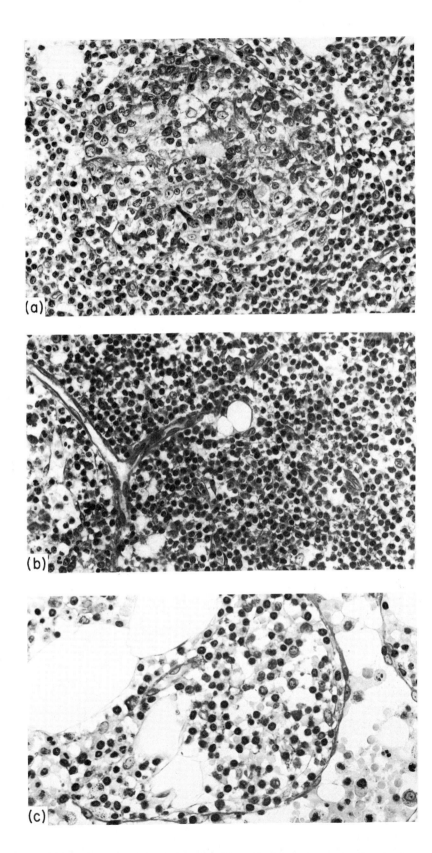

(a)

(b)

(c)

(Hashimoto *et al.*, 1957). When multiple nodules are found in a section, immunohistology is required to rule out or to confirm involvement by a neoplastic lymphoproliferative disorder.

2.6.2   *Plasma Cells*

These represent the final developmental stage of the B lymphocyte, and quite possibly, they are produced and mature in the bone marrow as well as at other sites in the body. Plasma cells have a cartwheel nuclear chromatin pattern, pale blue cytoplasm and frequently a perinuclear 'hof'. Transformed B lymphocytes (potential plasma cells) may leave the lymph nodes and mature in the bone marrow. The characteristic location of plasma cells is along the adventitia of small blood vessels (Fig. 2.8b), but they are also found singly and in small groups of 2 or 3 dispersed within the marrow. Plasma cells are a normal component of the cell population in the bone marrow.

2.6.3   *Mast cells*

These are thought to arise from the same granulocyte precursors which produce the basophilic leucocyte (Zucker-Franklin, 1980). Mast cells lie adjacent to the endothelial cells of sinusoids, at the endosteal surface of the trabecular bone, in the periosteum, in the walls of small arteries, scattered in the bone marrow, and frequently at the edges of lymphoid aggregates or nodules. Mast cells are characterized by oval to round nuclei and cytoplasm densely packed with bright red granules. Mast cells may be oval or spindle shaped, or thin and elongated resembling fibroblasts, in which case they are best identified in sections stained by toluidine blue and under high magnification as only few granules may be present. Small accumulations of mast cells and histiocytes (previously designated fibro-histiocytic lesions) may also be found in the bone marrow; their significance is unknown.

2.7   Bone marrow stroma

This provides the supporting framework for the haematopoiesis which takes place in the extravascular compartment and is supported by the reticular cells, fat cells, fibroblasts and their fibrils and by the extensive network of blood vessels including the sinusoids and their accompanying nerves (de Bruyn, 1981). Fat cells occupy about a third of the marrow volume in the iliac crest biopsy. They serve a supporting, filling and metabolic function as shown, for example by their ability to participate in steroid aromatization (Frisch *et al.*, 1980). There are close associations between the mesenchymal elements—the endothelium, the advential cells, fibroblasts and osteoblasts, and the endosteal lining cells as well as reticular cells and macrophages. Fibroblasts, elongated cells with elongated nuclei, may be indistinguishable from the so-called reticular cells. Fibroblasts produce the reticular fibres of which the normal bone marrow has few, mainly in association with blood vessels and endosteum.

2.7.1 Fibres

The normal bone marrow contains only thin reticular fibres best visualized by the Gomori stain for reticulin (Fig. 2.15) or similar stains and by polarized light. Fibrosis in the marrow may involve reticulin fibres only, or also collagen (i.e. bundles of reticulin). Myelofibrosis may occur in numerous conditions, which are described in the appropriate sections of this book, and shown schematically in Fig. 2.16. All these components, in various proportions constitute the micro-environment which provides the niches for the stem cells and the inductive influences which direct them to one or other line of differentiation.

2.7.2 Blood vessels

The medullary arteries enter via the cortical bone and branch within the marrow (Fig. 2.17) and the trabeculae, accompanied by nerve fibres (Plate If and Fig. 2.15b). The smaller branches divide into arterioles, and then into capillaries which frequently have a cuff of plasma cells around them, and lead into the sinusoids. These form a system of channels of variable width and length whose walls consist of a single layer of endothelial cells, an incomplete outer covering of adventitia and, when large, a loose network of reticulin fibres. The sinusoids in turn drain into the periosteal veins. The endothelial cells of post-capillary, or post-sinusoidal venules may be plump, with vesicular nuclei and distinct nucleoli. This layer forms the interface between the intra- and the extravascular compartments, which must be traversed by the blood cells for entry into the circulation. Thus a BMB provides a cut through the vascular system and may therefore supply additional information in diseases which affect it, such as arteriosclerosis, arteritis, amyloidosis, etc. Physiologically, portions of the sinusoidal channels are collapsed at any one time and the expansion and contraction of the vascular system within the rigid bony cage enclosing the marrow, contribute (together with quantitative changes in fat cells) to the extreme fluctuations in the production of blood cells of which the marrow is capable. When the need arises, an increase of up to ten-fold its usual capacity is possible. It should be remembered that the parenchyme of the bone marrow is at all times composed of a rapidly

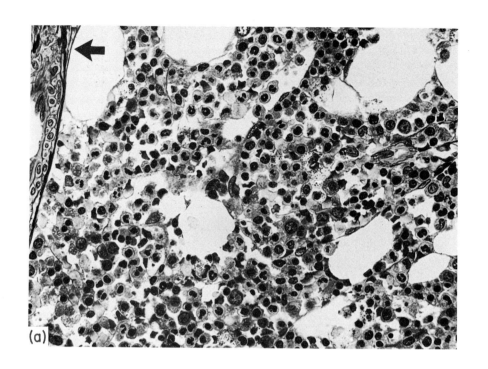

(a)

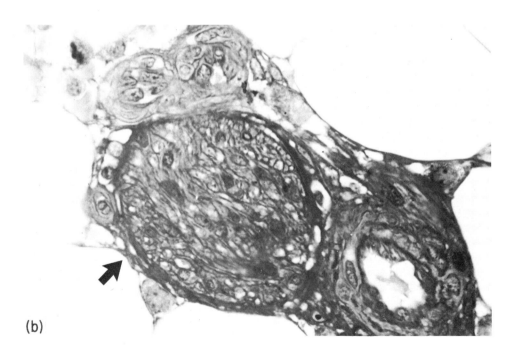

(b)

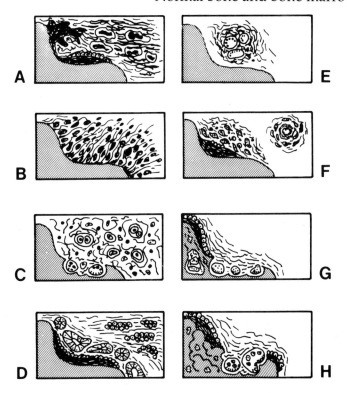

Fig. 2.16   Schematic outline of histogenesis of fibrosis in the bone marrow: A = myelofibrosis/osteomyelosclerosis, B = malignant lymphoma centrocytic, C = Hodgkin's disease, D = adenocarcinoma, E = granuloma, F = systemic mastocytosis, G = primary hyperparathyroidism, H = Paget's disease.

evolving, highly mobile population so that a section of a biopsy is comparable to a still of a motion picture. This helps to account for the great variety seen in biopsy sections, which are nevertheless within the 'normal' range. Moreover, many processes in the bone marrow are highly efficient and fast and leave few traces, as witness the disposal of normoblast nuclei and the trans-endothelial passage of reticulocytes and granulocytes which is so rarely observed.

Fig. 2.15   (a) Section of normal bone marrow stained for reticulin which is found around blood vessels (arrow) while little is evident in the stroma. × 250, Gomori. When examined by polarized light more reticulin fibres are evident; (b) arteries and nerve (arrow) in cross-section. Nerves are relatively rare in the marrow itself, though they may be more frequently encountered in the periosteal tissues. × 400, Giemsa.

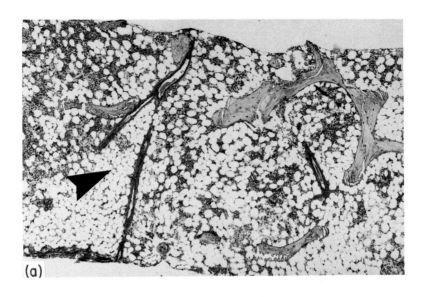

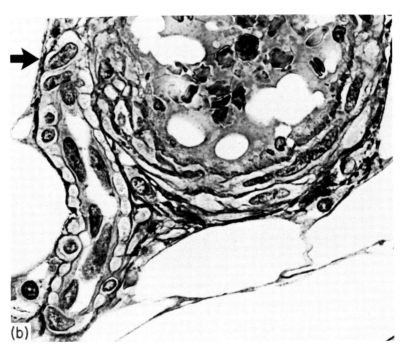

Fig. 2.17 (a) Bone biopsy of 70 year old patient after prostatectomy; no chemotherapy, no metastases; note partial hypoplasia and blood vessels crossing the section (arrow). × 400, Giemsa; (b) normal artery in bone marrow, near point of bifurcation (arrow). × 1000, Gomori.

References

Bruyn, P. P. de (1981), Structural substrates of bone marrow function. *Sem. Haemat.*, **18**, 179–93.

Chambers, T. J. (1980), Cellular basis of bone resorption. *Clin. Orthop.*, **151**, 283–93.

Crosby, W. H. (1977), Delivery of platelets by the marrow—the derivation of platelets. In *Topics in Haematology* (eds S. Seno, F. Takaku and S. Sirino), Excerpta Medica, Amsterdam, Oxford, pp. 416–19.

Dancey, J. T., Deubelbeiss, K. A., Harker, L. A. and Finch, C. A. (1976), Neutrophil kinetics in man. *J. clin. Invest.*, **58**, 705–15.

Ferrant, A., Rodham, J., Cordier, A. *et al.* (1980), Selective hypoplasia of pelvic bone marrow. *Scand. J. Haematol.*, **25**, 12–18.

Frisch, R. E., Canick, J. A. and Tulschinsky, D. (1980), Human fatty marrow aromatizes androgen to estrogen. *J. clin. Endocrin. Metab.*, **51**, 394–6.

Frost, H. M. (1962), Tetracycline labelling of bone and the zone of demarcation of Osteoid Seams. *Can. J. Biochem. Physiol.*, **40**, 485–9.

Furth, R. van., Raeburn, J. A. and Sweet, T. L. van (1979), Characteristics of human mononuclear phagocytes. *Blood*, **54**, 485–500.

Hashimoto, M., Masanori, H. and Tsukasa, S. (1957), Lymphoid nodules in human bone marrow. *Acta Pathol. Jap.*, **7**, 33–52.

Johnell, O. (1980), Bone marrow cell content and osteoclasts in crista biopsies. *Acta Orthop. Scand.*, **51**, 399–401.

Krause, J. R. and Stolc, V. (1980), Serum ferritin and bone marrow biopsy iron stores. *Amer. J. clin. Path.*, **74**, 461–4.

Levine, R. F., Hazzard, K. C. and Lamberg, J. D. (1982), The significance of megakaryocyte size. *Blood*, **60**, 1122–31.

Loutit, J. F. and Nisbet, N. W. (1982), The origin of osteoclasts. *Immunobiology*, **161**, 193.

Mauch, R., Botnick, L. and Hellman, S. (1981), Decline in marrow proliferative capacity as a function of age. *Blood*, **58**, Suppl.I, 113a.

Osmond, D. G., Fahlman, M. T. E., Fulop, G. M. and Rahal, D. M. (1981), Regulation and localization of lymphocyte production in the bone marrow. In *Microenvironments in Haemopoietic and Lymphoid Differentiation*, Pitman Medical, London. (Ciba Foundation Symposium 84, Pitman Medical, London, pp. 68–85).

Owen, M. (1980), Origin of bone cells in the post-natal organism. *Arthr. Rheumat.*, **23**, 1073–80.

Raisz, L. G. and Kream, B. E. (1983), Regulation of bone formation (second of two parts). *New Engl. J. Med.*, **309**, 83–9.

Rodan, G. A. and Martin, T. J. (1981), Role of osteoblasts in hormonal control of bone resorption—a hypothesis. *Calcif. Tissue Int.*, **33**, 349–51.

Rywlin, A. M., Ortega, R. S. and Dominguez, C. J. (1974), Lymphoid nodules of the bone marrow: normal and abnormal. *Blood*, **43**, 389–400.

Rywlin, A. M. (1976), *Histopathology of the Bone Marrow*, Little, Brown and Company, Boston.

Williams, L., Udupa, K. B. and Lipschutz, D. A. (1981), Age and erythropoiesis. *Clin, Res.*, **29**, 864A.

Zucker-Franklin, D. (1980), Ultra-structural evidence for common origin of human mast cells and basophils. *Blood*, **56**, 534–40.

3 The cytopenias: hypoplastic and aplastic marrows

3.1 Cytopenias

A peripheral cytopenia may be due to ineffective or decreased cell production, increased peripheral utilization and/or increased destruction without an adequately matching compensatory increase in production. The cause for the cytopenia may thus lie in the bone marrow, the periphery or both. Drugs in particular have been implicated (for review see Gordon-Smith, 1980) and in some cases these may induce cytopenias by an immunologic mechanism. Other causes include defects in the bone marrow microcirculation (Knospe and Crosby, 1971), endocrine dysfunction (Ferrari et al., 1976) alcohol abuse (Ballard, 1980), and multifactorial such as viral infections (Bannister et al., 1983) and the anaemia of chronic diseases. Alcohol is now one of the major causes of disease and death in industrialized countries (Saunders, 1983). The possible aetiologies of cytopenias (including anaemias) are far too numerous to be listed here, and they can be found in the many excellent textbooks of haematology available. This chapter will describe those conditions in which a BMB provides diagnostic or useful ancillary information.

3.2 Pancytopenias with reduction in the formed elements of the blood

3.2.1 Aplastic Anaemia

When hypoplasia or aplasia is suspected, a BMB should be performed to exclude other causes that might be responsible. These include refractory anaemias, malignant lymphomas, hairy cell leukaemia (and other leukaemias), myelofibrosis and metastatic carcinomas (Table 3.1); these conditions are considered in later chapters. The haematological effects of drugs, especially cytopenias, have been reviewed by Young and Vincent

Table 3.1 Bone marrow histology in patients with unexplained cytopenias

Bone marrow histology	Patients (number)	Percentage of total
Refractory anaemia	141	32
Aplastic anaemia	60	14
Malignant lymphomas (non-Hodgkin)	58	13
Acute leukaemia	50	11
Hairy cell leukaemia	45	10
Agnogenic myeloid metaplasia	40	9
Hodgkin's disease	14	3
Multiple myeloma	10	2
Preleukaemia (sequential biopsies)	5	1
Systemic mastocytosis	4	1
Malignant histiocytosis	3	1
Angioimmunoblastic lymphadenopathy	2	1

(1980). For a proper assessment of marrow cellularity a cylinder of at least 20–30 × 2 mm is required (Fig. 1.6). A representative bone marrow section in pancytopenia (aplastic anaemia) is shown in Fig. 3.1. There is a very heterogeneous group of possible aetiologies for aplastic anaemia (Camitta *et al.*, 1982; Gordon-Smith, 1980; Abdou *et al.*, 1981; Gutman *et al.*, 1978; Najean, 1981); in the majority of cases, the cause is not reflected in the bone marrow picture (Fischer and Fohlmeister, 1983). The haematopoietic tissue is drastically reduced, the number of sinusoids is decreased while fat cells are increased, and haemosiderin laden macrophages, mast cells, plasma cells and lymphocytes are scattered amongst the fat cells. When the lymphocytes show an absolute as well as a relative increase and/or are found in aggregates or nodules, an immunologic component to the cytopenia may be present. In a typical case of aplastic anaemia, isolated erythropoietic islands situated close to sinusoids and exhibiting maturation arrest and mitotic figures, dyerythropoiesis and erythrophagocytosis by histiocytes will also be present. Megakaryocytes may be absent, or there may be one or two small clusters. Small groups of myeloid precursors may also be found, as well as a few isolated neutrophils. In early cases, the marrow picture is characterized by interstitial oedema, necrotic cells and capillaries, and the presence of lipomacrophages. Though parameters of prognostic significance have been sought in BMB, the evidence so far is inconclusive, and no features of bone marrow histology have yet been identified which accurately predict the eventual outcome. Nevertheless, it appears that lymphocytic infiltrations and capillary necroses are usually absent or minimal in those cases who later recover. Moreover, complete or partial restitution takes place after aplasia caused by starvation or radiation therapy. There

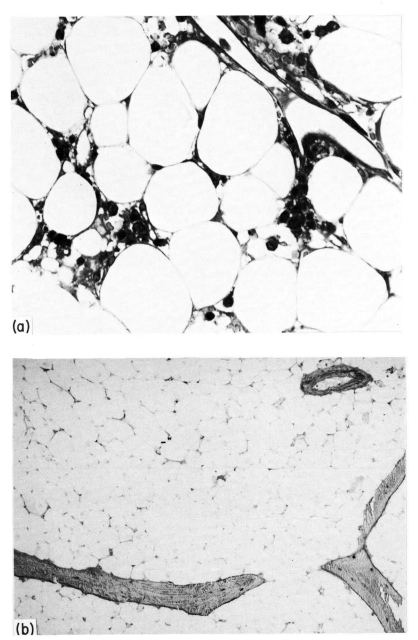

Fig. 3.1 (a) Patient with pancytopenia; no cause found other than chronic alcohol abuse. Bone biopsy showed only sparse, isolated foci of haematopoiesis. × 400, Giemsa; (b) patient with paraplegia due to space occupying lesion in spine; bilateral iliac crest biopsies showed total bone marrow aplasia. Blood count was normal. × 100, Giemsa.

appears to be a lesser risk of severe aplastic anaemia developing if the bone marrow histology shows partial atrophy only at the onset of disease, as opposed to a greater risk when complete replacement of haematopoiesis by fat cells is found *ab initio*. A quantitative reduction in erythropoiesis is frequently accompanied by a qualitative disturbance as well, i.e. dyserythropoiesis (see below). A reduction in trabecular bone volume (osteopenia) has also been observed in long-standing hypoplastic conditions, probably due to atrophy of nutrient blood vessels.

3.2.2   *Pure red cell aplasia*

On low magnification the marrow shows no striking alterations (Fig. 3.2). There may be a patchy replacement by fat cells together with areas of normal cellularity which, on closer inspection, contain no erythropoietic islands but only an isolated precursor or two. There are iron deposits in the stromal cells, aggregates of lymphoid cells (in many cases), macrophages containing cellular debris, mast cells and plasma cells, as well as megakaryocytes and granulopoiesis of normal aspect. Pure red cell aplasia has been ascribed to many different causes and has also been reported in lymphoproliferative and myeloproliferative disorders, in addition to other conditions with an immunologic background such as cold haemagglutinin disease (Cazzola *et al.*, 1983) or cases with an obscure aetiology (Table 3.2). Red cell aplasia has been associated with thymoma, with systemic lupus erythematosus, and with primary autoimmune hypothyroidism (Francis, 1982). In addition, excess of certain subsets of T-cells has been shown to interfere with the terminal differentiation of erythroid and granulocytic progenitors (Nathan and Sytkowski, 1983; Hocking *et al.*, 1983). Certain transient erythroblastopenias and aplastic anaemias of childhood may follow viral infections. The aplastic crisis in children with sickle cell anaemia has recently been shown to be associated with parvovirus infection (Editorial, *Lancet*, 1983).

3.2.3   *Granulocytopenia*

Few studies on BMB have been reported in this condition, especially in the acute phase. In this phase bone marrow histology is variable; it ranges from hypocellularity with extensive oedema and extravasation of erythrocytes from the disrupted sinusoids, to a reduction in myeloid precursors

---

Fig. 3.2   (a) Case of pure red cell aplasia; note absence of erythroid precursors, and small lymphoid cell infiltrate at arrow. × 250, Giemsa; (b) case of agranulocytosis, possibly drug-induced; note numerous erythroid islands, and lymphoid cell infiltrate (arrow). × 100, Giemsa.

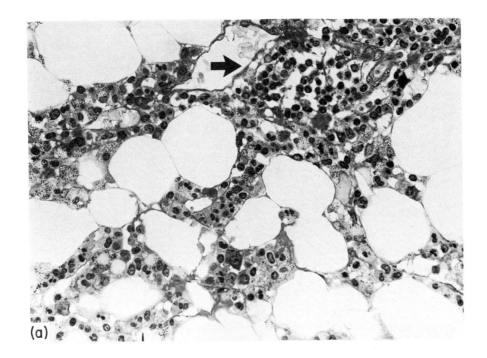

(a)

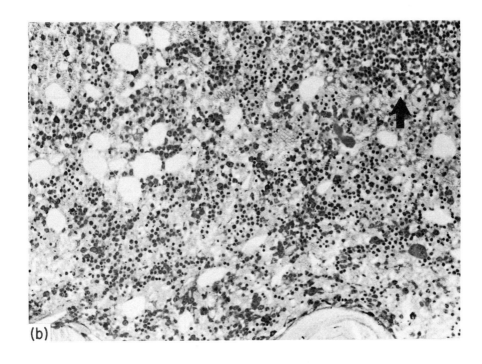

(b)

Table 3.2 Conditions with quantitative changes in erythropoiesis

Decreased	Increased	Neoplastic (increased)
Congenital	Congenital	MPD
Thymomas	CDAs	PV
Pure red cell aplasia	Haemoglobinopathies	CML
Aplastic crisis (PNH, etc.)	Haemorrhage	MF/OMS
Aplastic anaemia	Haemolysis	Erythroid malignancies
Infections	Megaloblastic anaemias	Preleukaemias
Chronic diseases	Iron deficiencies	
SLE	Secondary erythrocytosis	
Renal	Refractory anaemias	
Malignancies	Sideroblastic anaemias	
(preleukaemia hypoplastic		
phase)		
Unknown		

Abbreviations used in Tables:
CDA = congenital dyserythropoietic anaemias.   LPD = lymphoproliferative disorders
CML = chronic myeloid leukaemia.   MF/OMS = myelofibrosis/osteomyelosclerosis.
HD = Hodgkin's disease   MPD = myeloproliferative disorders.
IT = idiopathic (essential) thrombocythaemia.   PV = polycythaemia vera.
ITP = idiopathic thrombocytopenic purpura.   TTP = thrombotic thrombocytopenic purpura.

and/or maturation inhibition, while the other cell lines are not apparently affected (Fig. 3.2). When there is little or no reduction in the numbers of myeloid precursors, or even an apparent increase, together with profound maturation inhibition, the bone marrow picture may resemble that seen in promyelocytic leukaemias, due to the presence of the early precursors and the absence of the later maturational stages. In acute toxic conditions, haematopoiesis may be completely absent, the walls of the blood vessels appear damaged, and there is widespread precipitation of fibrinoid material. Drug-induced agranulocytosis has been reviewed by Young and Vincent (1980). Neutropenia together with a cellular bone marrow is also seen in autoimmune states, such as rheumatoid arthritis (Dancey and Brubaker, 1979), in Felty's syndrome (arthritis, splenomegaly and leukopenia) and in certain types of lymphoma (Kruskall et al., 1982; Balentine et al., 1983). Human cyclic neutropenia is probably due to abnormal regulation of production (Wright et al., 1981) and granulocyte precursors are reduced. In addition to the known causes of acquired neutropenia, pure white-cell aplasia may occur as a consequence of antibody mediated autoimmune inhibition of granulopoiesis (Levitt et al., 1983; Carmel, 1983), or T-lymphocyte mediated granulopoietic failure (Bagby et al., 1983). Conditions with quantitative alterations of granulopoiesis are listed in Table 3.3.

Table 3.3 Conditions with quantitative changes in granulopoiesis

Decreased	Increased	Neoplastic (increased)
Congenital	Congenital	MPD
Aplastic anaemia	Infections	PV
Drugs/radiation	Inflammations	IT
Infections	Trauma	CML
	Metabolic	MF/OMS
	Hypersensitivity	Acute leukaemias
	Hypersplenism	Preleukaemias
	Post-therapy	
	Malignancies	

For explanation of abbreviations see footnote to Table 3.2.

3.2.4   Thrombocytopenias

These may be primary or secondary. The primary group consists of hereditary or congenital types, and idiopathic thrombocytopenic purpura (ITP); the secondary group is due to many different causes (Table 3.4). Three main mechanisms may be distinguished: defective production, accelerated loss, destruction or utilization, and abnormal distribution. When thrombocytopenia occurs as part of a bi- or tri-cytopenia, and is due to decreased production, the picture in the biopsy is similar to those described above, and few or even no megakaryocytes are found. The same is true for the rare instances of megakaryocytic hypo- and aplasia (Stoll *et al.*, 1981). In cases with augmented peripheral consumption and/ or breakdown, an increase in megakaryocyte numbers is the rule. If the biopsy is taken in the acute stage, shortly after onset of thrombo-cytopenia, the normal range of megakaryocytes is found. In chronic states (such as ITP) there is a preponderance of young forms, though large ones are also present. Thrombocytopenia may be a presenting sign of

Table 3.4 Conditions with quantitative changes in megakaryopoiesis

Decreased	Increased	Neoplastic (increased)
Congenital	ITP	MPD
Aplastic anaemia	(TTP)	PV
Megaloblastic anaemia		Megakaryocytic myelosis
Drugs/radiation	Haemolysis	IT
LPD	Haemorrhage	CML
Other neoplasias	Hypersplenism	MF/OMS
	LPD	Preleukaemias
	HD	
	Malignancies	

For explanation of abbreviations see footnote to Table 3.2.

preleukaemia (Tricot *et al.*, 1982); and may occur in hypothermia (O'Brien *et al.*, 1982).

Thrombocytopenias in the myeloproliferative disorders and other haematopoietic neoplasias are considered below. A reduction in numbers of platelets in the peripheral blood with increased numbers of megakaryocytes in the bone marrow may also be found in patients with enlargement of the spleen due to non-neoplastic causes such as vascular disease. ITP must be distinguished from thrombocytopenia with decreased megakaryocytes as well as the immature form of megakaryocytic myelosis (see Chapter 8). Small or even micromegakaryocytes (as seen in dysplastic and some neoplastic conditions) may also occur in the bone marrows of patients with non-haematologic disorders, such as hepatic cirrhosis. Alcoholic liver disease is one of the main causes of illness and death in many industrialized countries (Saunders, 1983), frequently accompanied by cytopenias. Thrombocytopenia has been found in over 50% of patients with autoimmune thyroid disease (Hymes *et al.*, 1981).

A recent study of the spleen in a case of ITP has demonstrated transition of ceroid containing cells to foamy macrophages (Lasser, 1983). The author suggested that the sea-blue histiocytes phagocytose platelets and that they develop into foam macrophages when the ingested platelets are metabolized. A similar mechanism could account for the sea-blue histiocytes and foamy cells seen in the bone marrow, not only in ITP but also in other disorders such as the MPD, especially when interstitial deposition of platelets occurs.

3.2.5   *Thrombotic thrombocytopenic purpura*

Bone biopsies are rarely performed in this condition as tissue is usually taken from the buccal mucosa for diagnosis. In a case examined by us, clumps of platelets were found in small arterioles in the bone marrow (Fig. 3.3). The characteristic location for the platelet-fibrin deposits is at the arterio-capillary junctions. However, the hyaline thrombi in vessels usually associated with this condition were not observed in the bone marrow biopsy.

3.3   Pancytopenias with hypercellular marrow

3.3.1 ˙ *Refractory anaemias*

These are characterized by a hypercellular bone marrow in the presence of a peripheral cytopenia. Maturation inhibition in the bone marrow leads to accumulation of early precursors, usually in clusters. There is ineffec-

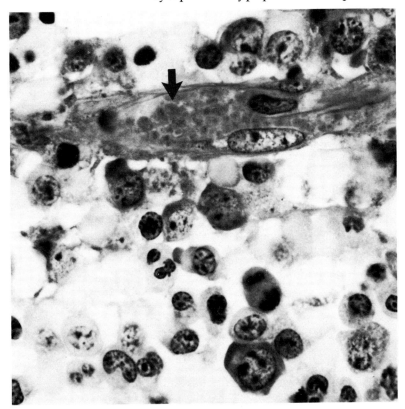

Fig. 3.3   Section of bone biopsy from patient with thrombotic thrombocytopenic purpura taken a week ante-mortem; note arteriole with plug of platelets (arrow). × 1000, Giemsa.

tive erythropoiesis, variable numbers of sideroblasts (Table 3.5) and there may be iron overload. These conditions are considered later with the myelodysplastic syndromes.

Table 3.5 Anaemias with a sideroblastic component

May occur in:	Alcohol abuse
	Megaloblastic anaemias
	Inflammatory diseases
	Myelodysplastic syndromes
	Myeloproliferative disease
	Lymphoproliferative disease
	Carcinomas

References

Abdou, N. I., Verdirame, J. D., Amare, M. and Abdou, N. L. (1981), Hetero-geneity of pathogenic mechanisms in aplastic anaemia: efficacy of therapy based on in-vitro results. *Ann. int. Med.*, **95**, 43–50.

Bagby, G. C., Lawrence, H. J. and Neerhout, R. C. (1983), T-lymphocyte mediated granulopoietic failure: in vitro identification of prednisone respon-sive patients. *New Eng. J. Med.*, **309**, 1073–8.

Balentine, L., Skikne, B. S., Park, C. H. and Lynch, S. R. (1983), Malignant lymphocytic lymphoma. Demonstration of a serum inhibitor and response to combination chemotherapy. *Cancer*, **52**, 35–8.

Ballard, H. S. (1980), Alcohol-associated pancytopenia with hypocellular bone marrow. *Am. J. clin. Pathol.*, **73**, 830–4.

Bannister, P., Miloszewski, K., Barnard, D. and Losowsky, M. S. (1983), Fatal bone marrow aplasia associated with non-A, non-B hepatitis. *Brit. med. J.*, **286**, 1314–15.

Camitta, B. M., Storb, R. and Thomas, E. D. (1982), Aplastic anemia (first of two parts). Pathogenesis, diagnosis, treatment and prognosis. *New Engl. J. Med.*, **306**, 645.

Carmel, R. (1983), An unusual case of auto-immune agranulocytosis with total absence of myeloid precursors. *Am. J. clin. Pathol.*, **79**, 611–15.

Cazzola, M., Barosi, G. and Ascari, E, (1983), Cold haemagglutinin disease with severe anaemia, reticulocytopenia and erythroid bone marrow. *Scand. J. Haematol.*, **30**, 25–9.

Dancey, J. T. and Brubaker, L. H. (1979), Neutrophil marrow profiles in patients with rheumatoid arthritis and neutropenia. *Brit. J. Haematol.*, **43**, 607–17.

Editorial, Lancet (1983), Bone marrow aplasia and parvovirus. *Lancet*, **2**, 21–2.

Ferrari, E., Ascari, E., Bossolo, P. A. and Barosi, G. (1976), Sheehan's syndrome with complete bone marrow aplasia: long term results of substitution therapy with hormones. *Brit. J. Haematol.*, **33**, 575–82.

Fischer, R. and Fohlmeister, I. (1983), Pathology of panmyelophthisis. *Verh. Dtsch. Ges. Path.*, **67**, 286–306.

Francis, D. A. (1982), Pure red-cell aplasia: association with systemic lupus erythematosus and primary autoimmune hypothyroidism. *Brit. med. J.*, **284**, 85.

Gordon-Smith, E. C. (Ed.) (1980), Haematological effects of drug therapy. *Clin. Haematol.*, **9**, (3).

Gutman, A., Frumkin, A., Adam, A., Bloch-Schtacher, N. and Rozenszajn, L. A. (1978), X-linked dyskeratosis congenita with pancytopenia. *Arch. Dermatol.*, **114**, 1667–71.

Hocking, W. G., Singh, R., Schroff, R. and Golde, D. W. (1983), Cell mediated inhibition of erythropoiesis and megaloblastic anemia in T-cell chronic lym-phopcytic leukemia. *Cancer*, **51**, 631–36.

Hymes, K., Blum, M., Lackner, H. and Karpatkin, S. (1981), Easy bruising, thrombocytopenia, and elevated platelet immunoglobin G in Graves' Disease and Hashimoto's Thyroiditis. *Ann. int. Med.*, **94**, 27–30..

Knospe, W. H. and Crosby, W. H. (1971), Aplastic anemia: a disorder of the bone-marrow sinusoidal microcirculation rather than stem-cell failure? *Lancet*, **1**, 20–2.

Kruskall, M. S., Weitzman, S. A., Stossel, T. P., Harris, N. and Robinson, S. H. (1982), Lymphoma with autoimmune neutropenia and hepatic sinusoidal infiltration: a syndrome. *Ann. int. Med.*, **97**, 202–5.

Lasser, A. (1983), Diffuse histiocytosis of the spleen and idiopathic thrombo-cytopenic purpura (ITP): histochemical and ultrastructural studies. *Am. J. clin. Pathol.*, **80,** 529–33.

Levitt, L. J., Ries, C. A. and Greenberg, P. L. (1983), Pure white-cell aplasia. Antibody-mediated autoimmune inhibition of granulopoiesis. *New Engl. J. Med.*, **308,** 1141–8.

Najean, Y. (1981), Long term follow-up in patients with aplastic anaemia. A study of androgen-treated patients surviving more than two years. *Am. J. Med.*, **71,** 543–51.

Nathan, D. G. and Sytkowski, A. (1983), Erythropoietin and the regulation of erythropoiesis. Editorial retrospective. *New Engl. J. Med.*, **308,** 520–2.

O'Brien, H., Amess, J. A. L. and Mollin, D. L. (1982), Recurrent thrombo-cytopenia, erythroid hypoplasia and sideroblastic anaemia associated with hypothermia. *Brit. J. Haematol.*, **51,** 451–6.

Saunders, J. B. (1983), Alcohol liver disease in the 1980s. *Brit. med. J.*, **287,** 1819–21.

Stoll, D. B., Blum, S., Pasquale, D. and Murphy, S. (1981), Thrombocytopenia with decreased megakaryocytes. Evaluation and prognosis. *Ann. int. Med.*, **94,** 170–5.

Tricot, G., Criel, A. and Verwilghen, R. L. (1982), Thrombocytopenia as present-ing symptom of preleukaemia in 3 patients. *Scand. J. Haematol.*, **28,** 243–350.

Wright, D. G., Dale, D. C., Fauci, A. S. and Wolff, S. M. (1981), Human cyclic neutropenia: clinical review and long-term follow-up of patients. *Medicine*, **60,** 1–13.

Young, G. A. R. and Vincent, P. C. (1980), Drug-induced agranulocytosis. *Clinics Haematol.*, **9,** 483–504.

4   The cytopenias: non-haematopoietic components

Stromal reactions in the bone marrow may accompany cytopenias. These are seen especially in the bone marrows of patients who suffer from various underlying clinical conditions, such as infection, sarcoidosis, diseases of collagen, Hodgkin's disease, malignant lymphomas and carcinomas, all without bone marrow involvement in the biopsy (Fig. 4.1). However, in many patients with cytopenias no aetiology or con-comittant disease is discovered, in spite of intensive investigation.

Bacterial and chemical toxins and radiation may all damage the components of the bone marrow stroma. The capillaries and sinusoids are especially vulnerable and liable to disruption, so that the intra- and extravascular compartments are no longer clearly separated.

The anaemia associated with chronic disorders occurs in infections including bacterial and fungal; chronic inflammatory, non-infectious conditions; malignant diseases; chronic hepatic and renal disorders. The anaemia in many of these conditions is thought to be due to impaired marrow response and defective iron metabolism.

Investigation of bone marrow biopsies may reveal infections in unusual situations, such as mycobacterium in acquired immune deficiency syndrome (AIDS) (Cohen *et al.*, 1983), Donovan bodies in Kala-Azar, Coxiella Burnetti in Q fever (Geddes, 1983), and the causative organism in leprosy (Lawrence and Schreiber, 1979). The bone marrow histology in one case of AIDS is shown in Fig. 4.2.

In severe cases there is disintegration of the sinusoids and degeneration of the walls of the small blood vessels—the larger ones are only affected when the noxae are overwhelming. In addition, such consequences may ensue as a result of allergic and autoimmune states.

Fig. 4.1   (a) Epithelioid cell granuloma in bone marrow of patient with sclerosing myelitis in case of SLE. × 400, Giemsa; (b) involvement of bone marrow in case of angio-immunoblastic lymphadenopathy (AILD) established by lymph node biopsy. × 600, Giemsa.

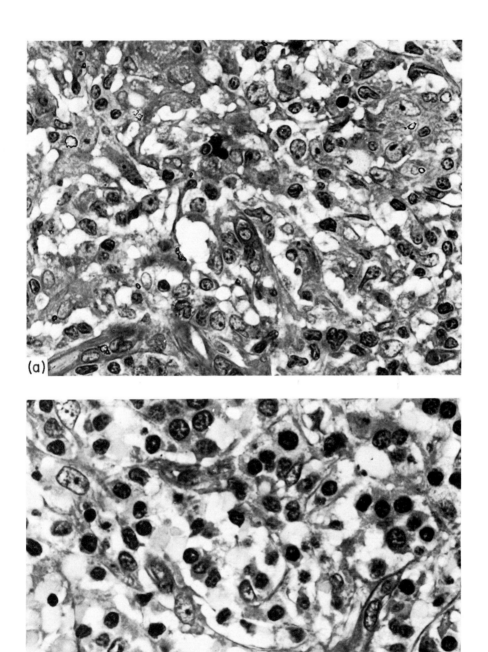

(a)

(b)

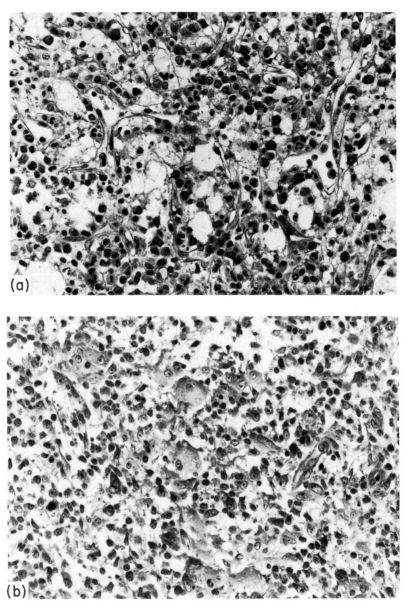

Fig. 4.2 Sections of biopsy of patients with acquired immune deficiency syndrome. (a) Lymphoid cells, histiocytes, fibroblasts and vascular proliferation; (b) another area from same section showing lymphoid cells and histiocytes. × 250, Giemsa.

In chronic inflammatory conditions haematopoiesis and fat cells are decreased and their place is taken by reticulin and collagen fibres, fibroblasts and capillaries, macrophages and other infiltrating cells (Fig. 4.3) (Schlag *et al.*, 1983). Thiele *et al.*, (1983) have described the distribution and size of megakaryocytes in inflammatory reactions. In long-standing hypoplasias there is a reduction in trabecular bone volume (osteopenia). Various toxins, including minerals, may also affect the trabecular bone; for example aluminium poisoning in renal dialysis patients (Wills and Savory, 1983). Such non-specific changes in the bone marrow may be roughly classified into 6 types:

(1) Acute inflammation, 'exudative' or 'necrotic' types: considerable residual haematopoiesis though necrosis of haematopoietic cells and capillaries is present, as well as oedema (Plate IIb), and there may be an increase in mature granulocytes. Necrosis of bone may be caused by chemotherapy with or without addition of steroids (Harper *et al.*, 1984).

(2) Chronic inflammation, 'atrophic type': little haematopoiesis remains; there is oedema, infiltration with lymphocytes, plasma cells and mast cells. The 'atrophic' type is also referred to as gelatinous transformation, serous atrophy, or exudative myelitis. Such changes in the bone marrow may be found in a large variety of diseases, including chronic infections, malignancies and poor nutrition. The marrow is hypocellular and fat cells are also reduced.

(3) Chronic inflammation, 'fibrotic type': haematopoiesis and fat reduced, increase in reticulin (sclerosing myelitis, Plate IIa) and development of collagen fibres, plasmacytosis, interstitial oedema, variable infiltration with lymphocytes and mast cells, and possibly osteoblastic new bone formation.

(4) Chronic inflammation, 'proliferative type': normocellular to hypercellular marrow, but with increases in plasma and mast cells, lymphocytes and eosinophils.

(5) Chronic inflammation, 'leukaemoid type': normocellular to hypercellular marrow with increases in neutrophil or eosinophil granulocytes or megakaryocytes (Plate IIf).

(6) Chronic inflammation, 'granulomatous type': characterized by the presence of giant cell granulomas (Fig. 4.4) or lipid granulomas, or epithelioid cell granulomas (with or without accumulation of lymphocytes), or mast cell granulomas (Plate IIc). Granuloma is the name applied to a special pattern of chronic inflammation. Granulomas are nodular (usually) aggregates of inflammatory cells, consisting mainly of modified macrophages also called epithelioid cells, because of their shape. Coalescence or fusion of macrophages gives rise to the multi-nucleated giant cells (Langhan's cells) whose nuclei often form a ring at the

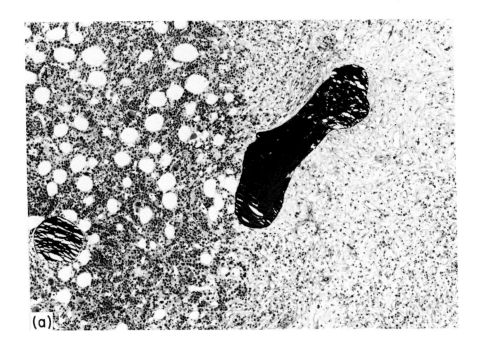

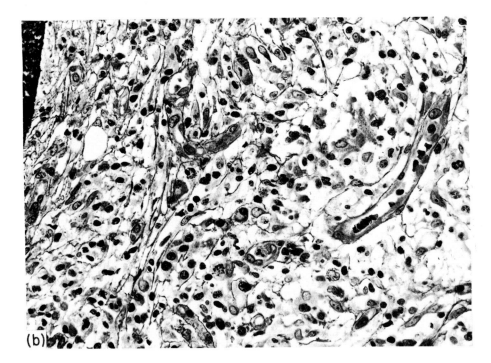

periphery of the cell mass. The giant cells may reach 300 μm in diameter, with numerous (more than 30) nuclei. The inclusion bodies (Schauman's, asteroid, or residual bodies) within giant cells are the non-specific products of metabolism and secretion in various stages of breakdown. Other cells such as fibroblasts, plasma cells, lymphocytes, and neutrophils, may be found in and around a granuloma.

The types of reaction seen in groups 1–5 have already been dealt with above. With reference to granulomas, it should be stressed that these are not unusual in the bone marrow (Schnaidt et al., 1980), and they may be found in hypocellular, normocellular or hypercellular marrow (Table 4.1). Granuloma formation occurs in response to numerous agents including mycobacterium, fungi, toxoplasma, histoplasma, malignant lymphomas and multiple myeloma (Falini et al., 1982), Hodgkin's disease, regional ileitis, sarcoidosis (Browne et al., 1978), as a reaction to non-haematologic neoplasms, in patients with primary biliary cirrhosis, in Q fever (Okun et al., 1979), in infectious mononucleosis (Martin, 1977), and in association with mitochondrial antibodies (Fagan et al., 1983). Granulomas come in various sizes and are of variable composition: they may be large or small, inter- or para-trabecular, single or multiple, consist of isolated giant cells or of giant cells and lymphocytes, plasma cells, histiocytes, epithelioid cells, eosinophils, mast cells and capillaries, fibroblasts and fibres, in varying proportions (Adler, 1980; Spector, 1980). The description of granulomas in the bone marrow in sarcoidosis serves as an example (see below). Granulomatous bone marrow disease has been reviewed by Bodem et al. (1983).

Table 4.1 Granulomas in bone marrow biopsies (no. 156)

Conditions	% of total
Unknown	22
Systemic mastocytosis	21
Hodgkin's disease	14
Malignant lymphomas	10
Tuberculosis	9
Sarcoidosis	8
Infections	5
Cancers	5
Collagen diseases	4
Polycythaemia vera	2

Fig. 4.3   (a) Patchy fibrosis in bone marrow of patient with autoimmune disease; note absence of megakarocytes in the fibrotic area. × 100, Gomori; (b) high power of area from section above; showing replacement of haematopoietic and fat cells by connective tissue containing capillaries, fibroblasts, reticulin fibres, lymphocytes and plasma cells. × 400, Gomori.

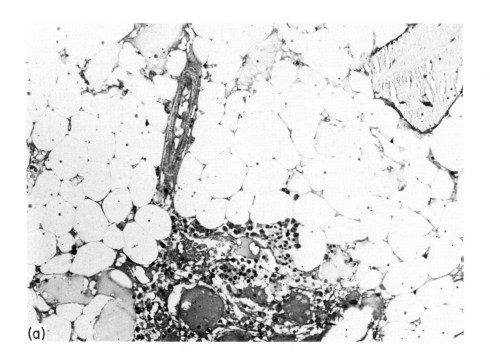

(a)

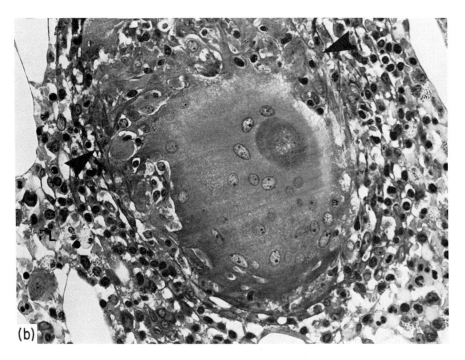

(b)

4.1   Lipid granulomas

These consist of lipid-laden macrophages, and there may be a small aggregate, or large accumulations. Lymphocytes, plasma cells and eosinophils, occasional giant cells, epithelioid cells and fibroblasts may be associated with lipid granulomas.

4.2   Sarcoidosis

About 30% of patients with sarcoidosis have characteristic granulomas in their bone marrow biopsies (Fig. 4.4). These granulomas are composed of epithelioid cells and giant cells, surrounded by lymphocytes together with fibres and amorphous eosinophilic material; very rarely Schauman or asteroid bodies are found. The giant cells may reach a size of 300 μm and contain 30 or so nuclei; the cytoplasm contains inclusion bodies which are the non-specific end-products of the cells' activities. Necrosis is not observed, in contrast to granulomas in the bone marrow in tuberculosis, which are otherwise similar to those in sarcoidosis (Table 4.2). Increased osteoclastic bone resorption may cause hypercalcaemia in sarcoidosis.

Table 4.2 Incidence of bone marrow involvement in granulomatous disorders

Patients No.	Condition	% involvement
75	Systemic mastocytosis	80%
44	Miliary tuberculosis	41%
43	Sarcoidosis	30%

4.2.1   Non-specific reactions in the bone marrow

It should be remembered that the bone marrow, as the source of reactive cells, has the capacity to react promptly and strongly to stimuli; that many such reactions are transitory (as are the stimuli which evoke them) and are followed by complete regeneration and restoration of the normal aspect of the bone marrow. To give but one example—in anorexia nervosa the pancytopenia is due to hypoplasia and exudative myelitis which are completely reversible on resumption of normal nutrition. However, other cases of exudative myelitis, morphologically similar but due to different

---

Fig. 4.4   (a) Pancytopenia of unknown aetiology, epithelioid cell granuloma in atrophic marrow. × 250, Giemsa; (b) granuloma in bone marrow in case of sarcoidosis; note giant cell with inclusion body, epithelioid cells (arrows) and outer rim of lymphoid cells. × 400, Giemsa.

causes, may terminate in myelofibrosis or even complete aplasia if repair of the damaged stroma is not effected. Though little data are available, it appears that the nature of aetiologic agent and possibly its persistence, influence the eventual outcome.

4.3   Blood vessels in cytopenias

Marrow atrophy (hypoplasia, fatty atrophy, replacement of the haematopoietic tissue by fat cells) may occur whenever pathologic alterations affect the blood vessels (Plate IIIc), such as in arteriosclerosis (Fig. 4.5), thrombosis and vasculitis. Such changes may also be found in diabetes accompanied by hypoplasia and osteopenia in the affected areas. Giant cell arteritis has also been detected by bone biopsy (Enos *et al.*, 1981).

4.4   Amyloidosis

Amyloid, a fibrillar material, is deposited extracellularly, and it is found first in the walls of the small blood vessels (Fig. 4.5).

The two main types are (a) 'amyloid of unknown origin' (though possibly derived from a plasma protein) and (b) amyloid of immunoglobulin origin, derived from the light chains of immunoglobulins. The first is the classic type of secondary amyloidosis which may develop in some chronic inflammatory diseases and in cancers. The second occurs in about 15% of patients with multiple myeloma or other plasma cell dyscrasia, as well as in some cases of so-called primary amyloidosis in which no predisposing cause is found. There are also rare forms of genetically determined amyloidosis.

Vascular amyloidosis has been described in the bone marrow in many and various conditions, mostly chronic, and though interstitial amyloidosis also occurs in the bone marrow, it is extremely rare. Amyloid is readily observed in Giemsa stained sections, though other stains such as Congo red are often applied for confirmation. It appears as a homogeneous bluish deposit, usually localized within the arterial walls. Extensive studies have shown that amyloid fibrils are formed by proteolysis of delta chains at an acid pH. Light chains are not processed by monocytes.

Deposits of amyloid in the walls of blood vessels are as readily detected in the bone marrow of patients with vascular amyloidosis, as in biopsies

Fig. 4.5   (a) Artery showing amyloid deposition (arrow) in wall, surrounded by plasma cells. × 800, Giemsa; (b) section showing hypoplastic bone marrow and blood vessel with thickened wall. × 100, toluidine blue; (c) sclerotic vessels in patient with diabetes. × 400, Gomori.

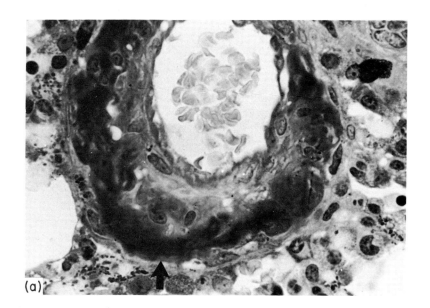

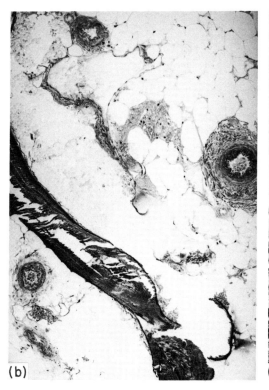
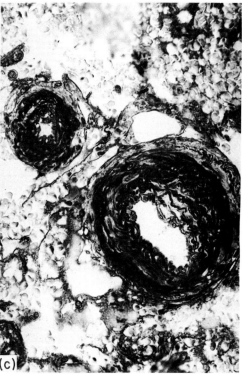

of the rectal mucosa (Krause, 1977). Interstitial amyloidosis, on the other hand, is infrequent in the bone marrow. Both have deleterious effects on haematopoiesis and the stroma, and lead to hypoplasia and osteopenia.

4.5   Bone marrow necrosis

As noted above, this may be found in the acute phase after thrombosis of a vessel, as ischaemic necrosis of bone in systemic lupus (Zizic *et al.*, 1980), in infections such as bacterial endocarditis (Eide, 1982), in Q fever (Brada and Bellingham, 1980), in streptococcal infections (Terheggen and Lampert, 1979), in other severe toxic and inflammatory states (Fig. 4.6), in rapidly growing leukaemias and lymphomas (Cowan *et al.*, 1980), and in the vicinity of expanding metastases (Conrad and Carpenter, 1979; Granot *et al.*, 1980; Hughes *et al.*, 1981; Frisch *et al.*, 1984). Necrosis in the bone marrow has also been observed in sickle cell disease: obstruction of vessels leads to ischaemia and necrosis of haematopoietic tissue. Fat embolism has also been implicated. When extensive, bone marrow necrosis causes bone pain.

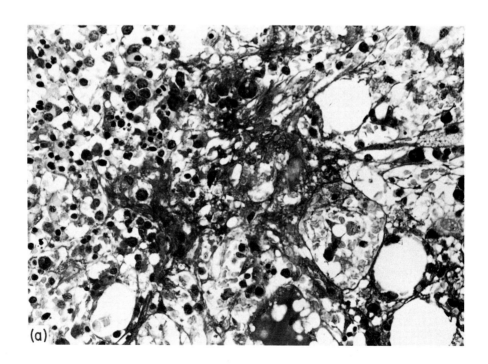

(a)

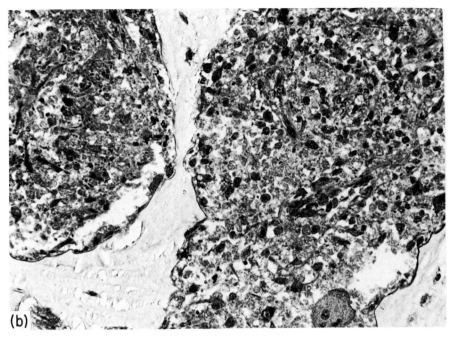

Fig. 4.6 (a) Exudative myelitis in sepsis; note 'Fibrinfaser-Sterne' stellate deposits of fibrin and incipient fibrosis of the bone marrow. × 400, Gomori; (b) sepsis with necrosis of bone marrow; cell outlines blurred and only nuclear smudges remain. × 250, Giemsa.

4.6   Osteomyelitis

This may result from haematogenous spread of organisms which then settled in the bone marrow. The organisms may gain entrance from contamination of fractures, from surgical operations, or from other more unobtrusive (or even unnoticed) inflammatory lesions. The typical lesion in the bone marrow is necrosis (in the acute cases), of both marrow and bone. This is accompanied by an intense reaction of polymorphonuclear leucocytes. This phase is sometimes called suppurative destructive necrosis. Subsequently, there is the phase of reactive reparative response, especially osteoblastic activity, which may eventually give rise to a dense sclerosis (Garrés sclerosing osteomyelitis), due to fibrous and bony repair of the destructive lesions (Plate IIe).

References

Adler, C. P. (1980), Granulomatous diseases of bone. In: *64th Verh. Dtsch. Ges. Path.* (ed. G. Dhom), Gustav Fischer Verlag, Stuttgart, pp. 359–60.

Bodem, C. R., Hamory, B. H., Taylor, H. M. and Kleopfer, L. (1983), Granulomatous bone marrow disease. A review of the literature and clinicopathologic analysis of 58 cases. *Medicine*, **62**, 372–83.

Brada, M. and Bellingham, A. J. (1980), Bone marrow necrosis and Q fever. *Brit. med. J.*, **281**, 1108–9.

Browne, P. M., Sharma, O. P. and Salkin, D. (1978), Bone marrow sarcoidosis. *J. Am. med. Assoc.*, **240**, 2654–55.

Cohen, R. J., Samoskuk, M. K., Busch, D. and Lagios, M. (1983), Occult infections with M. intracellulare in bone-marrow biopsy specimens from patients with AIDS. *New Engl. J. Med.*, **308**, 1475–6.

Conrad, M. E. and Carpenter, J. T. (1979), Bone marrow necrosis. *Am. J. Haemat.*, **7**, 181–9.

Cowan, J. D., Rubin, R. N., Kies, M. S. and Cerazo, L. (1980), Bone marrow necrosis. *Cancer*, **46**, 2168–71.

Eide, J. (1982), Bone infarcts in bacterial endocarditis. *Human Pathol.*, **13**, 631–4.

Enos, W. F., Pierre, W. V. and Rosenblatt, J. E. (1981), Giant cell arteritis detected by bone marrow biopsy. *Mayo Clinic Proc.*, **56**, 381–3.

Fagan, E. A., Moore-Gillon, J. C. and Turner-Warwick, M. (1983), Multiorgan granulomas and mitochondrial antibodies. *New Engl. J. Med.*, **308**, 572–5.

Falini, B., Tabilio, A., Velardi, A., Cernetti, C., Aversa, F. and Martelli, M. F. (1982), Multiple myeloma with a sarcoidosis-like reaction. *Scand. J. Haematol.*, **29**, 211–16.

Frisch, B. Bartl, R., Mahl, G. and Burkhardt, R. (1984), Scope and value of bone marrow biopsies in metastatic cancer. *Invasion Metastis 4*, Suppl. **1**, 12–30.

Geddes, A. M. (1983), Q fever. *Brit. med. J.*, **287**, 927–8.

Granot, H., Polliack, A. and Metzner, T. (1980), Bone marrow necrosis as the only manifestation of disseminated carcinomatosis. *Acta Haemat. (Basel)*, **64**, 232–5.

Harper, P. G., Trask, C. and Souhami, R. L. (1984), Avascular necrosis of bone caused by combination chemotherapy without corticosteroids. *Brit. med. J.*, **288**, 267–8.

Hughes, R. G., Islam, A., Lewis, S. M. and Catovsky, D. (1981), Spontaneous remission following bone marrow necrosis in chronic lymphocytic leukaemia. *Clin. lab. Haematol.*, **3**, 173–84.

Kaltwasser, J. P., Hubner, K., Bergmann, L., Schalk, K. P., Schneider, M. and Mitrou, P. S. (1983). Bone marrow histology and T-cell subsets as indicators of immunopathogenesis in aplastic anaemia and pure red cell anaemia. *Verh. Dtsch. Ges. Path.*, **67**, 307–12.

Krause, J. R. (1977), Value of bone marrow biopsy in the diagnosis of amyloidosis. *South. Med. J.*, **70**, 1072–4.

Lawrence, C. and Schreiber, A. J. (1979), Leprosy's footprints in bone-marrow histiocytes. *New Engl. J. Med.*, **300**, 834–5.

Martin, M. F. R. (1977), Atypical infectious mononucleosis with bone marrow granulomas and pancytopenia. *Brit. med. J.*, **2**, 200.

Okun, D. B., Sun, N. C. J. and Tanaka, K. R. (1979), Bone marrow granulomas in Q fever. *Am. J. clin. Pathol.*, **71**, 117–21.

Schlag, R., Burkhardt, R., Bartl, R. and Kettner, G. (1983), Acute and chronic inflammatory changes in the bone marrow. *Verh. Dtsch. Ges. Path.*, **67**, 474–7.

Schnaidt, U., Vyukupil, K. F., Thiele, J., Scheller, S. and Georgii, A. (1980), Granuloma-like lesions of the bone marrow. In *Verhandlungen der Deutschen Gesellschaft für Pathologie* (ed. G. Dhom), Gustav Fischer Verlag, Stuttgart, pp. 21–4.

Spector, W. G. (1980), The morphology, kinetics and fate of granulomas. In *Verhandlungen der Deutschen Gesellschaft für Pathologie* (ed. G. Dhom), Gustav Fischer Verlag, Stuttgart, pp. 21–4.

Terheggen, H. G. and Lampert, F. (1979), Acute bone marrow necrosis caused by streptococcal infection. *Eur. J. Paed.*, **130,** 53–8.

Thiele, J., Holgado, S., Choritz, H. and Georgii, A. (1983), Density distribution and size of megakarocytes in inflammatory reactions of the bone marrow (myelitis) and chronic myeloproliferative diseases. *Scand. J. Haematol.*, **31,** 329–41.

Wills, M. R. and Savory, J. (1983), Aluminium poisoning: dialysis encephalopathy, osteomalacia and anaemia. *Lancet*, **2,** 29–33.

Zizic, T. M., Hungerford, D. S. and Stevens, M. B. (1980), Ischemic bone necrosis in systemic lupus erythrematosus. *Medicine*, **59,** 134–42.

5 Qualitative abnormalities of erythropoiesis

5.1 Dyserythropoiesis

This incorporates both morphological and kinetic aspects of erythropoiesis, and recognizes the fact that even when erythroblasts are functionally abnormal some survive and mature, and so reach circulation, albeit that they are abnormal and their descendent erythrocytes are likely to have a shortened life span (Lewis and Verwilghen, 1977). Thus, dyserythropoiesis includes both quantitative and qualitative anomalies of erythropoiesis. A certain degree of morphological dyserythropoiesis may be seen whenever hyperplasia (or perhaps accelerated production) occurs, but this is transitory, lasting only until equilibrium has been re-established, and as such might be considered 'physiological dyserythropoiesis'.

Two broad categories of pathological dyserythropoiesis are recognized: congenital and acquired. Included in the first are the Congenital Dyserythropoietic Anaemias, i.e. CDA I, II (Hempas) and III and their variants; the thalassaemic syndromes, the haemoglobinopathies; congenital sideroblastic anaemias, Fanconi's anaemia and others (Table 5.1). Bone marrow biopsies are rarely performed in these conditions as they are usually diagnosed by biochemical and haematological tests. They are characterized by hyperplastic and ineffective erythropoiesis with a haemolytic component of variable magnitude, and associated disturb-

Table 5.1 Disturbance of haemoglobin synthesis

1. Disorders of iron metabolism
2. Disorders of globin synthesis
   Thalassaemia syndromes
   Other haemoglobinopathies
3. Disorders of porphyrin and haem synthesis
4. Drug-induced

ances in iron metabolism. Frequently the trabecular bone is affected by the hyperplastic marrow so that varying degrees of osteodystrophy and osteomalacia result (Pootrakul *et al.*, 1981). The second category embraces a wide range of conditions including nutritional deficiencies (e.g. vitamin B_{12}, folate, iron), the myelodysplastic syndromes, haematological malignancies involving the red cell series directly, and those which affect erythropoiesis by altering the micro-environment. Only the CDAs will be described in detail in this chapter; others will be discussed in appropriate sections elsewhere.

5.2   Megaloblastic (and megaloblastoid) erythropoiesis

This is due to deficiency of vitamin B_{12} or folic acid or both, and similar morphological changes are observed whatever the cause, such as increased demand, defective absorption, insufficient supply, lack of intrinsic factor, effects of drugs, such as anticonvulsants, some oral contraceptives, antitubercular drugs, and large doses of other antibiotic agents (Table 5.2). The erythroid cells are larger than normal, with large

Table 5.2 Megaloblastic or megaloblastoid maturation

1. Defective DNA synthesis (acquired)
   Deficiency of vitamin B_{12} and/or folate
     Dietary GI tract anomalies
     Increased demand drugs
2. Accelerated haematopoiesis due to
   (1) Haemolysis
   (2) Haemorrhage
3. Congenital anomalies of erythropoiesis
4. Of uncertain origin
   Acquired sideroblastic anaemia
   Myelodysplastic syndromes
   Accompanying other malignancies
5. Neoplastic alterations
   Myeloproliferative disorders

nuclei which have a much finer chromatin pattern than erythroblasts undergoing normoblastic maturation, and there are proportionally many more immature erythroid cells than late forms. In addition, the other cell lines also show disturbed maturation such as giant bands (metamyelocytes) in the neutrophilic series, hypersegmented polymorphs and multinucleate megakaryocytes. There is increased iron in the stromal cells (Table 5.3) unless iron deficiency is also present. The bone marrow is frequently hypercellular with reduction in fat cells.

Table 5.3 Conditions with quantitative changes in iron stores

Decreased	Increased
Deficiencies	Congenital haemoglobinopathies
Diet	Sideroblastic anaemia
Vegetarians	Congenital dyserythropoietic anaemias
Utilization	Haemochromatosis
Pregnancy	Acquired sideroblastic anaemias
Lactation	Chronic diseases
Loss	Collagen
Haemorrhage	Renal
Varices	Storage diseases
Diagphragmatic hernia	In older age groups
Parasites	Erythroid malignancies
Malignancies	Myelofibrosis/osteomyelosclerosis
Polycythaemia vera	Other malignancies
	Haemosiderosis
	Transfusion overload

5.2.1   Iron deficiency

Iron deficiency is still very prevalent throughout the world. The bone marrow shows hyperplasia of the erythroid series, the cells are small, there are many late forms with pale cytoplasm due to insufficient haemoglobinization, and the cytoplasmic edges are ragged. There is a considerable degree of ineffective erythropoiesis, with intramedullary destruction. In some cases of marked iron deficiency, the marrow may even be hypocellular.

5.3   Congenital dyserythropoietic anaemias

The diagnosis is usually made by smears of aspirates of bone marrow and by electron microscopy, by means of which and in conjunction with other biochemical and haematological investigations the types and their variants are distinguished. Bone marrow biopsy sections show a hypercellular marrow with an extreme degree of erythropoietic hyperplasia and corresponding reduction in fat cells (Fig. 5.1). At high magnification some characteristic nuclear aberrations are seen even in the light microscope although their detailed structure requires electron microscopy (Lewis and Verwilghen, 1977). These include bi-nuclearity, multi-nuclearity, internuclear bridges, and nuclear budding, fragmentation and degeneration (karyorrhexis) and a variety of atypical mitotic figures. Cytoplasmic abnormalities include vacuolation, basophilic stippling, and iron containing granules (ringed sideroblasts also occur) and

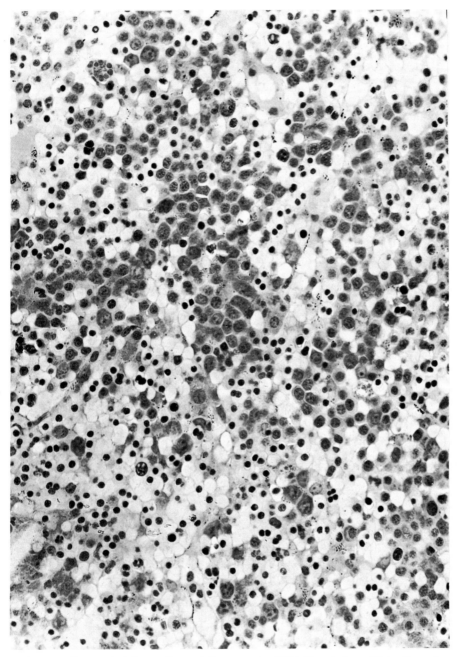

Fig. 5.1 Congenital dyserythropoietic anaemia, CDA II; note loss of fat cells and extreme erythroid hyperplasia. × 400, Giemsa.

intercellular cytoplasmic connections. Not all erythroid precursors are affected so that apparently normal ones are seen alongside the dyserythropoietic cells.

Macrophages with engulfed erythroblasts and nuclear debris are prominent; in some cases of CDA II Gaucher-like histiocytes have been observed in the bone marrow. As in most situations with augmented and ineffective erythroid turnover, iron stores are increased and deposits are found (in severe cases) in reticular, endothelial and endosteal cells and, if transfusion overload occurs, even in the osteoid seams. In long-standing cases, the trabecular bone is osteopenic with increased osteoid, and normal or increased bone turnover.

5.4   Porphyrias

These comprise a group of disorders classified as either erythropoietic or hepatic according to the site of occurrence of the metabolic defect. The bone marrow shows erythroblastic hyperplasia. There may be a dimorphic population, with the presence of macroblasts due (possibly) to folate deficiency, because of increased requirement and consumption and therefore a relative lack. The pathological population of erythroid precursors exhibits marked dyserythropoietic features.

5.5   Haemolytic anaemias

Bone biopsies are generally not of much diagnostic significance. The congenital haemolytic anaemias are due to inborn errors of erythrocyte metabolic enzymes and unstable haemoglobins; the only feature to be seen in a biopsy, may be increased erythroid hyperplasia. In acquired haemolytic anaemias biopsies may help in the differential diagnosis, especially when involvement by malignant conditions is a contributing factor. Abnormal antibodies together with proliferation of the RES with augmented phagocytosis may be involved in the haemolytic episodes in these cases. Among the acquired haemolytic anaemias, paroxysmal nocturnal haemoglobinuria (PNH) is of special interest (Schreiber, 1983). The increased sensitivity of erythrocytes to complement-mediated lysis is due to a membrane defect which has also been found in granulocytes, platelets and in colony forming units, suggesting that PNH results from a change at the level of the pluripotent stem cells (Dessypris et al., 1983). The bone marrow is usually hyperplastic, but hypoplasia may occur, and even an 'aplastic crisis', in which there is a transient failure of red cell production.

Crises in haemolytic conditions may be precipitated by infections, especially those of the upper respiratory tract. Some aplastic crises in haemolytic anaemias have recently been ascribed to a parvovirus (Davies, 1983). In severe haemolysis, the bone marrow fat cells are replaced by hyperplastic normoblastic erythropoiesis (Plate Ve) with a predominance of early erythroblasts (Fig. 5.2); many mitotic figures are seen as well as macrophages with nuclear remains. These are also found in other situations, such as the aplastic crisis of PNH in which erythropoietic activity is reduced. Increased erythropoiesis due to haemorrhage is also characterized by an imbalance in favour of immature erythroblasts, perhaps due to accelerated passage and release into the circulation. In addition, there is a concomitant increase in megakaryocytes, due to loss and increased utilization of platelets. In chronic haemolytic anaemias, extension of haematopoiesis into shafts of the long bones and even into the liver and spleen may occur.

5.6   Sideroblastosis

Anaemias with a sideroblastic component may occur in alcoholics, megaloblastic anaemias, inflammatory diseases, haematological malignancies, myelodysplastic syndromes and miscellaneous other conditions (Table 5.4).

Haemosiderosis is defined as accumulation of iron in cells of the reticuloendothelial system, especially the liver. When this is extensive, it leads eventually to fibrosis in the affected tissues.

In iron overload, iron may be found in macrophages and reticular cells, in sinus endothelial cells, in endosteal cells, and even deposited in osteoid on the surface of the trabecular bone; and in osteocytic lacunae (Fig. 5.3 and Plate IXf). After staining with Prussian blue (or any other iron stain) iron present in cells appears as a pale cytoplasmic 'wash' and as fine to coarse clumps in intracellular granules. When considerable haemosiderin is present it will also be seen as brownish-yellow intracellular deposits in the Giemsa stain. Bone marrow iron stores are better assessed in sections than in smears of aspirates which may not contain sufficient stromal elements to be representative.

Haemosiderosis is usually due to transfusion overload in hereditary conditions such as the thalassaemias, sickle cell disease, spherocytosis, red cell enzyme deficiencies, or in acquired conditions such as aplastic anaemia and myelofibrosis. The clinical consequences of transfusional iron overload have been detailed by Schafer *et al.* (1981).

5.7   Haemochromatosis

This may occur as a familial (or primary, or idiopathic) entity, or in association with a variety of hepatic disorders (secondary), and in con-

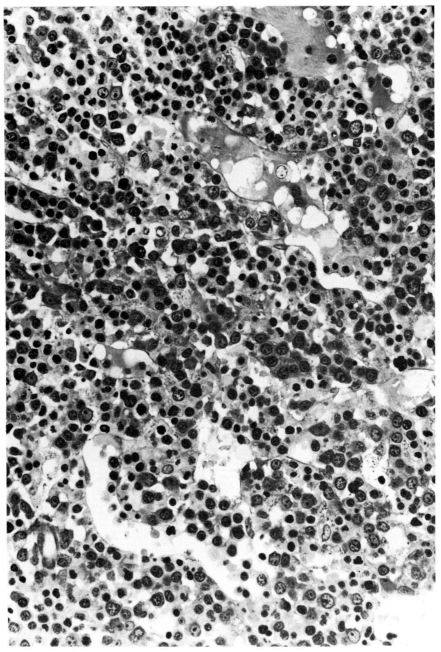

Fig. 5.2 Biopsy section of patient with haemolytic anaemia, drug induced, showing erythroid hyperplasia, but no increase in megakaryocytes. × 400, Giemsa.

Table 5.4 Sideroblastic erythropoiesis

Hereditary	Enzyme deficiencies
Acquired	'Idiopathic'
	Drugs
	Alcohol abuse
	Connective tissue diseases
	Inflammatory diseases
	Haematological malignancies
	Other malignancies

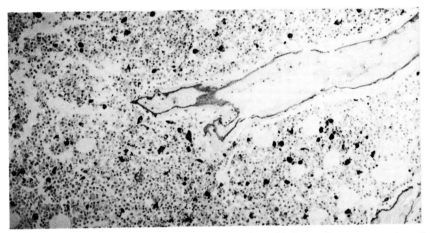

Fig. 5.3   Section of bone biopsy of patient with multiple myeloma, anaemia and transfusional iron overload; the black dots represent macrophages loaded with haemosiderin, and the trabecular bone is outlined by iron deposited on the osteoid tissue. × 60, Berlin blue.

genital transferrin deficiency. In the primary form, there may be less deposition of haemosiderin in the cells of the reticulo-endothelial system. However, osteoporosis and even collapse of a vertebral body have been noted, usually ascribed to ascorbic acid deficiency which in turn is secondary to the oxidative effects of the body iron. Another mechanism, and possibly a more direct one, is the inhibitory effect on osteoblasts due to the deposition of iron in endosteal cells and osteoid seams.

Recent studies have shown that determination of the erythrocyte ferritin content is a useful non-invasive test to distinguish haemo-chromatosis from alcoholic liver disease with iron overload (van der Weyden *et al.*, 1983).

References

Davies, L. R. (1983), Aplastic crises in haemolytic anaemias: the role of a parvovirus-like agent. *Brit. J. Haematol.*, **55**, 391–3.

Dessypris, E. N., Clarke, D. A., McKee, Jr. L. C. and Krantz, S. B. (1983), Increased sensitivity to complement of erythroid and myeloid progenitors in paroxysmal nocturnal hemoglobinuria. *New Engl. J. Med.*, **309**, 609–3.

Lewis, S. M. and Verwilghen, R. L. (eds) (1977), *Dyserythropoiesis*, Academic Press, London, p. 5.

Pootrakul, P., Hungsprenges, S., Fucharoen, S., Baylink, D., Thompson, E., English, E., Lee, M. and Finch, C. (1981), Relation between erythropoiesis and bone metabolism in thalassemia. *New Engl. J. Med.*, **304**, 1470–6.

Schafer, A. I., Cheron, R. G., Dluhy, R., Cooper, B., Gleason, R. E., Soeldner, J. S. and Bunn, H. F. (1981), Clinical consequences of acquired transfusional iron overload in adults. *New Engl. J. Med.*, **304**, 319–24.

Schreiber, A. D. (1983), Paroxysmal nocturnal hemoglobinuria revisited. *New Engl. J. Med.*, **309**, 723–4.

Weyden, M. B. van der, Fong, H., Salem, H. H., Batey, R. G. and Dudley, F. J. (1983), Erythrocyte ferritin content in idiopathic haemochromatosis and alcoholic liver disease with iron overload. *Brit. med. J.*, **286**, 752–4.

6 Hyperplastic reactions

6.1 Erythrocytosis

Erythrocytosis or secondary polycythaemia, without leucocytosis or thrombocytosis, may occur when erythropoiesis is stimulated by raised levels of erythropoietin. This occurs as a result of abnormal mutant haemoglobins with increased oxygen affinity and also in acquired conditions in which erythrocytosis occurs as a result of 'appropriate' stimuli such as high altitude, pulmonary or cardiovascular disease; or 'inappropriate' when excess erythropoietin production is due to non-physiologic causes such as renal carcinoma, cerebellar adenomas and uterine myomas. The causes of a quantitative increase in erythropoiesis are listed in Table 3.2. The diagnosis of the cause of the erythrocytosis is made by appropriate clinical investigation. The appearance of the bone marrow is similar irrespective of cause: normal architectural pattern, normocellular to increased cellularity with numerous foci of erythropoiesis exhibiting all maturational stages. In some cases, the parenchyme to fat ratio may be unaltered, or exceptionally even increased. In the absence of iron deficiency, iron stores are not depleted and there is normal reticulin. There may be a discrepancy between the erythrocytosis in the peripheral blood and the apparent activity in the bone marrow—an expression of its reserve capacity and the efficiency and speed with which it can compensate. Chronic erythroid hyperplasia may be accompanied by accelerated bone turnover (Weinstein, 1981). The blood count may be elevated, normal or even low.

An elevated blood count is also seen in relative polycythaemia (also referred to as 'pseudo' or 'stress' polycythaemia). This is due to a reduced plasma volume. The red cell mass is not increased and the bone marrow is normal.

6.2   Leukaemoid reactions

This refers to peripheral blood values and pictures resembling those seen in certain leukaemias, notably CML. They may be elicited by numerous conditions (Table 3.3), including infections, bacterial and viral, inflammatory diseases, necroses, allergic reactions, haemolytic anaemias, burns, drugs, toxins and neoplasms. Characteristically, and most frequently, there is leucocytosis involving the neutrophilic granulocytes with a shift to the left, though other cell lines may also be implicated; thus, eosinophils are present in parasitic, allergic and dermatologic conditions, in connective tissue diseases and drug reactions (Table 6.1), lymphocytes in whooping cough, chicken pox and infectious mononucleosis, and monocytes in some granulomatous disorders. Marked lymphocytosis suggesting chronic lymphocytic leukaemia has been observed in hyposplenism (Wilkinson *et al.*, 1983). Eosinophilia has been described in lymphoblastic leukaemias and lymphomas (Catovsky *et al.*, 1980).

Table 6.1 Causes of eosinophilia

Allergic disorders (bronchial asthma, etc.)
Skin diseases
Parasitic infections
Loeffler's syndrome
Primary hypereosinophilic syndrome
'Tropical' eosinophilia
Infections
Myelo- and lymphoproliferative disorders
Malignancies (esp. with metastases, necrosis)
Post-radiation
Immune and collagen diseases
Hodgkin's disease
Mastocytosis

The histological differentiation between a leukaemoid reaction and CML in the bone marrow may not be possible. The same holds for eosinophilic CML and a marked eosinophilic reaction or the hypereosinophilic syndrome. However, in the reactive conditions overall cellularity is increased proportionately (Figs 6.1, 6.2). In bacterial sepsis, granulocytic precursors may replace the fat completely, with numerous polymorphonuclear leucocytes scattered throughout the marrow. Macrophages with crystalloid inclusions are rare but Charcot–Leyden crystal containing cells may be found whenever there is eosinophilic hyperplasia (Fig. 6.2); perivascular plasmacytosis may be pronounced, granulocytic hyperplasia is perivascular and intertrabecular rather than the marked

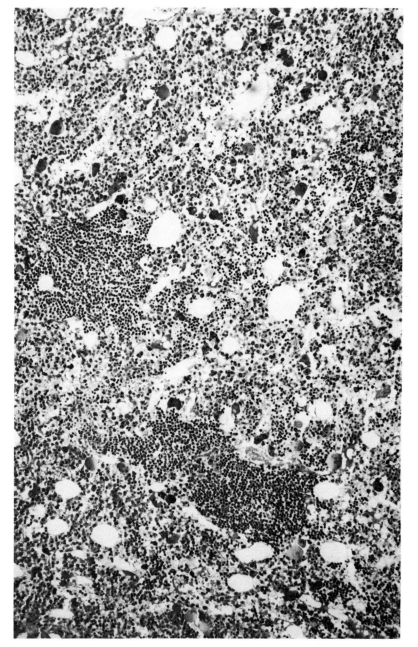

Fig. 6.1 Bone biopsy section of patient with CML and leukaemoid reaction. × 250, Giemsa.

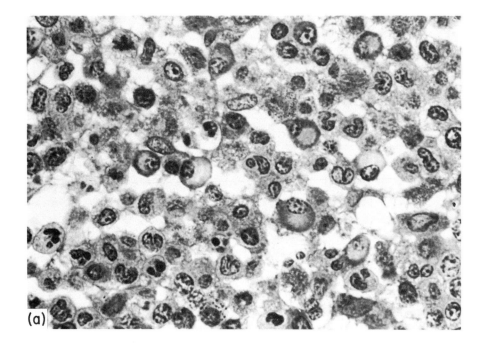

(a)

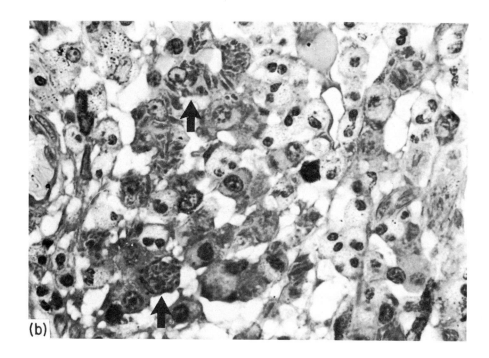

(b)

paratrabecular localization seen in CML. Megakaryocyte numbers vary, with no atypical features, and micromegakaryocytes are absent. When the peripheral blood counts are very high the bone marrow picture may resemble that of promyelocytic leukaemia. In leukaemoid reactions the hyperplasia involves mainly the neutrophilic and eosinophilic lines while in CML basophils are also involved, as reflected by the increased basophil count in the peripheral blood.

In infectious mononucleosis the marrow is hypercellular with increases in all haematopoietic elements as well as reticular cells; granulomas may also be present. Hypercellularity with an increase in histiocytes showing erythrophagocytosis is also seen in Kawasaki's disease (Marsh *et al.*, 1980; Kato *et al.*, 1983).

6.3 Thrombocytosis

Elevated platelet count may occur as a temporary phenomenon post-splenectomy, in acute or chronic inflammations after haemorrhage, in iron deficiency and post-operatively (see Table 3.4). It is also seen in patients with Hodgkin's disease, malignant lymphomas, and car-cinomas; in the last group it may represent a non-specific proliferative response to tissue necrosis as well as resulting from stimulation by specific factors. In these secondary thrombocytoses the bone marrow shows a normal architectural pattern, with normal to increased cellularity (depending on the aetiology), and an increase in megakaryocytes, but without the marked polymorphism, atypia, clustering and presence of pyknotic forms which characterize neoplastic megakaryocyte prolifer-ations, except in occasional cases with very severe infections. It should be stressed that very high platelet counts ($1000 \times 10^9/l$ or higher) in reactive conditions may be found in the absence of striking megakaryo-cytic hyperplasia or hypertrophy in the bone marrow (Fig. 6.3). Localized megakaryocytic increases may be found in the vicinity of metastases in the bone marrow (see p. 259 and Fig. 12.17).

6.4 Plasmacytosis

Plasmacytosis in the bone marrow (reactive plasmacytosis) may occur in

---

Fig. 6.2 (a) Bone marrow biopsy of patient with leukaemoid reaction due to retroperitoneal tumour (malignant inflammatory histiocytoma); note granulo-cytic hyperplasia and numerous plasma cells. The WBC was $18.0 \times 10^9/l$. $\times 600$, Giemsa; (b) eosinophilic reaction with multiple myeloma; note numerous crystal-containing histiocytes (arrows), presumably breakdown products of eosinophils. $\times 600$, Giemsa.

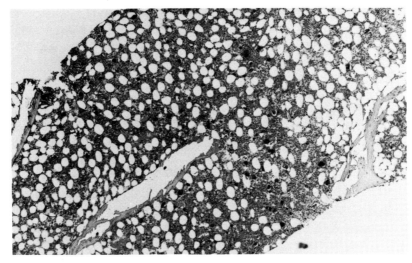

Fig. 6.3 Biopsy section of patient with diabetes and platelet count of $1000 \times 10^9/l$. Reaction to infection; no evident hyperplasia of megakaryocytes. $\times$ 40, Giemsa.

numerous conditions, especially those involving antigenic stimulation, allergic and autoimmune states and as an accompanying phenomenon of immunoproliferations elsewhere, for example in the immunoproliferative disease of the small intestine (Khojasteh *et al.*, 1983). Bone marrow plasmacytosis also occurs in leukaemoid reactions and in the presence of other malignancies (see p. 259). In these cells the plasma cases are dispersed throughout the marrow and clustered around capillaries (Fig. 6.2).

6.5   Mast cells

Increases in mast cells in the bone marrow may occur in allergic and autoimmune conditions, hypoplastic anaemias (both relative and absolute increases), lymphoproliferative disorders (Yoo *et al.*, 1978), as in lymphoplasmacytoid malignant lymphomas and in hairy cell leukaemia, vascular diseases, osteoporosis, myelodysplasias and preleukaemias; mast cells are also found in the neighbourhood of metastatic carcinoma, in myelofibrosis, and in mastocytosis.

References

Catovsky, D., Bernasconi, C., Verdonck, P. J., Postma, A., Hows, J., van der Does-van den Berg, A., Rees, J. K. H., Castelli, G., Morra, E. and Galton, D. A. G. (1980), The association of eosinophilia with lymphoblastic leukaemia or lymphoma: a study of seven patients. *Brit. J. Haematol.*, **45**, 523–34.

Kato, H., Inoue, O., Koga, Y., Shingu, M., Fujimoto, T., Kondo, M., Yamamoto, S., Tominaga, K. and Sasaguri, Y. (1983), Variant strain of propionibacterium acnes: a clue to the aetiolology of Kawasaki disease. *Lancet,* **2,** 1383–8.

Khojasteh, A., Haghshenass, M. and Haghighi, P. (1983), Immunoproliferative small intestinal disease. A 'Third-World Lesion'. Current concepts. *New Engl. J. Med.,* **308,** 1404–5.

Marsh, W. C., Bishop, J. W. and Koenig, H. M. (1980), Bone marrow and lymph node findings in a case of fatal Kawasaki's disease. *Arch. Pathol. Lab. Med.,* **104,** 563–7.

Weinstein, R. S., Hutson, M. S., Ide, L. F. and Lutcher, C. L. (1981), Chronic erythroid hyperplasia and accelerated bone turnover. *Clin. Res.,* **29,** 864A.

Wilkinson, L. S., Tang, A. and Gjested, A. (1983), Marked lymphocytosis suggesting chronic lymphocytic leukaemia in three patients with hyposplenism. *Am. J. Med.,* **75,** 1053–6.

Yoo, D., Lessin, L. S. and Jensen, W. C. (1978), Bone marrow mast cells in lymphoproliferative disorders. *Ann. int. Med.,* **88,** 753–7.

7 Osteopathies

The function of the skeleton is at least three-fold: (1) it constitutes the means for direct locomotion and movement, providing support and a protective covering for softer, vulnerable tissues; (2) it participates in the homeostasis of minerals; and (3) it houses the bone marrow which provides the formed elements of the blood.

The osteon (see Chapter 2) is the functional unit of cortical and compact bone, and the osteons carry out remodelling throughout life. Remodelling of the cancellous bone in the axial skeleton is carried out from the endosteal surface by osteoblasts which lay down lamellae of appositional osteoid and by the osteoclasts which resorb bone at the trabecular surface forming Howship's lacunae. Parathyroid hormones, calcitonin and metabolites of vitamin D are among the most important of the numerous substances participating in the intricate mechanisms controlling calcium metabolism and the integrity of bone.

Parathyroid hormone is the principal polypeptide hormone controlling calcium metabolism in the human.

Metabolites of vitamin D. The manner in which these participate in the control of osseous remodelling is not yet completely identified (Fraser, 1983; McCarthy *et al.*, 1984).

Calcitonin is involved in the regulation of calcium and bone metabolism. The rate of secretion of calcitonin is a function of the level of calcium in the plasma. Calcitonin inhibits resorption of mineral from bone; it acts on the osteoclasts, its action being mediated through the adenylate cyclase cyclic AMP system. Concepts on the regulation of bone formation and resorption (Parfitt, 1982) and the maintenance of the equilibrium between the two have expanded rapidly during recent years by advances made at the biochemical, molecular, cellular and tissue organizational levels. Moreover, the close association between bone and marrow and the interdependence and interactions of these two organs have only recently been fully appreciated (see reviews by Raisz, 1981; Vaughan, 1981); it has long been known that diseases of marrow affect the bone (e.g. hair-on-end skull in thalassaemia, and osteolysis in multiple myeloma), and disorders

88

of bone affect the marrow (anaemia in osteopetrosis and in Paget's disease). In addition, disturbances of connective tissue components affect both bone and marrow, such as haematopoietic hypoplasia and osteopenia in angiopathies; finally, both tissues may be profoundly altered by pathological changes in other organs such as anaemia and osteodystrophia in renal disease and erythrocytosis in pulmonary disorders. As this brief survey implies, trabecular bone is vulnerable and may be affected to varying degrees in a wide variety of diseases, either primary or secondary. In many of these a BMB is indicated, as anomalies of formation, resorption and mineralization may be diagnosed by the histological findings well before they are evident on X-rays. Moreover, with the introduction of fluorescent tetracycline markers, quantitation of basic kinetic variables of osseous remodelling is now feasible (Fallon and Teitelbaum, 1982). However, it is not possible in this chapter to deal with all of these aspects, and only the major entities will be considered.

7.1 Osteoporotic syndromes

These are defined as conditions in which a decrease in trabecular bone (Fig. 7.1) and to some extent in cortical bone values occurs to levels below those required for mechanical support (Meunier et al., 1979; Nordin et al., 1980). In addition to primary (idiopathic) osteoporosis, it occurs as a secondary event in a wide variety of conditions (Gruber, 1981). Some parts of the skeleton are far more liable to osteopenia than others, for example, the vertebrae and the femoral neck (Avioli and Raisz, 1981; Frisch et al., 1982). In iliac crest biopsies the osteopenia may be accompanied by a decrease in haematopoietic tissue, an increase in fat cells, a decrease in paratrabecular sinusoids, and an increase in mast cells (Fallon et al., 1983). Functionally one defect is thought to be a disturbance of the balance between formation and resorption in favour of the latter, but, especially in the so-called primary (idiopathic, age related, senile, post-menopausal) osteoporosis, the cause is most likely to be multifactorial (Darby, 1981; Nordin et al., 1981; Lips et al., 1982; Parfitt, 1982; Milhaud et al., 1983). It should be stressed that osteoporosis is the most common bone disease, affecting especially women past the menopause (Whedon, 1981; Stevenson and Whitehead, 1982). In bone biopsies osteoclastic activity may be observed, particularly if rarefied trabeculae with resorption lacunae are present—in serial sections the osteoclasts will also be found (Frisch et al., 1982). Osteoblasts and osteoid seams are few and far between. The formation of trabecular bone in osteoporosis has been studied by Darby and Meunier (1981). Generalized osteopenia also accompanies systemic mastocytosis (Fallon et al., 1981) and, rarely, calcitonin deficiency (Stevens et al., 1982).

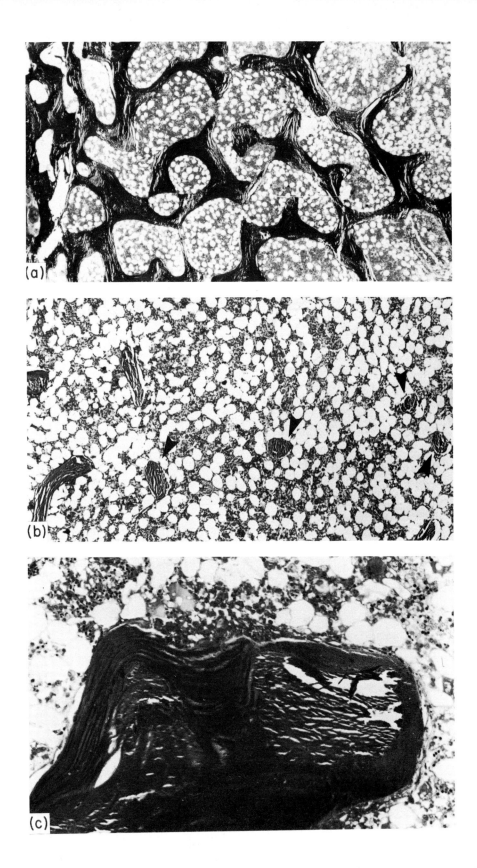

There is an association between osteoporosis and activity; physically active people, including post-menopausal women, are less likely to become osteoporotic. Exercise may have a beneficial effect even in established osteoporosis, as shown by an increase in density of the lumbar vertebrae. There appears to be an increased risk of femoral neck fractures in patients with renal insufficiency receiving fluorides (Gerster *et al.*, 1983).

Recent work indicates that osteoporosis occurs in different forms; in some cases the cortical bone is more effected, in others the cancellous, or both (Dixon, 1983). Osteoporosis also occurs in men (Seeman *et al.*, 1983). Recent studies have demonstrated that involutional osteoporosis can be divided into two distinct syndromes differing with respect to epidemiology, patterns of trabecular and cortical bone loss, parathyroid function and cause (Riggs and Melton, 1983).

7.2 Endocrine osteoporosis

Osteopenia may occur in hyperpituitarism, hyperthyroidism, hyperparathyroidism, and increased production (or administration) of steroids (Muls *et al.*, 1982). Glucocorticoid induced osteoporosis has been documented in patients treated for asthma and rheumatoid arthritis (Baylink, 1983). Bone marrow biopsies taken at the time of initial diagnosis provide base lines for monitoring the progression of disease and the effects of therapy. The picture observed is one of rarefaction of the trabecular bone without or with only very slightly increased osseous remodelling.

7.3 Miscellaneous causes of osteoporosis

These are manifold and include prolonged administration of large quantities of heparin, localized immobilization, 'disuse' osteoporosis (Stout, 1982) and 'juvenile' osteoporosis, which must be distinguished from congenital osteogenesis imperfecta (Herbage *et al.*, 1982), and metabolic osteoporosis as in diabetes which may affect adults and children (Shore *et al.*, 1981). Trabecular bone thickness is reduced in alcohol abuse (Schnitzler and Solomon, 1982).

Fig. 7.1 (a) Section of bone biopsy of young adult, illustrating normal trabecular bone structure. × 25, Gomori; (b) 'Idiopathic' osteoporosis in elderly patient, showing drastic reduction in volume percentage of trabecular bone; isolated trabecular profiles indicated by arrows. × 40, Giemsa; (c) biopsy section of patient with osteomalacia, the broad osteoid seams extend across the whole trabecular width in some places. × 250, toluidine blue.

Osteoporosis may also occur in iron overload, and in metabolic disorders in the presence of vascular changes, for example, microangiopathies of the marrow vessels (see Fig. 4.5). Osteoporosis, especially in the pelvic region, has also been described in Mönckeberg's arteriosclerosis (Amos and Wright, 1980).

7.4   Myelogenous osteopathies

Alterations in trabecular bone volume have been observed in all haematological malignancies (Burkhardt et al., 1984) as well as in non-neoplastic alterations in the cellularity of the bone marrow (Table 7.1) and

Table 7.1 Myelogenous osteodysplasia (MOD)

Conditions	No. patients	MOD,%
Osteomyelosclerosis	350	100
Multiple myeloma	710	70
Hodgkin's disease	130	61
Myelofibrosis	620	50
Aplastic anaemia	155	40
Chronic myeloid leukaemia	710	40
Polycythaemia vera	800	25
Malignant lymphomas	1255	20
Acute leukaemias	895	10
*Congenital haemolytic conditions		
*Storage diseases		

*Only few cases in these groups examined; all had some degree of osteodysplasia.

with benign lymphoid hyperplasia (Vigorita et al., 1983). Recent studies have shown that myeloid leukaemia cells produce a bone resorbing factor (Gewirtz et al., 1981). Rarefaction of trabecular bone is seen in conditions associated with hypercellularity as well as hypocellularity. When the cells of the intramedullary haematological malignancies are loosely packed with a connective tissue component, there may be paratrabecular fibrosis and even new bone formation. If considerable osteosclerosis is induced and mineralization delayed there will be a high incidence of osteomalacia. This situation may occur, for example, in bone marrow metastases of prostatic carcinoma (Charhon et al., 1983). However, it should be borne in mind that when bone marrow abnormalities which are accompanied by reductions in trabecular bone are found in older people, especially women, these could have been superimposed on some degree of pre-existing osteopenia. Osteopathies caused by metastases are considered in the section on non-haematological malignancies (pp. 264–7).

7.5 Osteodystrophies

These occur in congenital disorders of connective tissue, cartilage and bone, in vitamin D resistant rickets, in vitamin D dependent rickets, in gastro-intestinal and hepatic disorders, chronic metabolic acidosis (Cunningham *et al.*, 1982), and as a consequence of drug administration, e.g. anti-convulsant therapy (Kragstrup *et al.*, 1982). Classic examples are primary hyperparathyroidism and renal osteodystrophy (secondary hyperparathyroidism).

7.6 Osteomalacia

This may be a component of any of the disorders mentioned above. Osteomalacia (Fig. 7.1c) arises when newly formed bone matrix is inadequately mineralized (Plate IVb). About 24% of the trabecular surface covered by osteoid is considered the upper limit of normal; higher values suggest osteomalacia. Islands of non-mineralized bone matrix may also be found within the trabeculae (Fig. 7.1c). Increased osteoid seams and osteoid width and augmented remodelling (together with anomalies of tetracycline labelling as revealed by bone biopsies) are generally required for diagnosis (Frame and Parfitt, 1978; Avioli and Raisz 1981). Since X-rays cannot distinguish osteoid tissue, a bone biopsy is mandatory if osteomalacia is suspected on biochemical or clinical grounds. Osteomalacia may ensue from vitamin deficiencies resulting from hepatic (Dibble and Losowsky, 1982), renal (Brown *et al.*, 1982) or intestinal disease, from dietary insufficiencies and from drugs. Sub-clinical osteomalacia may be more frequent in the elderly than previously suspected, and can be diagnosed only by bone biopsy (Hosking *et al.*, 1983). It may occur in Turner's syndrome (Shore *et al.*, 1982) and as a result of intramedullary malignancies or during their treatment (Okita and Block, 1979). It is also seen in patients after uretero-sigmoidostomy; healing occurs by correction of the acidosis (Siklos *et al.*, 1980). In many cases a direct cause is a decrease in serum calcium or phosphorus, or both. Resistant osteomalacia may develop in patients on haemodialysis (Hodsman *et al.*, 1981). Initially there is an increase in osteoid plus a slight rise in the number of osteoblasts—later osseous remodelling and paratrabecular fibrosis may develop and the picture is then similar to that in secondary hyperparathyroidism. It is not possible to distinguish the histological picture in osteomalacia due to various other causes from that seen in renal osteodystrophy. In the latter the bone may be osteoporotic, osteomalacic, or resemble that in primary hyperparathyroidism. However, in malabsorption, osteoblasts tend to be more in evidence as opposed to osteoclasts in HPT. It should be emphasized that a wide range in the extent of remodelling may be observed in these conditions, from small localized patches to extensive stretches of the trabecular surface.

7.7   Other rare conditions

(a) Gorham's vanishing bone disease is possibly due to immune or other activation of osteoclasts, whose unopposed activity is responsible for the vanishing bone. (b) In marble bone disease (osteopetrosis), in which osteoblastic bone formation is not balanced by osteoclastic resorption, the osteoclasts are present on the cancellous bone, but apparently are not able to resorb it. This disease has recently been successfully treated by transplantation of monocytes from compatible donors (Coccia *et al.*, 1980); in the recipient these were transformed into osteoclasts which were able to restore the balance between formation and resorption, and thus a cure was effected. (c) Fluorosis, due to prolonged intake of fluorides, may cause a combination of osteosclerosis and osteomalacia. (d) Hypophosphataemic osteomalacia, in the presence of benign haemangiomas may be due to the action of a humoral agent, which increases the renal clearance of phosphate.

7.8   Osteodystrophy

7.8.1   Hyperparathyroid osteodystrophy

Osteodystrophy occurs in hyperparathyroidism (HPT); it is generally acquired (Mundy and Fisher, 1980), and rarely congenital (Law *et al.*, 1983). In both primary and secondary HPT, osseous remodelling is augmented, and there is a lack of orderly arrangement and balance between formation and resorption (Fig. 7.2). Both osteoblastic and osteoclastic activities are closely associated with the blood vessels, especially the sinusoids and their endothelia. There is paratrabecular fibrosis in the affected areas and a reduction in haematopoiesis (Fig. 7.2). Mild, asymptomatic hyperparathyroidism is not rare, and may lead eventually to skeletal disease. When the condition is severe, the fibrosis may be extensive and replace the haematopoietic elements. In primary HPT and in disequilibrium hypercalcaemia (Hosking, 1983) osteoclastic remodelling usually outpaces osteoblastic bone production so that the trabeculae may become excavated with cystic formations as well as exhibiting areas

Fig. 7.2   (a, b and c) Bone biopsy section of patient with primary hyperparathyroidism showing distortion of trabecular bone structure, typical excavating bone lesions with osteoclasts (arrows), paratrabecular coarse fibrosis extending into the marrow cavities, and hypo-cellular marrow. (a) × 4, (b) × 60, (c) × 250, Gomori.

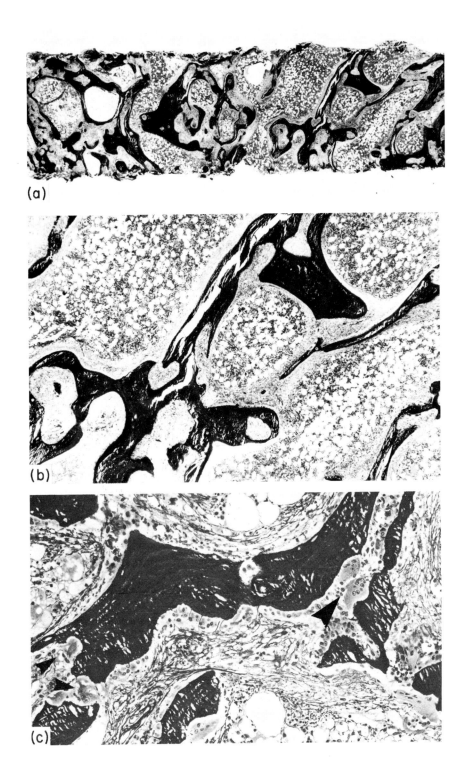

(a)

(b)

(c)

of rarefaction (Plate IVc) and of widened osteoid seams (osteomalacia) (Amelin *et al.*, 1979).

Accumulations of osteoclasts associated with haemosiderin-laden macrophages (as a result of haemorrhage) together with fibrosis constitute the so-called 'brown tumours' which may also be found in the bone marrow biopsy. Occasionally, osteoblastosis and fibrosis may predominate.

In primary HPT, two types of bone changes have been reported in some studies: striking lesions in patients without renal calculi, and minimal effects in those with kidney stones (Beil *et al.*, 1974).

Primary HPT may also occur in infants (Eftekhari and Yousefzadeh, 1982); and in cases of suspected or biochemically and radiologically supported HPT, a bone biopsy will reveal the exact type of osteodystrophy involved.

Giant cell tumour of bone (also called osteoclastoma) must be considered in the differential diagnosis of histological findings in the bone biopsy interpreted as 'brown tumour' due to hyperparathyroidism. The clinical picture and biochemical spectrum must always be taken into account. The great majority of giant cell tumours occur in the long bones, but rare instances of their occurrences in other locations, including the pelvis, have been reported (Vanel *et al.*, 1983). In addition, metastasis of giant cell tumours may be found in that region. Caballes (1981) has discussed the classification and the mechanisms of metastases of the so-called giant cell tumours of bone.

7.8.2   Renal osteodystrophy

This is due to derangements in metabolic and homeostatic control of minerals; usually it represents a progressive form of bone disease which presents histologically as a mixture of osteosclerosis, osteoporosis, osteomalacia and osteitis fibrosis cystica. Thus renal osteodystrophy presents a variable picture which includes osteoporosis, osteomalacia and 'osteitis fibrosa cystica' (Plate IVd); and reduction in haematopoiesis; fibrosis and oedema of the marrow contribute to the anaemia of chronic renal disease. In any individual patient different aspects may predominate, and identification of the type by bone biopsy enables appropriate therapy to be instituted (Maloney *et al.*, 1982). Special types of osteodystrophies have been observed in renal patients undergoing dialysis (see above). Many studies have reported on quantitative bone histology in patients with renal disease (e.g. Eastwood, 1982). The findings in bone oxalosis and renal osteodystrophy have been described by Gherardi *et al.*, (1980).

In areas of very active HPT there may be no residual haematopoietic tissue, its place having been taken by stimulated connective tissue and blood vessels, particularly arterioles. However, such mesenchymal activation is not exclusive to primary and secondary hyperparathyroidism, as it may occur in Paget's disease of bone, in osteomyelitis, in malignant lymphomas, in myelomas, and in metastatic carcinomas (Table 7.2). In many instances there is a prominent population of infiltrating cells such as lymphocytes, plasma cells, macrophages, and mast cells, especially in association with the angiogenesis and the osteogenesis which characterize the activated mesenchyme.

Table 7.2 Blood vessels in bone biopsies in various diseases

	Arteries	Arteriol.	Capill.	Sinus
Normal	2 0–26	26 4–81	101 38–208	1700 910–2520
Hyperparathyroid (HPT)	14 0–39	53 10–173	568 330–1196	2076 817–1996
Osteoporosis	3 0–3	24 8–48	75 48–90	976 518–1342
Paget's disease	25 10–48	285 82–410	1130 412–2110	2330 1320–3100
Polycythaemia vera	23 6–45	66 48–97	307 230–412	3756 2490–4910
CML	16 1–29	58 26–86	1055 410–1812	2460 1868–3112
Myelofibrosis/ Osteomyelosclerosis	39 2–49	183 125–250	2126 1280–3340	2073 1412–2938
Aplasia	2 0–4	73 32–168	229 91–355	1000 335–1420
Multiple myeloma	16 1–23	126 81–190	654 310–854	1737 1110–2025

40 cases in each group.
All upper numbers are mean values /100 mm²; lower numbers indicate range.

7.9 Paget's disease of bone

Though a number of speculations have been put forward as to the aetiology of Paget's disease of bone none has yet been proved (Frame and Marel, 1981; Hosking, 1981). However, it appears to be primarily a disease of osteoclasts, whose unrestrained activity also stimulates the osteoblasts so that greatly increased overall osseous remodelling results (Plate IVa) with an overgrowth of bone formation (Meunier *et al.*, 1980; Krane, 1980). Bone scan is used to diagnose and document the extent and activity of the disease process (McKillop and Fogelman, 1984). Inclusion bodies, similar to the nucleocapsids of the measles virus group, have been found by electron microscopy in both nucleus and cytoplasm of the osteoclasts (Editorial, *Lancet*, 1982), indicating that Paget's disease may be due to a viral infection, but possibly other co-factors are also required for overt disease to develop. The osteoclasts are hyperplastic and hypertrophic—their size may reach many times that of the normal osteoclasts. The number of nuclei per cell varies greatly—as many as one hundred have been counted and the nucleoli are also large and prominent. Bone resorption is accelerated as a consequence, which, in turn, stimulates rapid bone formation. This is accompanied by vascular hyperplasia and fibrosis, which together with the enlarged trabeculae encroach on the marrow cavities and thereby cause a reduction in haematopoietic tissue, and the anaemia which is frequently observed in these patients. Both cortical and cancellous bone are involved, and the final result is structurally altered and abnormal bone (Fig. 7.3) which is unable to withstand mechanical stress, and therefore gives rise to the typical deformities in the severely affected patients. In early lesions, the osteoclastic activities and the overall picture may resemble that of primary hyperparathyroidism (Fig. 7.4). The osteoblasts and the osteocytes show no morphological abnormalities, though the bone which is produced is both woven and lamellar and has the mosaic pattern pathognomonic for Paget's disease. The mosaic pattern (Fig. 7.3) is due to the cement lines of the newly formed bone which is randomly deposited by the osteoblasts to fill the cavities left by the osteoclasts. The osteoclasts, in addition to their size and large number of nuclei, have intranuclear and cytoplasmic vacuoles and inclusions, while degenerating cells with pyknotic nuclei are also usually present. There is generally a focal involvement of the pelvis, femur, skull, tibia, clavicles and ribs, in decreasing order of frequency (Guyer, 1981). A common symptom is bone pain. With the introduction of the diphosphonates and calcitonin, effective modalities of treatment appear to be available (Krane, 1982). BMB are therefore indicated both for establishing the diagnosis as early as possible and to monitor the effects of therapy. The incidence of Paget's disease is high—an estimated 4% of the general population in some countries

---

Fig. 7.3   (a) Section of bone biopsy of patient with Paget's disease; the trabecular bone shows the typical mosaic pattern (small arrows); note giant osteoclasts (arrow in centre) and large stretches of the trabecular surface covered by osteoblasts. The intertrabecular cavities are filled with connective tissue to the exclusion of haematopoiesis. × 300, Giemsa; (b) lymphoplasmacytoid lymphoma (immunocytoma) in patient with Paget's disease of bone; note mosaic bone pattern and marrow cavity occupied by lymphoid cells. × 300, Giemsa.

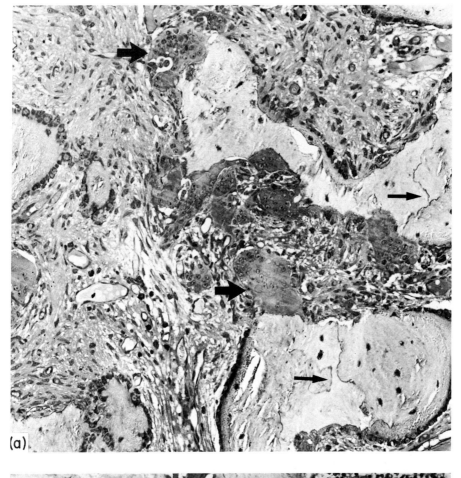

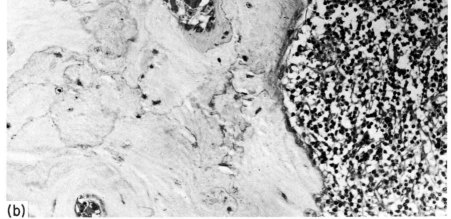

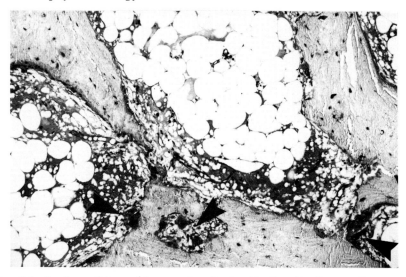

Fig. 7.4 Section of bone biopsy of patient with Paget's disease diagnosed radiologically, biopsy taken from area near focus of affected bone; note increased remodelling, osteoclasts (arrows) and paratrabecular fibrosis, but no typical mosaic bone pattern. × 100, Giemsa.

(Barker, 1981; Detheridge *et al.*, 1982, 1983), with low rates in young adults but increasing numbers in the older age groups. The pelvis is nearly always affected, so that in a high proportion of the patients an early bone biopsy is diagnostic.

The development of osteosarcoma in pre-existing lesions in Paget's disease has been reported. Other conditions, especially those affecting the older age groups, may occur in patients with Paget's disease. The chance occurrence of osteogenesis imperfecta and Paget's disease in a single patient has recently been described (Shapiro *et al.*, 1983).

7.10   Osteogenesis imperfecta

Osteogenesis imperfecta is one of the most common inherited bone diseases. It is due to an hereditary defect or defects in collagen metabolism, whose precise nature has not yet been clarified. Morphologically the bones of the skeleton are delicate, the cortices thin and porous, and the trabeculae few and far between (Plate IVe). The osteocytes and osteoblasts show no apparent alterations but the matrix produced is defective. Osteogenesis imperfecta represents a heterogeneous group of diseases and the severity varies from lethal (Pope *et al.*, 1984) to relatively mild (Shapiro *et al.*, 1983). Various abnormalities in collagen chains have been demonstrated (Nichols *et al.*, 1984).

7.11   Osteopetrosis (marble bone disease)

This disease derives its name from the extreme thickening of the cancellous bone, due to excessive and unbalanced bone formation, leading to widening of the cortices as well as trabecular sclerosis. Progressive encroachment on the intertrabecular cavities results in diminution of the amount of space required for effective haematopoiesis, as well as causing neurologic and other difficulties. Cases with varying degrees of severity have been described (Kaibara *et al.*, 1982; Shapiro *et al.*, 1980). The defect lies in the osteoclasts, which do not function properly. Transplantation with compatible bone marrow has led to dramatic improvement when repopulation with donor cells has occurred and when these produced osteoclasts able to resorb bone normally and thus restore the equilibrium between formation and resorption (Coccia *et al.*, 1980). At least two forms of osteopetrosis have been described, an early rapidly progressive and a delayed, more benign form (Kaibara *et al.*, 1982). The histological, ultrastructural and biochemical findings in osteopetrosis have been reviewed by Shapiro *et al.* (1980).

7.12   Hyperostosis

Disorders of ossification may also result from long term administration of drugs, e.g. retinoid hyperostosis is associated with 13-cis-retinoic acid administered for refractory ichthyosis (Pittsley and Yodes, 1983). Since the observation that there appears to be a lower risk of various types of epithelial carcinomas associated with increased intake of natural or synthetic retinoids, these substances are coming into widespread use. Consequently, in view of the above findings, more work is indicated on their mechanism of action and their effects on the formation and resorption of bone.

7.13   Fibrous dysplasia

Fibrous dysplasia is presumed to be a developmental disorder of the mesenchyme of the osseous tissues, of unknown aetiology, which is characterized by the replacement of bone and marrow by masses of fibrous tissues, sometimes containing islands of immature (woven) bone and cartilage. It occurs most frequently in girls, between the ages of 5 and 15 years, though any age may be affected. Three main types have been described: monostotic, in which a single bone is involved; polyostotic in which lesions are found in many bones; and as part of Albright's syndrome associated with skin pigmentation and endocrinopathies.

The defects affect both cortical and cancellous bone, and range in size

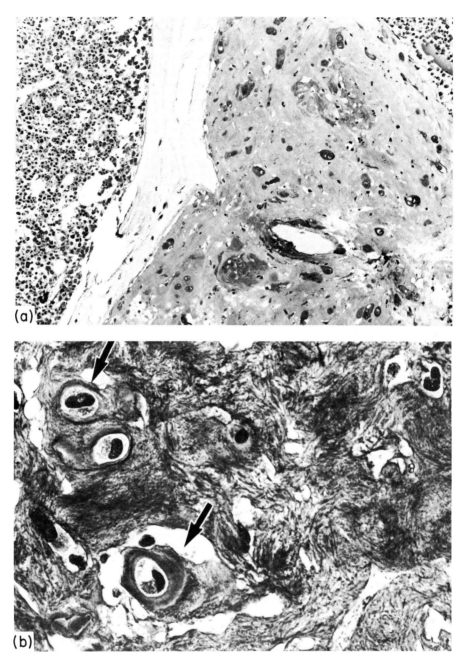

Fig. 7.5 (a) Chondrosarcoma; note trabecular bone with normal bone marrow on the left side and the tumour on the right. × 100, Giemsa; (b) high power view of the tumour cells within their cartilaginous matrix (arrows). × 600, Giemsa.

from a few millimetres to large areas, causing distortion of the normal contour of the bone involved. The fibrous dysplasia appears to arise in the marrow cavity; it varies in cellularity and in vascularization; there are few osteoblasts and osteoclasts, and little change occurs with the passage of time. Removal of parathyroid adenomas has no influence on the fibrous dysplasia (Ehrig and Wilson, 1972).

Chondrosarcoma is the second most common cancer of bone next to osteosarcoma, and in about half of the cases the pelvic bones may be involved (Huvos et al., 1983; Spjut and Ayala, 1983). When centrally located the chondrosarcoma may spread within the marrow cavities (Fig. 7.5) replacing the normal tissues by cartilaginous-like masses (Plate IVf), and the aspect of the cells within these masses is very important for the diagnosis (which may be difficult). The cells are not arranged in columns, and their nuclei may be hyperchromatic, multiple, or contain many lobes, or have bizarre shapes, and many mitotic figures may be seen. Ossification may take place, and when it does, it starts within the cartilage. Some chrondrosarcomas may also contain myxomatous areas.

7.13.1   *Differential diagnosis of osteosarcoma, chondrosarcoma and fibrosarcoma of bone*

Sanerkin (1980) has proposed that these may best be defined by the origin of the tumour cell and by the presence or absence of alkaline phosphatase activity. Osteosarcoma, arising from osteoblasts, is alkaline phosphatase positive, chondrosarcoma arising from chondroblasts is alkaline phosphatase negative, and fibrosarcoma, which has its origin in fibroblasts, is also alkaline phosphatase negative. According to the author, this would obviate the necessity of using the presence of osteoid as a criterion.

References

Amelin, A. Z., Vantsevich, L. M., Slutski, L. I. and Sosaar, V. B. (1979), Biopsy used in the diagnosis of parathyroid osteodystrophy. *Klin. Med. Mosk.*, **57**, 81–4.

Amos, R. S. and Wright, V. (1980), Mönckeberg's arteriosclerosis and metabolic bone disease. *Lancet*, **2**, 248–9.

Avioli, L. V. and Raisz, L. G. (Eds.) (1980), Metabolic bone disease. *Clinics in Endocrin. and Metab.*, **9**, 177–206.

Barker, D. J. R. (1981), The epidemiology of Paget's disease. *Metab. Bone Dis. Rel. Res.*, **4 & 5**, 231–4.

Baylink, D. J. (1983), Glucocorticoid-induced osteoporosis. *New Engl. J. Med.*, **309**, 306–8.

Beil, E., Prechtel, K., Bartl, R. and Kronseder, A. (1974), Histomorphometrical studies of iliac crest biopsies and parathyroid glands with primary hyperparathyroidism. *Verh. Dtsch. Ges. Path.*, **58**, 344–7.

104   Biopsy Pathology of Bone and Bone Marrow

Brown, D. J., Ham, K. N., Dawborn, J. K. and Xipell, J. M. (1982), Treatment of dialysis osteomalacia with desferrioxamine. *Lancet*, **2**, 343–5.

Burkhardt, B., Frisch, B., Bartl, R., Jäger, K., Schlag, R. and Hill, W. (1984), Myelogenous osteodysplasia: diagnosis and development. *Virchows Archives* (in press).

Caballes, R. L. (1981), The mechanism in the so-called 'benign cell tumor of bone'. *Human Pathol.*, **12**, 762–7.

Charhon, S. A., Chapuy, M. C., Delvin, E. C., Valentin-Opran, A., Edouard, C. M. and Menier, P. J. (1983), Histomorphometric analysis of sclerotic bone metastases from prostatic carcinoma with special reference to osteomalacia. *Cancer*, **51**, 918–24.

Coccia, P. F., Krivit, W., Cervenka, J., Clawson, C., Kersey, J. H., Kimm., T. H., Nesbit, M. E., Ramsay, N. K. G., Warkentin, P. E., Teitelbaum, S. L., Kahn, A. J. and Brown, D. M. (1980), Successful bone-marrow transplantation for infantile malignant osteopetrosis. *New Engl. J. Med.*, **302**, 701–8.

Cunningham, J., Fraher, L. J., Clemens, T. L., Revell, P. Q. and Papapoulos, S. E. (1982), Chronic acidosis with metabolic bone disease. Effect of alkali on bone morphology and vitamin D metabolism. *Am. J. Med.*, **73**, 199–204.

Darby, A. J. (1981), Bone formation and resorption in postmenopausal osteoporosis. *Lancet*, **2**, 536.

Darby, A. J. and Meunier, P. J. (1981), Mean wall thickness and formation periods of trabecular bone packets in idiopathic osteoporosis. *Calcif. Tissue Int.*, **33**, 199–204.

Detheridge, F. M., Guyer, P. B. and Barker, D. J. P. (1982), European distribution of Paget's disease of bone. *Brit. med. J.*, **285**, 1005–7.

Detheridge, F. M., Baker, D. J. P. and Guyer, P. B. (1983), Paget's disease of bone in Ireland. *Brit. med. J.*, **287**, 1345–6.

Dibble, J. B. and Losowsky, M. S. (1982), Osteomalacia in chronic liver disease. *Brit. med. J.*, **285**, 157–8.

Dixon, A. St. J. (1983), Non-hormonal treatment of osteoporosis. *Brit. med. J.*, **286**, 999–1000.

Eastwood, J. (1982), Quantitative bone histology in 38 patients with advanced renal failure. *J. clin Pathol.*, **35**, 125–34.

Editorial (1982), Viruses and Paget's disease of bone. *Lancet*, **2**, 1198–9.

Eftekhari, F. and Yousefzadeh, D. K. (1982), Primary infantile hyperparathyroidism: clinical, laboratory and radiographic features in 21 cases. *Skeletal Radiol.*, **8**, 201–8.

Ehrig, V. and Wilson, D. R. (1972), Fibrous dysplasia of bone and primary hyperparathyroidism. *Ann. int. Med.*, **77**, 234–8.

Fallon, M. D., Whyte, M. P. and Teitelbaum, S. L. (1981), Systemic mastocytosis associated with generalized osteopenia: Histopathological characterization of the skeletal lesion using undecalcified bone from two patients. *Human Pathol.*, **12**, 813–20.

Fallon, M. D. and Teitelbaum, S. (1982), The interpretation of fluorescent tetracycline markers in the diagnosis of metabolic bone diseases. *Human Pathol.*, **13**, 416–7.

Fallon, M. D., Whyte, M. P., Craig, R. B. and Teitelbaum, S. L. (1983), Mast-cell proliferation in postmenopausal osteoporosis. *Calcif. Tissue Int.*, **35**, 29–31.

Frame, B. and Parfitt, A. M. (1978), Osteomalacia: current concepts. *Ann. int. Med.*, **89**, 966–82.

Frame, B. and Marel, G. M. (1981), Paget's disease: a review of current knowledge. *Radiology*, **141**, 21–4.

Fraser, D. R. (1983), The physiological economy of Vitamin D. *Lancet*, **1**, 969–71.

Frisch, B., Eventov, J., Salama, R. and Burkhardt, R. (1982), Histologic studies on femoral neck biopsies from patients with fractures of the proximal femur. In *Osteoporosis* (eds J. Menczel *et al.*), John Wiley and Sons, New York, pp. 237–47.

Gerster, J. C., Charon, S. A., Jaeger, P., Boivin, G., Briancon, D., Rostan, A., Baud, C. A. and Meunier, P. J. (1983), Bilateral fractures of femoral neck in patients with moderate renal failure receiving fluoride for spinal osteoporosis. *Brit. med. J.*, **287**, 723–5.

Gewirtz, A., Viguery, A., Stewart, A. and Hoffman, R. (1981), Production of a bone resorbing factor by human myeloid leukemia cells. *Blood*, **58**, Supplement 1, 139A.

Gherardi, G., Poggi, A., Sisca, S., Calderaro, V. and Bonucci, E. (1980), Bone oxalosis and renal osteodystrophy. *Arch. Pathol. Lab. Med.*, **104**, 105–11.

Gruber, H. E., Stauffer, M. E., Thompson, E. R. and Baylink, D. J. (1981), Diagnosis of bone disease by core biopsies. *Sem. Haemat.*, **18**, 258–78.

Guyer, P. B. (1981), Paget's disease of bone: the anatomical distribution. *Metab. Bone Dis. Rel. Res.*, **4 & 5**, 239–42.

Herbage, D., Borsali, F., Buffevant, Ch., Flandin, F. and Aguercif, M. (1982), Composition, cross-linking and thermal stability of bone and skin collagens in patients with osteogenesis imperfecta. *Metab. Bone Dis. Rel. Res.*, **4**, 95–101.

Hodsman, A. B., Sherrard, D. J., Wong, E. G. C. *et al.* (1981), Vitamin D resistant osteomalacia in hemodialysis patients lacking secondary hyperparathyroidism. *Ann. int. Med.*, **94**, 629–37.

Hosking, D. J. (1981), Paget's disease of bone. *Brit. med. J.*, **283**, 686–8.

Hosking, D. J. (1983), Disequilibrium hypercalcaemia. *Brit. med. J.*, **286**, 326–7.

Hosking, D. J., Kemm, J. R., Knight, M. E., Campbell, G. A., Cotton, R. E. and Beryman, R. (1983), Screening for subclinical osteomalacia in the elderly: normal ranges or pragmatism. *Lancet*, **2**, 1290–2.

Huvos, A. G., Rosen, G., Dabska, M. and Marcove, R. C. (1983), Mesenchymal chrondrosarcoma. A clinicopathologic analysis of 35 patients with emphasis on treatment. *Cancer*, **51**, 1230–7.

Kaibara, N., Katsuki, I., Hotokebuchi, I. and Takagashi, K. (1982), Intermediate form of osteopetrosis with recessive inheritance. *Skeletal Radiol.*, **9**, 47–51.

Kragstrup, J., Melsen, F. and Mosekilde, L. (1982), Reduced wall thickness of completed remodelling sites in iliac trabecular bone following anticonvulsant therapy. *Metab. Bone Dis. Rel. Res.*, **4**, 181–5.

Krane, S. M. (1980), Skeletal metabolism in Paget's disease of bone. *Arthritis and Rheumatism*, **23**, 1087–94.

Krane, S. M. (1982), Etidronate disodium in the treatment of Paget's disease of bone. *Ann. int. Med.*, **96**, 619–25.

Law, W. M., Hodgson, S. F. and Heath, H. (1983), III. Autosomal recessive inheritance of familial hyperparathyroidism. *New Engl. J. Med.*, **309**, 650–3.

Lips, P., Netelenbos, J. C., Jongen, M. J. M., Ginkel, F. C. van, Althius, A. L., Schaik, C. L. van, Vijgh, W. J. F. van der, Vermeiden, J. P. W. and Meer, C. van der (1982), Histomorphometric profile and vitamin D status in patients with femoral neck fracture. *Metab. Bone Dis. Rel. Res.*, **4**, 85–93.

Maloney, N. A., Ott, S. M. and Sherrard, D. J. (1982), Renal osteodystrophy revisited. *Calcif. Tissue Int.*, Supp. N1, **34**, S33.

McCarthy, D. M., Hibbin, J. A. and Goldman, J. M. (1984), A role for 1,25-dihydroxyvitamin D_3 in control of bone-marrow collagen deposition? *Lancet*, **1**, 78–80.

McKillop, J. H. and Fogelman, I. (1984), Regular review: bone scintigraphy in benign bone disease. *Brit. med. J.*, **288**, 264–6.

Meunier, P. J., Courpron, P., Edouard, C., Alexandre, C., Bressot, C., Lips, P. and Boyce, B. F. (1979), Bone histomorphometry. In *Osteoporotic States: Osteoporosis II* (ed. U.S. Barrel), Grune and Stratton, New York.

Meunier, P. J., Coindre, J. M., Edouard, C. M. and Arlot, M. E. (1980), Bone histomorphometry in Paget's disease. *Arthritis and Rheumatism*, **23**, 1095–1103.

Milhaud, G., Christiansen, C., Gallagher, C., Reeve, J., Seeman, E., Chesnut, C. and Parfitt, A. (1983), Pathogenesis and treatment of postmenopausal osteoporosis. *Calcif. Tissue Int.*, **35**, 708–11.

Muls, E., Bouillon, R., Boelaert, J., Lamberigts, G., Imschoot, S. van., Daneels, R. and Moor, P. de. (1982), Etiology of hypercalcemia in a patient with Addison's disease. *Calcif. Tissue Int.*, **34**, 523–6.

Mundy, G. R. and Fisher, R. (1980), Primary hyperparathyroidism. *Lancet*, **1**, 1317–20.

Nichols, A. C., Pope, F. M. and Craig, D. (1984), An abnormal collagen: a chain containing cysteine in autosomal dominant osteogenesis imperfecta. *Brit. med. J.*, **288**, 112–13.

Nordin, B. E. C., Peacock, M., Aaron, J., Crilly, G. G., Heyburn, P. J., Horsman, A. and Marshall, D. H. (1980), Osteoporosis and osteomalacia. *Clin. Endocrin. Met.*, **9**, 177–206.

Nordin, B. E. C., Aaron, J., Speed, R. and Crilly, R. G. (1981), Bone formation and resorption as the determinants of trabecular bone volume in osteoporosis. *Lancet*, **2**, 277–9.

Okita, K. and Block, M. (1979), Osteomalacic new bone formation during therapy of acute granulocytic leukemia. *Am. J. clin. Pathol.*, **71**, 645–50.

Parfitt, A. M. (1982), The coupling of bone formation to bone resorption: a critical analysis of the concept and of its relevance to the pathogenesis of osteoporosis. *Metab. Bone Dis. Rel. Res.*, **4**, 1–6.

Pittsley, R. A. and Yoder, F. W. (1983), Retinoid hyperostosis: skeletal toxicity associated with long term administration of 13cis retinoic acid for refractory ichthyosis. *New Engl. J. Med.*, **208**, 1012–14.

Pope, F. M., Cheah, K. S. E., Nicholls, A. C., Price, A. B. and Grosveld, F. G. (1984), Lethal osteogenesis imperfecta congenita and a 300 base pair gene deletion for an α1(I)-like collagen. *Brit. med. J.*, **288**, 431–4.

Raisz, R. G. (1981), What marrow does to bone. *New Engl. J. Med.*, **304**, 1485–6.

Riggs, B. L. and Melton, J., III (1983), Evidence for two distinct syndromes of involutional osteoporosis. *Am. J. Med.*, **75**, 898–901.

Sanerkin, N. G. (1980), Definitions of osteosarcoma, chondrosarcoma and fibrosarcoma of bone. *Cancer*, **46**, 178–85.

Schnitzler, C. M. and Solomon, L. (1982), Bone morphometry after alcohol abuse. *Calcif. Tissue Int.*, Supp. N1, **34**, S35.

Seeman, E., Melton, L. J., O'Fallon, W. M. and Riggs, B. L. (1983), Risk factors for spinal osteoporosis in men. *Am. J. Med.*, **75**, 977–83.

Shapiro, F., Glimcher, M. J., Holtrop, M. E., Tashjian, A. H., Brickley-Parsons, D. and Kenzora, J. E. (1980), Human osteopetrosis. A histological, ultrastructural and biochemical study. *J. Bone Jt Surg.*, **62A**, 384–99.

Shapiro, J. R., Triche, T., Rowe, D. W., Munabi, A., Cattell, H. S. and Schlesinger, S. (1983), *Arch. int. Med.*, **143**, 2250–7.

Shore, R. M., Chesney, R. W., Marzess, R. B., Rose, P. G. and Bargman, G. J. (1981), Osteopenia in juvenile diabetes. *Calcif. Tissue Int.*, **33**, 455–7.

Shore, R. M., Chesney, R. W., Marzess, R. B., Rose, P. G. and Bargman, G. J. (1982), Skeletal demineralization in Turner's syndrome. *Calcif. Tissue Int.*, **34**, 519–22.

Siklos, P., Davie, M., Jung, R. T. and Chalmers, T. M. (1980), Osteomalacia in uretero-sigmoidostomy: healing by correction of the acidosis. *Brit. J. Urology*, **52**, 61–2.

Spjut, H. J. and Ayala, A. G. (1983), Skeletal tumours in children and adolescents. *Human Pathol.*, **14**, 628–42.

Stevenson, J. C. and Whitehead, M. I. (1982), Postmenopausal osteoporosis. *Brit. med. J.*, **285**, 585–8.

Stevenson, J. C., White, M. C., Joplin, G. F. and MacIntyre, I. (1982), Osteoporosis and calcitonin deficiency. *Brit. med. J.*, **285**, 1010–11.

Stout, S. D. (1982), The effects of long-term immobilization on the histomorphology of human cortical bone. *Calcif. Tissue Int.*, **34**, 337–42.

Vanel, L., Contesso, G., Rebibo, G., Zafrani, B. and Masselot, J. (1983), Benign giant-cell tumours of bone and pulmonary metastases and favourable prognosis. Report on two cases and review of the literature. *Skeletal Radiol.*, **10**, 221–6.

Vaughan, J. (1981), Osteogenesis and haematopoiesis. *Lancet*, **2**, 133–6.

Vigorita, V. J., Suda, M. K. and Lane, J. M. (1983), Osteoporosis with idiopathic nodular lymphoid hyperplasia of the marrow. *Arch. Pathol. Lab. Med.*, **107**, 276–7.

Whedon, J. D. (1981), Osteoporosis. *New Engl. J. Med.*, **7**, 397–9.

8 Myeloproliferative disorders

8.1 Haematological malignancies

Haematological malignancies are derived from precursors of the myeloid or lymphoid cell lines, or from a precursor common to both (Fig. 8.1) which may give bi-phenotypic leukaemias. The haematological malignancies are characterized by alterations in the architecture, the topography, the relative proportions of the bone marrow constituents, and in some cases the more or less striking cytological features of the cell lines directly concerned, as well as concomitant alterations in the others. In the evaluation of biopsies with hyperplasias or proliferations of haematopoietic elements, a number of specific questions should be systematically considered:

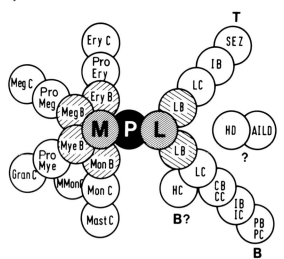

Fig. 8.1 Schematic representation of the derivation of myelo- and lymphoproliferative disorders. P = pluripotent stem cell; M = early myeloid precursors; L = early lymphoid precursors; shaded circles = committed precursors; clear circles = differentiated cell lines.

(1) Is there a hyperplasia or proliferation outside normal limits?

(2) What is the cytology of the cells comprising the hyperplasia?

(3) Is it monomorphic? or does it contain more than one cytological type?

(4) Is there a particular spatial arrangement? Is the growth nodular or diffuse? Does it form a pattern? How much of the marrow cavities does it occupy?

(5) Note the presence or absence of fibres (sclerosis); is there oedema or exudation between the cells?

(6) Note the presence or absence of histiocytes, macrophages, and other cells such as lymphocytes and mast cells.

(7) Is there an effect on the haematopoietic and fat tissues?

(8) Is there an effect on the bone and bone cells?

(9) Are there changes in blood vessels, or stimulation of neo-angiogenesis?

The differential diagnosis of the myelo- and lymphoproliferative disorders is listed in Table 8.1.

Table 8.1 Differential diagnosis in lympho- and myeloproliferative diseases

Reactive hyperplasias	*Granulomas*
Infections	Infections
Immune diseases	Sarcoidosis
Malignancies	Malignancies
Splenic disorders	Drugs
Hepatic disorders	Allergic/immune/rheumatic
Pulmonary disorders	AIDS
Hypertension	Unknown
Hyperplasia of unknown aetiology	Fibrosis of bone marrow
Hypo- and aplasias	Metastatic carcinoma
Enzyme deficiencies	Hyperparathyroidism
Storage diseases	Osteoporosis
Eosinophilic syndromes	Osteomalacia
Mastocytosis	
Autoimmune lymphoproliferative disease	

Myeloproliferative disorders (MPD) include the disorders listed in Table 8.2, as well as the variant, transitional and intermediate forms (Dameshek, 1951; Gilbert, 1973; Laszlo, 1975; Frisch *et al.*, 1984a, b). The MPD are haematological neoplasias of clonal origin (Boggs, 1981; Fialkow *et al.*, 1981; Castro-Malaspina *et al.*, 1982), and as such are primary disorders of the bone marrow. It is of interest that the erythrocytic, granulocytic, megakaryocytic and lymphocytic cell lines have all been identified as belonging to abnormal clones in the MPD, but no entity has

Table 8.2 Histological classification of the myeloproliferative diseases

Clinical diagnosis	Bone marrow histopathology
Acute Leukaemia†	*Myeloblastic (hyper and hypo-cellular forms) Monoblastic Erythroblastic Megakaryoblastic Mixed (acute myelofibrosis AMF) Lymphoblastic, BC‡
Subacute Leukaemia (smouldering)	**Promyelocytic Myelomonocytic *Proerythrocytic Promegakaryocytic **Mixed
CML (CGL)	*Granulocytic Granulo/megakaryocytic
MF/OMS/(AMF)	*Myelofibrotic *Osteomyelosclerotic
PV/IT	Megakaryocytic Erythro/megakaryo/granulocytic Erythro/megakaryocytic **Erythro/granulocytic **Erythrocytic
Myelodysplasia Preleukaemia	Mixed cellularity

Criteria for classifying: cell line(s), degree of cellular differentiation, presence and degree of fibrosis.

*In borderline cases, reactive alterations with similar histological pictures must be excluded.

**Further clinical data and/or sequential biopsies are necessary for establishing the histological diagnosis.

†In some cases cytochemistry and/or EM are required for phenotype identification of the cell lineage of the 'blasts' in the blast crisis.

‡BC = blast crisis.

AMF is listed twice as it is acute, the cells are very immature, and there is extensive fibrosis.

yet been described with proliferation or involvement of the osteoclast, though it is thought also to be derived from the haematopoietic pluripotent stem cell, via the monocytic series. Though leukaemic transformation represents clonal evolution from a neoplastic stem cell, it is capable (for variable periods of time) of producing differentiated progeny. In spite of this, the clone is inherently unstable and susceptible to maturation disturbances. Transformations to a blastic crisis or to myelofibrosis or osteomyelosclerosis (MF/OMS) have been documented in all the chronic MPD. Initially at least, there are no unequivocal histological characteristics which distinguish the chronic MPD from their normal counterparts in the bone marrow. The MPD are characterized by anomalies in growth which result in a steadily increasing number of haematopoietic cells in the absence of an appropriate stimulus. In most cases the bone marrow is infiltrated diffusely and extensively so that a considerable tumour burden has accumulated before the disorder is diagnosed. Moreover, a 'normal' marrow cellularity may represent an increase in a previously hypocellular area, and does not exclude an MPD when other indications are present (Table 8.3). Nevertheless, the overall histological pattern is almost invariably altered, and thereby permits reliable interpretation and diagnosis. Experience with a large number of biopsies in the MPD has shown that when the bone marrow histology does not appear to reflect a clinically evident MPD in the first biopsy (Plate Vc), it will do so subsequently. In the evaluation of the histological features of the bone marrow in patients with MPD the values given in Table 1.1 serve as base lines for the estimation of increases or decreases in the parameters investigated. As the bone marrow is the source of myeloid cells, a bone marrow biopsy should be included in the investigation of all patients with MPD, and not only when a dry tap is obtained. Moreover, as far as polycythaemia vera and its transformation is concerned, the criteria of the PV Study Group cannot always be met, so that early, borderline, variant and transitional cases may be excluded from consideration in therapeutic protocols, comparative studies and clinical trials. The PV Study Group has recommended that a bone biopsy be taken at diagnosis and once annually thereafter.

Histological recognition and classification is accomplished by means of three criteria: recognition of the predominant proliferative cell lines, the degree of its differentiation, and the fibrotic reaction. Identification of a cell line as proliferative takes into consideration cytological, histological

Table 8.3 Non-representative bone-marrow histology in initial biopsies in myeloproliferative diseases (% of each group)

Clinical diagnosis	No. *	Non-repr.** histology	Increase in*** fat cells
PV	732	9%	6%
IT	188	10%	16%
CML	544	2%	0%
AMM	641	1%	18%
MPD (?)	668	14%	22%

*No. of patients in each group is taken as 100%.
**Non-representative.
***Either diffuse, or patchy hypoplasia.
AMM = agnogenic myeloid metaplasia.
MPD (?) = type of MPD not classifiable by clinical criteria alone.
PV = polycythaemia vera.
IT = idiopathic (essential) thrombocythaemia.

and histotopographical criteria. This classification by means of clearly defined characteristics enables categorization of bone marrow biopsies of most patients who may therefore be assigned (in some cases tentatively or temporarily) to a clinical entity. This histological evaluation has yielded five main groups as shown in Fig. 8.2.

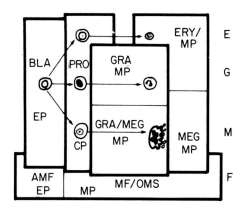

Fig. 8.2 Histological groups in myeloproliferative disorders: EP = early precursors—no maturation in bone marrow; CP = committed precursors—partial maturation in bone marrow; MP = mature progeny produced; AMF = acute myelofibrosis; BLA = blastic phase, acute leukaemia; PRO = sub-acute; GRA = granulocytic; MEG = megakaryocytic; ERY = erythroid; E = erythropoiesis; G = granulopoiesis; M = megakaryopoiesis; F = fibrosis.

It should be emphasized that these groups are not sharply divided; they overlap, and the position of any particular case within the group will depend, at least to some extent, on the criteria of the investigator (Table 8.4). The same holds true for the division of the major entities into subgroups (see below). A special requisite of a classification of the MPD is

Table 8.4 Clinical diagnoses and their underlying histopathology in the myeloproliferative diseases

Clinical diagnosis No.*	†NORM	Bone marrow histopathology (% of each group)							
		ERY	MEG	GRA/ MEG	GRA	MF	OMS	PRO	BLA
PV (732)	2	90	1	2	0	3	1	1	0
IT (188)	1	8	60	15	2	4	4	5	1
CML (544)	0	1	1	26	43	9	8	7	5
AMM (641)	0	1	3	4	2	42	38	5	5
MPD(?) (668)	0	3	7	7	9	30	15	25	4

* The No. patients in each group is taken as 100%.
† Headings indicate predominant proliferative cell lines(s), or fibrosis.
See Table 8.3 and Fig. 8.2 for explanation of abbreviations.

that it incorporates the possibility of indicating the subsequent course of the disease; these considerations underline the fact that a single biopsy represents only an instance in a constantly evolving process which may move in any one of several directions. The histological transformations observed in serial biopsies are shown in Fig. 8.3 and Table 8.5. Concur-

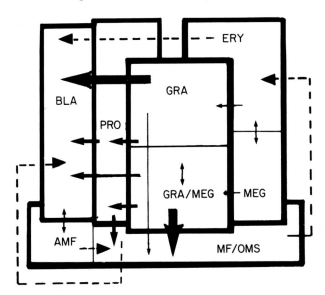

Fig. 8.3 Histological metamorphosis in myeloproliferative disorders: arrows indicate direction of evolution, and their thickness indicates the relative frequency, broken lines = rare occurrence. Abbreviations, as in Fig 8.2.

Table 8.5 Histological evolution of myeloproliferative disease in the bone marrow

First biopsy	No.[+]	NORM	ERY	MEG	GRA/ MEG	GRA	MF	OMS	PRO	BLA[†]
					Sequential biopsies (% of each group)					
NORM	(12)	25*	50	—	—	17	—	—	8	—
ERY	(240)	3	86*	1	3	0·5	3	1	2	0·5
MEG	(36)	3	7	71*	10	—	3	7	—	—
GRA/MEG	(46)	—	2	2	20*	12	27	12	15	10
GRA	(60)	2	—	2	3	52*	5	4	12	20
MF	(63)	—	2	—	2	3	49*	30	3	11
OMS	(36)	—	—	3	—	—	3	89*	—	5
PRO	(41)	2	2	—	2	5	12	7	51*	18
BLA	(21)	5	—	—	—	14	5	—	5	71*

Mean time interval = 23 months, * = no change from initial histologic findings.
+ No. of patients in each group is taken as 100%.
† Headings refer to predominant proliferative cell line(s), or fibrosis.
See Fig. 8.2 for explanation of abbreviations.

rent occurrence of myelo- and lymphoproliferative disorders occurs (Manoharan *et al.*, 1981; Papayannis *et al.*, 1982). It was also observed in our material (see Chapter 10). Moreover, benign lymphoid infiltrates are not uncommon in the myeloproliferative disorders (Jäger *et al.*, 1983), (Fig. 8.4).

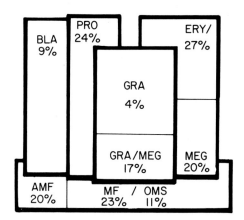

Fig. 8.4 Frequency of benign lymphoid nodules in the bone marrow in myeloproliferative disorders, % = percentage of biopsies with lymphoid nodules in each group. Abbreviations as in Fig. 8.2.

8.2   Polycythaemia vera (PV)

The first of the 5 groups represents the clinical entities of polycythaemia vera (PV) and idiopathic thrombocythaemia (IT) (Fig. 8.5). The cell

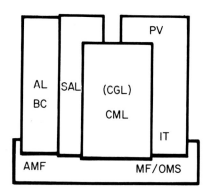

Fig. 8.5   Clinical entities in myeloproliferative disorders. AL = acute leukaemias; BC = blast crisis; SAL = sub-acute (smouldering) leukaemias; CGL = chronic granulocytic leukaemia; CML = chronic myeloid leukaemia; PV = polycythaemia vera; IT = idiopathic (essential) thrombocythaemia.

populations show progressive development to mature elements (Fig. 8.6). PV is not diagnosed from histology alone, but this provides a valuable additional parameter. The bone marrow in PV shows an increase in the overall cellularity (Ellis and Peterson, 1979; Vykoupil *et al.*, 1980; Lucie and Young, 1983) with a corresponding decrease in fat cells. The hyperplastic cell lines are found in their normal topographic locations: erythroid in the parasinusoidal zones, granulocytic in the paratrabecular and perivascular regions, and megakaryocytes in the intertrabecular areas, except when greatly increased in numbers, in which case they are also found along the endosteum, i.e. heterotopia (Plate Va and b). When greatly hyperplastic the megakaryocytes exhibit extreme polymorphism (Thiele *et al.*, 1983), with variable nuclei—small and round to highly convoluted—and variable cytoplasmic density (Table 8.6). There is an apparent increase in all the marrow blood vessels especially the sinusoids; iron stores are depleted; a variable increase in reticular fibres, rarefaction of the trabecular bone, and infiltrations of lymphocytes and plasma cells complete the picture. Extension of haematopoietic tissue into the lower extremities may occur (Kurnick *et al.*, 1980). However, this full-blown picture may not yet be present in early PV and the picture may then resemble that seen in haemolysis or secondary erythrocytosis. The situation is usually clarified in follow-up biopsies.

The bone marrow histology in PV can be further divided into 4 sub-types as follows:

(1) The classic trilinear type as described above, in which there is hyperplasia of the erythrocytic, megakaryocytic and granulocytic cell lines (Fig. 8.6).

(2) The bi-linear type involving the erythrocytic and megakaryocytic lines (Fig. 8.7).

(3) The bi-linear type involving the erythrocytic and granulocytic lines (Fig. 8.7).

(4) The unilinear type in which only the erythroid line exhibits hyperplasia in the bone marrow histology.

When 'spent' (or burned out) PV occurs, the peripheral blood levels begin to fall. The bone marrow then presents a mixed picture: partially fibrotic, as in early MF, with increased fibroblasts and blood vessels, large erythroid islands consisting predominantly of immature cells, reduced granulopoiesis and dysplastic megakaryocytes. The marrow may even resemble that in some forms of aplastic anaemia. Though an increase in reticulin is part of the disease picture (McBrine *et al.*, 1980), extensive myelofibrosis develops almost exclusively in cases with marked proliferation of megakaryocytes. Reorganization of erythropoiesis into PV has been recorded following splenectomy for myelofibrosis (Barosi *et al.*, 1984).

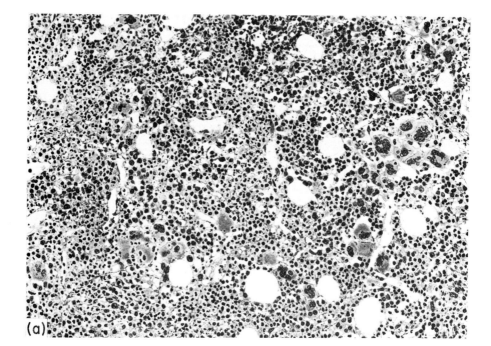

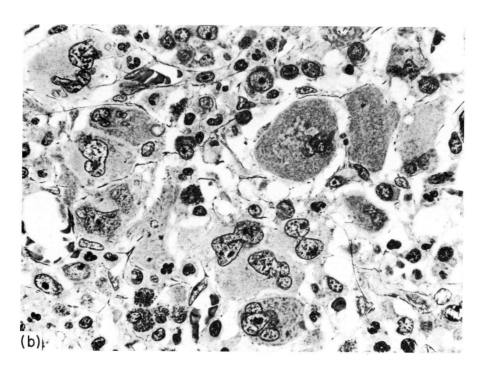

Table 8.6 Assessment of megakaryocytes in myeloproliferative disease

Biopsies	Histology	Megas[+]	◎	◉	◕	✿	🦋
240	ERY/MEG/GRA	5240			+	++	+++
54	MEG	20 410		+	++	++	+++
77	GRA/MEG	8364		+	++	++	++
65	GRA	632		+	++		
48	PROMEG	28 380	+	+++	++	+	
21	MEG-BLAST	36 710	+++	+			

[+]Mean of megakaryocytes per 100 mm² bone marrow.
See Fig. 8.2 for explanation of abbreviations.

8.2.1   Differential diagnosis

In secondary erythrocytosis there is hyperplasia of the erythroid series only, and the other characteristic histological features of PV are absent. Megakaryocytes are not affected, fat cells are not markedly reduced, iron stores are not depleted (unless there is an identifiable cause of iron deficiency) and reticulin is not increased. In some haemolytic conditions, hepatic diseases and refractory anaemias, the marrow may also be hypercellular almost to the exclusion of fat cells, but the other histological features should indicate the diagnosis (Plate Vf).

8.3   Idiopathic thrombocythaemia (IT)

Primary, idiopathic or essential thrombocythaemia is a mature type of megakaryocytic myelosis, characterized by sustained increase in the platelet count at a level of $1000 \times 10^9/l$ or more.

Recent evidence indicates that it is a clonal disorder with origin in a multi-potent stem cell (Fialkow et al., 1982). Platelets, erythrocytes and granulocytes are involved (Gaetani et al., 1982; for review, see Harker and Zimmerman, 1983).

There is progressive maturation of the megakaryocytes, with production of platelets and their release into the bloodstream. The bone marrow may be hypo-, normo- or hyper-cellular with hyperplasia of the mega-karyocytes (Fig. 8.8). These frequently form clusters of polymorphic cells, ranging in size from micro to gigantic forms and they also include pyknotic cells. The nuclei range from small, round and single to con-voluted masses. The normal architectural pattern of the bone marrow may be preserved or effaced. The erythroid and myeloid precursors may

Fig. 8.6   Polycythaemia vera: (a) trilinear proliferation; note reduction in fat cells and polymorphic megakaryocytes. × 250, Giemsa; (b) trilinear proliferation; pleomorphic megakaryocytes surrounded by fine reticular fibres. × 600, Gomori.

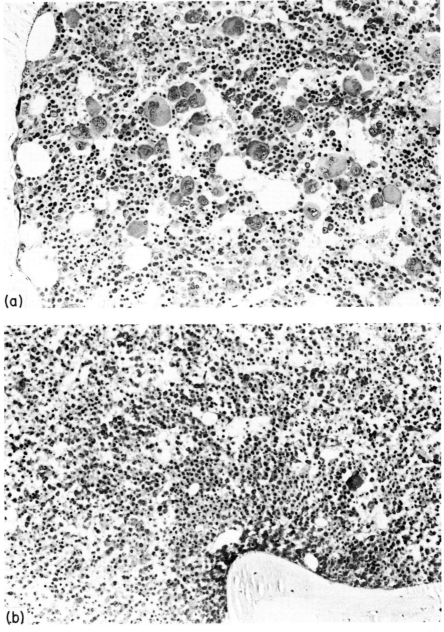

Fig. 8.7 Bone marrow histology in polycythaemia vera: (a) erythrocytic and megakaryocytic proliferation; (b) erythrocytic and granulocytic proliferation. Both × 250, Giemsa.

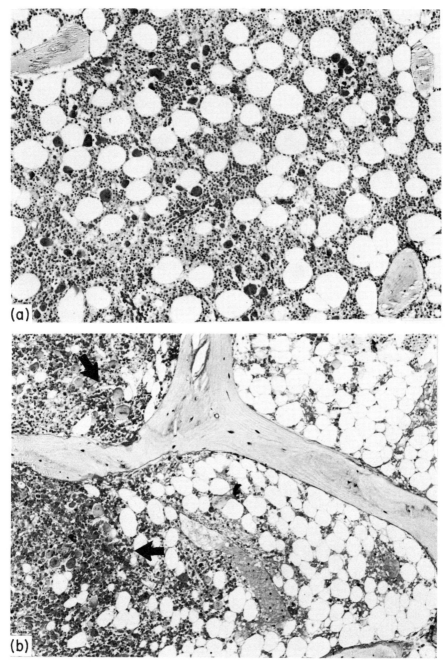

Fig. 8.8 (a) Mature megakaryocytic myelosis without increased cellularity. × 250, Giemsa; (b) immature megakaryocytic myelosis; note variability in cellularity of intertrabecular cavities, clusters of megakaryocytes at arrows. × 250, Giemsa.

be reduced and at times show striking dysplastic features (Plate VIe). Macrophages may be prominent, some with cellular debris and crystalline inclusions. Characteristic for IT is the localization of the megakaryocytes at the walls of the sinusoids, or projecting into their lumina (Fig. 8.9). The different bone marrow histological pictures which were found in a survey of patients, under the clinical syndrome of thrombocythaemia are shown in Fig. 8.10; this clearly demonstrates that IT is a syndrome with a variable underlying bone marrow histopathology and that it corresponds to a typical megakaryocytic myelosis in only 60% of cases. Though IT generally has a slow and static course, the megakaryocytic hyperplasia may lead to fibroblastic stimulation and development of MF at any time (Plate Vd).

Criteria of IT recently published by the PV Study Group (Laszlo et al., 1983) are as follows: platelet counts $>1000 \times 10^9/l$; megakaryocytic hyperplasia in the bone marrow, but a trilinear hyperplasia may also be present; Ph chromosome negative (but occasional cases may be Ph chromosome positive (Verhest and Monsieur, 1983)); absence of prominent fibrosis, but reticulin may be increased; absence of myeloid metaplasia; no increase in red cell mass; no iron deficiency; no previous myelosuppressive therapy; splenomegaly and hepatomegaly may be present. Thus, bone marrow biopsy is important for establishing the diagnosis.

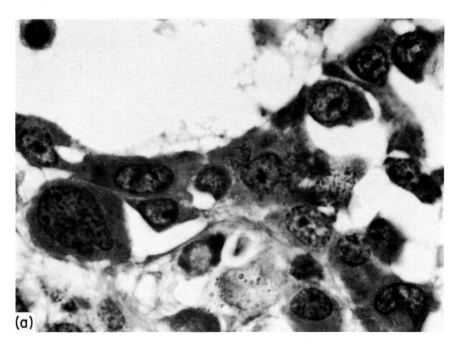

(a)

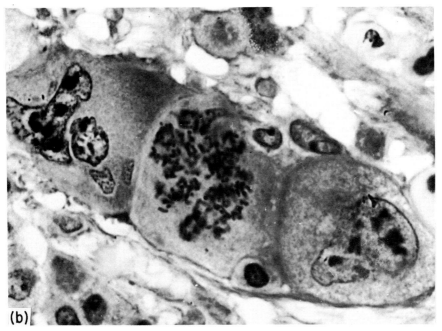

Fig. 8.9 (a) Micromegakaryocytes in myeloproliferative disorders. × 1000; (b) giant megakaryocytes in MPD, mitotic figure in centre. × 1000, Giemsa.

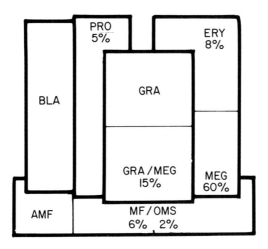

Fig. 8.10 Bone marrow histology in survey of patients with the clinical syndrome of idiopathic (essential) thrombocythaemia. % = percentage of patients in each group. Abbreviations as in Fig. 8.2.

8.4   Chronic myeloid leukaemia (CML)

Chromosome studies have demonstrated that granulocytes, erythroid cells, megakaryocytes and lymphocytes all contain the characteristic chromosome (Kersey, 1983). Staging of CML and evaluation of prognostic factors has not included bone biopsies in recent studies (Tura and Baccarini, 1981; Gomez et al., 1982). Nor are bone marrow biopsies routinely performed in patients with CML (Goldman and Lu, 1982; Koffler and Golde, 1981) though they provide useful information (Georgii et al., 1980; Bartl et al., 1982). Studies of BMB of patients with clinically established CML have shown that it may be divided, broadly speaking, into two groups: the granulocytic and the mixed granulocytic and megakaryocytic, i.e. a uni- or bi-cellular proliferation (Fig. 8.11). In the former there is hyperplasia of the white cells, the eosinophil precursors often appear prominent (Fig. 8.12) with endosteal seams and perivascular cuffs of granulopoiesis which show increasing maturation towards the central parts of the marrow cavities. The proportion of immature to mature cells may be higher in the bone marrow than in the peripheral blood. Asynchronous maturation is evidenced by early cytoplasmic granulation and hyposegmentation of the nucleus (Pelger–Huet anomaly). Eosinophils and basophils may be increased. In the mixed type, hyperplasia of both myeloid and megakaryocytic elements is seen (Fig. 8.13). The megakaryocytes exhibit polymorphism and heterotopia in some cases and numerous small and micromegakaryocytes in others (Branehog et al., 1982). The marrow in both types of CML is densely packed, with few residual fat cells. In addition, there may be macrophages with crystalloid inclusions; plasma and mast cells, and lymphocytes in variable numbers are usually present. Ineffective erythropoiesis with maturation arrest is found in many patients with CML. There is some rarefaction of the cancellous bone (occasionally thick trabeculae especially in sub-cortical regions alternate with attenuated ones or with occasional areas of circumscribed osteolysis), a moderate (mainly perivascular) increase in reticulin, as well as in blood vessels are also fairly constant features. Reversal of even severe bone marrow fibrosis has been achieved following bone marrow transplantation in CML (Islam et al., 1981; McGlave et al., 1982; Oblon et al., 1983). Cases have been described with predominant hyperplasia of one of the three series—neutrophilic, eosinophilic, basophilic—or involvement of one of the three to a greater extent than the others in individual patients with

Fig. 8.11 Bone biopsy sections of CML. Gran. = granulocytic; Gran./Meg. = mixed granulocytic megakaryocytic. Thickness of arrows indicates tendency to transformation: F = MF/OMS; B = blastic crisis; A = aplasia, therapy induced. Reproduced with permission from Bartl et al. (1984).

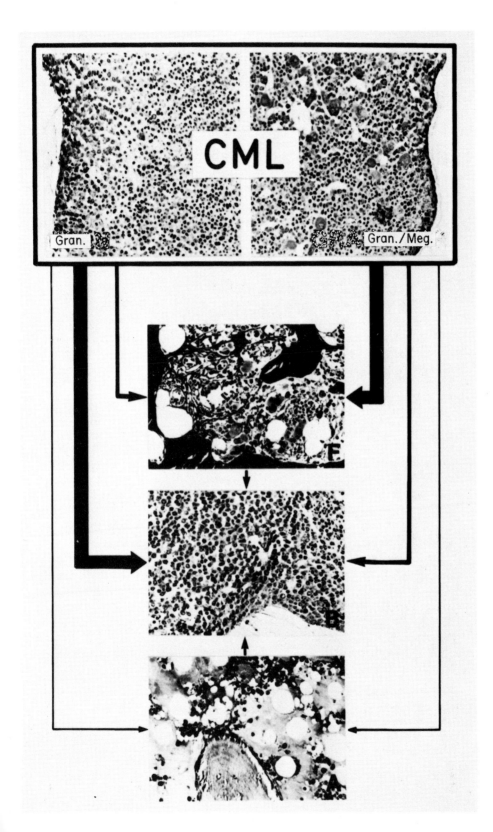

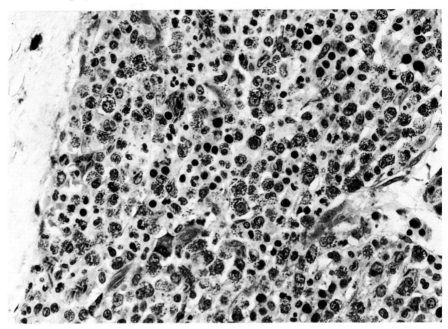

Fig. 8.12   CML with strong eosinophilic component; differentiation from hyper-eosinophilic syndrome not possible on biopsy histology alone. × 600, Giemsa.

CML, and sub-groups may be identified on this basis (Feremans *et al.*, 1983). Whether these have any clinical or prognostic significance has not yet been established. In addition, basophil production may be increased just before and during blastic transformation (Denburg *et al.*, 1982). Recent studies indicate that eosinophilia in the myeloproliferative disorders is an intrinsic part of the disease process (Crowley and Myers, 1983; Flaum *et al.*, 1981).

As the disease progresses, it is thought that intra-clonal mutation leads to changes in tempo, character and uncoupling of growth from differentiation. When this occurs, progressively wider osteoid seams of immature precursors herald the onset of blastic crisis (Fig. 8.14). Classification of transformation in CML has so far only been made on smears of aspirates (Spiers, 1979; Alimena, 1982). However, more information may be obtained from bone biopsies especially on the likelihood of imminent transformation as this is more frequently observed in the granulocytic

Fig. 8.13   (a) CML, mixed granulocytic and megakaryocytic. Trabecular bone at left; note numerous megakaryocytes. × 400, Giemsa; (b) CML, development of myelofibrosis; haematopoiesis reduced except for dysplastic megakaryocytes. × 400, Gomori.

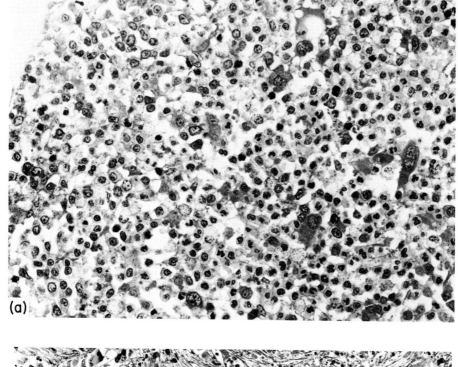

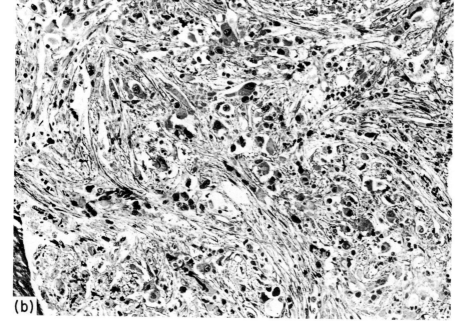

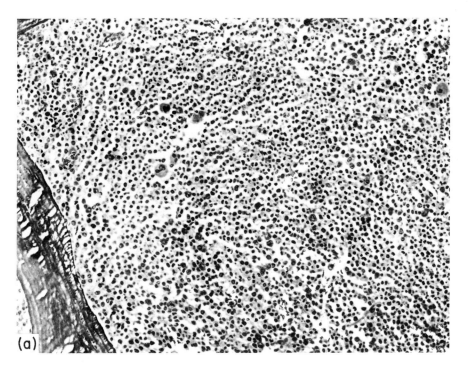

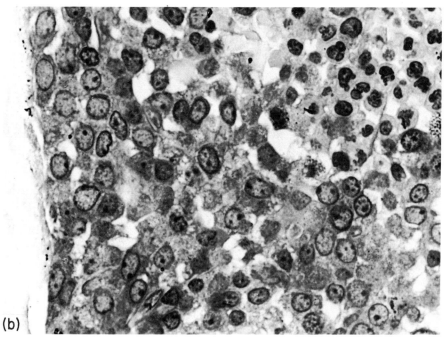

type of CML, while the mixed type has a greater tendency to develop into MF/OMS (Bartl *et al.*, 1982; Georgii, 1983; Frisch *et al.*, 1984b). Blastic transformation to cells of the myeloid and lymphoid cell lines has been demonstrated in CML (Williams, 1982). After aggressive chemotherapy, a hypo-cellular, even aplastic phase, may ensue (Fig. 8.11).

Important for therapy is the observation that normal haematopoietic precursors are present in the bone marrow in patients with Ph positive CML, though special techniques may be required to detect them (Coulombel *et al.*, 1983).

Histological studies in CML in blast transformation, after ablative therapy, and after bone marrow autografting, have shown that bone biopsies are required for differential diagnosis, for detection of residual blasts, for assessment of overall cellularity and to monitor regeneration of haematopoiesis.

8.5 Myelofibrosis/osteomyelosclerosis (MF/OMS)

These will be considered together, as the separation between them is to some extent artificial. These terms are somewhat loosely used in the following sense: myelofibrosis means an increase in the reticular content in the bone marrow, in severe cases to the exclusion of haematopoietic tissue (Hernandez-Nieto, 1978; Duhamel and Stachowiak, 1981; Burkhardt *et al.*, 1982; Manoharan *et al.*, 1982; Bartl *et al.*, 1982, Frisch *et al.*, 1984b). An increase in reticulin is relatively easy to demonstrate as with the commonly used stains for reticular fibres viewed in polarized light normal bone marrow shows very few, apart from some fibres near the bone and around some of the blood vessels. Myelosclerosis refers to a marrow which has collagen fibres in the stroma, in addition to the reticular fibres described above, while osteomyelosclerosis implies the presence of newly formed bone in addition to the reticulin and the collagen fibres (Plate Ve). This bone is both appositional and sprouting, that is both lamellar and woven. With respect to their occurrence, when large biopsies are carefully examined (if necessary, several sections at different levels) all three processes will generally be found, though one or the other predominates. The bone marrow to some extent reflects the development of the disease, and three main phases (corresponding to three main types of histology) have been described. The hyper-cellular phase (Figs 8.15, 8.16) in which peripheral blood count values may be

---

Fig. 8.14 CML: (a) dense cellularity with absence of fat cells, trabecular bone at left, seam of immature cells extending into central marrow cavity: blast crisis. × 300, Gomori; (b) higher magnification of (a) to show immature myeloid precursors. × 1000, Giemsa.

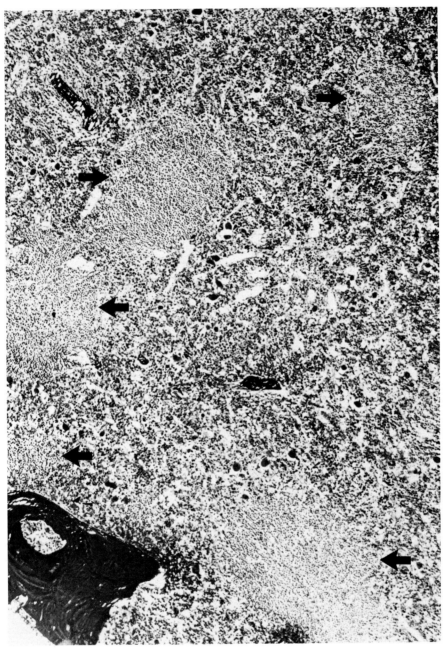

Fig. 8.15 Bone biopsy section of patient with myelofibrosis, cellular phase and multiple lymphoid nodules (arrows) requiring follow-up in case of development of a lymphoproliferative disorder. × 100, Gomori.

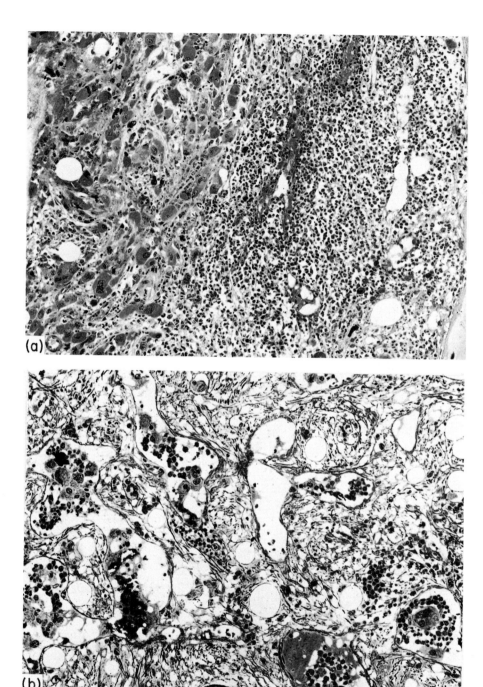

Fig. 8.16 Myelofibrosis: (a) cellular phase, effacement of normal bone marrow architecture and compartmentalization of haematopoiesis; dysplastic megakaryocytes, upper centre and left; granulopoiesis, right and centre. × 100, Giemsa; (b) oedema and fibrosis of marrow, sclerosis of vessel walls, residual haematopoietic cells confined to intravascular spaces. × 100, Gomori.

relatively high, the patchy phase with alternating areas of fibrosis and haematopoiesis, and low or normal peripheral blood count values, and the phase of obliterative sclerosis (Fig. 8.17), which is reflected in pancytopenia usually with increasing transfusion requirements. However, these phases are not sharply separated, clinically or histologically, and overlap occurs between them. They need not be sequential and

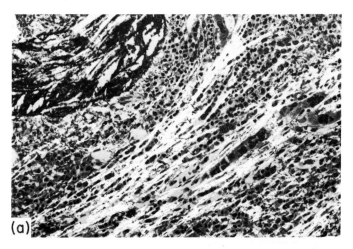

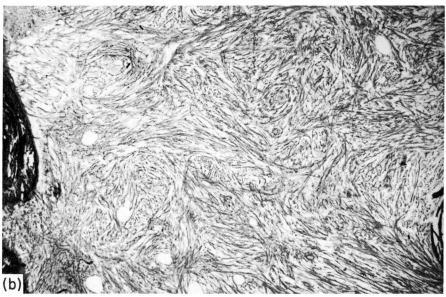

Fig. 8.17   Myelofibrosis: (a) residual haematopoiesis between strands of fibrous tissue. × 100, Gomori, polarized light; (b) obliterative phase, fibrotic, almost acellular marrow. × 400, Gomori.

therefore may be found simultaneously in different parts of the skeleton, or even of the same section. This indicates spatial discordance in the evolution of the disease process. From the point of view of haematopoiesis they could be described as: (1) haematopoietic hyperplasia, and (2) haematopoietic hypoplasia; both phases show a reduction in fat cells, increase in blood vessels and in fibroblasts, but when few cells remain in the obliterative phase there are clusters of polymorphic megakaryocytes (Fig. 8.18) with interstitially deposited platelets near them (Fig. 8.19),

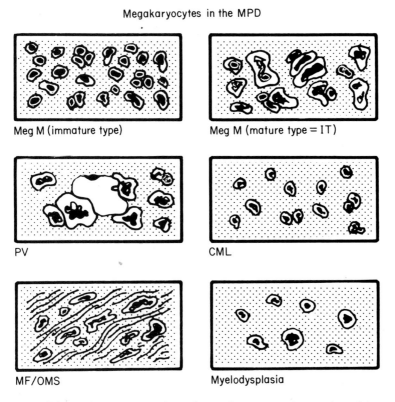

Fig. 8.18 Schematic representation of megakaryocytes in myeloproliferative disorders, to indicate differences in size and in nuclear configuration.

areas of oedema, gelatinous degeneration and infiltration with lymphocytes, plasma and mast cells, as well as macrophages containing haemosiderin or crystalloids and prominent islands of immature haematopoietic cells (Figs 8.19, 8.20). Characteristic for MF are the megakaryocytes, which may still be discerned within the dense fibrous tissue even when the other haematopoietic elements have disappeared

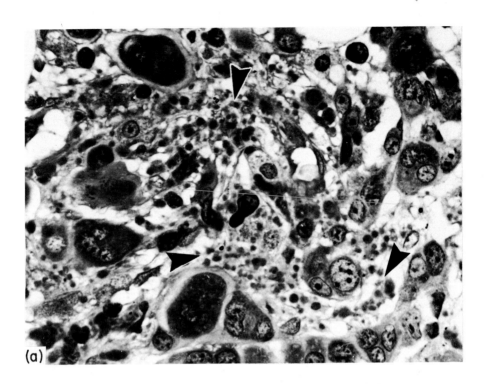

(a)

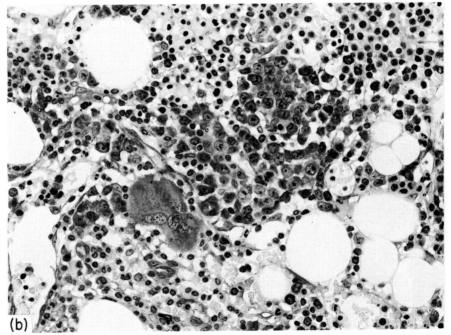

(b)

(Fig. 8.21). Frequently, naked nuclear masses are found, presumably remnants of megakaryocytes; little is known about how long they survive, or how they are eventually disposed of; in contrast to red cell nuclei which vanish rapidly into the voracious RES. Radley and Haller (1983) described phagocytosis of megakaryocyte nuclear remnants in mice. However, this is rarely observed in the human bone marrow, even in conditions with hyperplasia of megakaryocytes. Naked nuclei may be seen in the sinusoids and possibly they are washed away and disintegrate in the bloodstream. With progression of the disease process, networks of reticulin merge with bundles of collagen dividing the marrow into compartments, and causing sclerosis of the sinus walls, which no doubt is one reason for the appearance of intravascular islands of haematopoietic precursors (Plate VIf), frequently observed in bone biopsies in both MF and OMS, in the cellular as well as in the fibrotic phases.

In MF the overall trend is trabecular rarefaction, though occasional foci of hyperplasia with osteoclastic activity may also be found, while in OMS appositional new bone (Fig. 8.22) as well as irregular spicules of woven bone (Fig. 8.23) contribute to the progressive diminution of the marrow cavities (Fig. 8.22 and Plate Ve), the contents of which, however, are often not so densely fibrotic as in obliterative MF; and some residual haematopoietic function is retained (Fig. 8.23). Agnogenic myeloid metaplasia is the term applied to MF/OMS when the cause or the preceding disease is unknown, and there is extramedullary haematopoiesis in liver and spleen. It is now thought that most (if not all) cases are a consequence of a preceding MPD.

Some of the histopathological aspects and the clinical features with special reference to prognostic variables predicting survival, have been reviewed by Varki et al. (1983).

8.5.1   Pathogenesis of MF

Recent experimental evidence has supported earlier speculations on the association of megakaryocytes with myelofibrosis (Hickling, 1937; Burkhardt et al., 1975). It has been shown that megakaryocytes and platelets are capable of producing a growth factor (which is mitogenic for fibroblasts) as well as Factor 4, an inhibitor of collagenase (Castro-Malaspina and Moore, 1982; Moore, 1982). In normal thrombogenesis whole megakaryocytes, fragments of their cytoplasm or platelets are shed directly into the bloodstream via the sinusoids, hence the high platelet

---

Fig. 8.19 Myelofibrosis: (a) megakaryocytes and platelets in the interstitial spaces (arrows). × 1000, Giemsa; (b) osteomyelosclerosis; islands of immature erythropoiesis (centre). × 400, Giemsa.

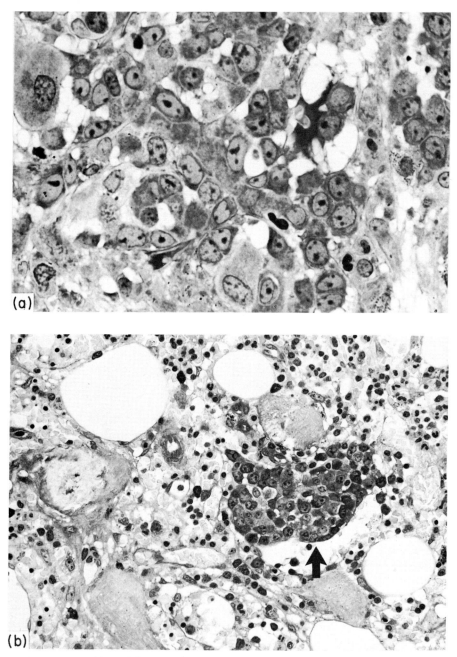

Fig. 8.20 Myeloproliferative disease: (a) large clusters of megakaryoblasts and promegakaryocytes. × 600, Giemsa; (b) islands of erythroid precursors. × 400, Giemsa. In both cases not to be mistaken for metastases.

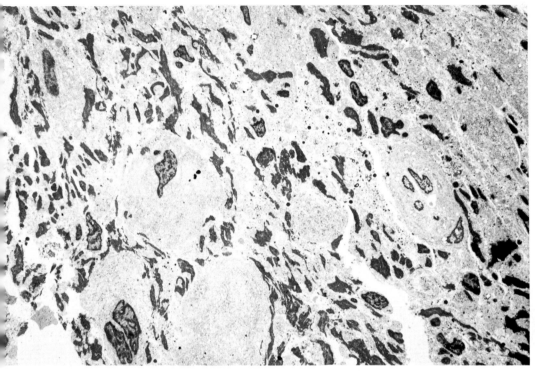

Fig. 8.21 Electron micrograph showing fibrotic phase of myelofibrosis and dysplastic megakaryocytes. × 1000.

counts in the chronic MPD when there is hyperplastic and effective megakaryopoiesis in the bone marrow. In contrast 'ineffective' megakaryopoiesis may stimulate fibrosis: when hyperplasia of megakaryocytes involves disintegration of large numbers within the marrow in the interstitial spaces instead of release into the bloodstream, these intramedullary megakaryocyte and platelet components are released and stimulate fibroblasts and fibrillogenesis. This is by no means the only (or exclusive) mechanism. Lymphocytes, granulocytes, monocytes and mast cells may all produce growth factors. The last-named, especially, are observed near the surface of osseous trabeculae during new bone formation (Fig. 8.23). (This is a somewhat paradoxical situation, as mast cells adjacent to trabeculae have also been implicated in osteoporosis.) Ineffective haematopoiesis with intramedullary destruction of immature precursors (Fig. 8.24) including megakaryocytes is characteristic in MF. An autoimmune reaction mediated by circulating immune complexes has also been implicated (Caligaris-Cappio *et al.*, 1981; Gordon *et al.*, 1981).

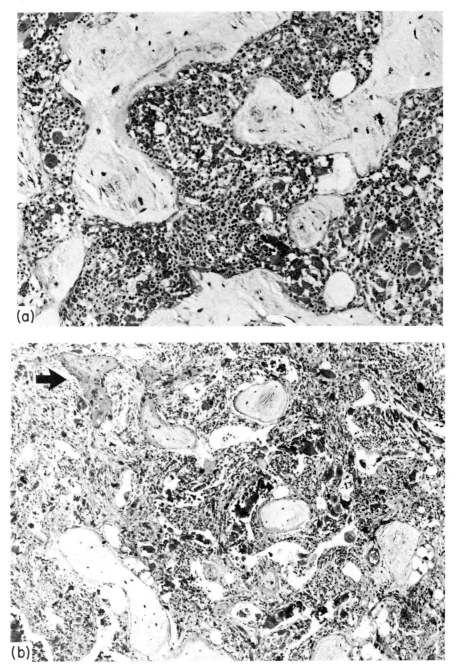

Fig. 8.22 (a) Bone biopsy of a case of clinical PV showing developing osteo-myelosclerosis; increase in trabecular bone, but no fibrosis of marrow. × 250, Giemsa; (b) further stage in development of OMS; woven bone at arrow upper left; note fibrosis of marrow and clusters of megakaryocytes. × 100, Giemsa.

8.5.2   Transformation in MF/OMS

A blast crisis may develop in any of the entities in the MPD, including MF/
OMS (Fig. 8.24b and Plate VIa–d). Moreover, transition of MF to PV has
also been observed (Hasselbach and Berild, 1983). The bone marrow
picture in blast crisis may differ from that in acute leukaemia: the
histology is less uniform and monotonous; increasing and widening
endosteal seams of immature precursors may precede blastosis in the
peripheral blood. When megakaryoblasts are involved, they are more
numerous in the marrow than in the blood and require marker techniques
for identification (Williams and Weis, 1982). A special feature in the bone
marrow of patients with MPD is the occurrence of lymphoid nodules.
These may be multiple and in most cases represent benign lymphoid
hyperplasia; their frequency is given in Fig. 8.4.

Concurrent MPD and LPD also occur and this has been observed in 128
cases in our series. 19% had a primary LPD, 7% had a primary MPD and
in the remaining 74% the primary disorder could not be ascertained. The
frequency of the histological groups, and the median survivals of the
patients, are given in Fig. 8.25.

8.5.3   Differential diagnosis of MF

There are numerous conditions that may induce fibrosis in the bone
marrow. These include the lymphoproliferative disorders, Hodgkin's
disease, metastatic carcinoma, and sclerosing myelitis due to various
kinds of injury and toxic agents, as well as unknown causes. All are
accompanied by a reduction in haematopoiesis which affects the
megakaryocytes also. In most cases, if the fibrosis is due to one of the
lymphoproliferative disorders or metastatic carcinoma, the corresponding cells will be recognized. But in some instances there may be a fibrotic
marrow with only un-identifiable hyper-chromatic nuclei present. If at
the same time trabecular alterations similar to those in MF/OMS are also
present, a second biopsy from another site is warranted, to clarify the
diagnosis. The possibility of two concurrent pathological conditions
should also be considered. These may be two haematological malignancies or myelofibrosis together with a non-haematological disorder,
such as the nephrotic syndrome (Karcher et al., 1982).

The effects of therapy on bone marrow histology should be borne in
mind when biopsies of patients after treatment are interpreted (Fig. 8.26).

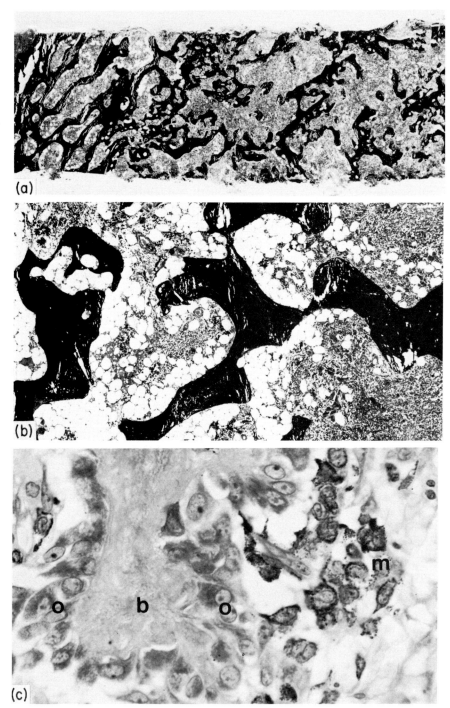

Fig. 8.23 Osteomyelosclerosis: (a) note patchy distortion of trabecular bone. ×
10, Gomori; (b) altered trabecular bone structure; the marrow has fatty, fibrotic
and cellular areas. × 100, Giemsa; (c) association of mast cells (cluster indicated by
m) with new bone formation (b), osteoblasts (o). × 1000, Giemsa.

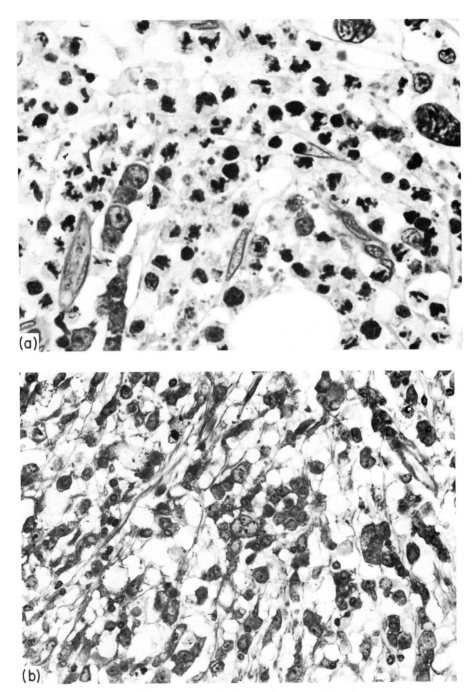

Fig. 8.24 (a) Myelofibrosis; necrosis of granulocytic cells in the marrow. × 600. Giemsa; (b) blast crisis in MF; section showing immature cells and fibres. × 400, Giemsa.

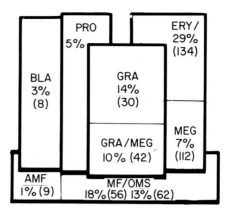

Fig. 8.25 Frequency and median survival of patients in the histological groups in the MPD; ( ) = median survival in months; % = percentage of patients in each group. Abbreviations as in Fig 8.2.

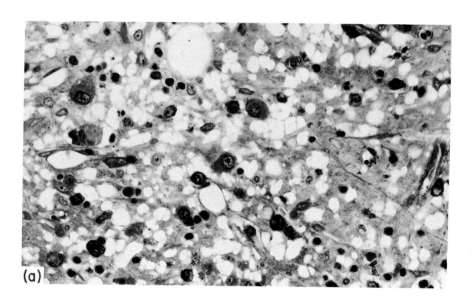

(a)

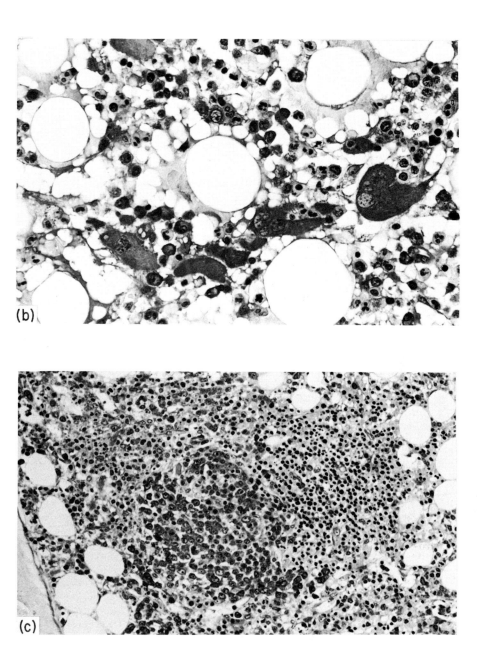

Fig. 8.26 Features of bone marrow after intensive chemotherapy: (a) oedematous stroma, regenerating fat cells and widely scattered haematopoietic cells. × 400; (b) cluster of megakaryocytes in oedematous stroma containing plasma cells and lymphocytes. × 400; (c) later regenerative phase; large erythropoietic islands in largely reconstituted marrow. × 250, Giemsa.

References

Alimena, G., Dallapiccola, B., Gastaldi, R., Mandelli, F., Brandt, L., Mitelman, F. and Nilsson, P. G. (1982), Chromosomal, morphological and clinical correlations in blastic crisis of chronic myeloid leukaemia. A study of 69 cases. *Scand. J. Haematol.*, **28**, 103–17.

Barosi, G., Baraldi, A., Cazzola, M., Fortunato, A., Palestra, P., Polino, G., Ramella, S. and Spriano, P. (1984), Polycythaemia following splenectomy in myelofibrosis with myeloid metaplasia. A reorganization of erythropoiesis. *Scand. J. Haematol.*, **32**, 12–18.

Bartl, R., Frisch, B. and Burkhardt, R. (1982), *Bone Marrow Biopsies Revisited. A New Dimension for Haematologic Malignancies*, Karger, Basel.

Bartl, R., Frisch, B. and Burkhardt, R. (1984), *Bone Marrow Biopsies Revisited*, 2nd edn, Karger, Basel.

Boggs, D. R. (1981), Clonal origin of leukemia: site of origin in the stem cell hierarchy and the significance of chromosomal changes. *Blood Cells*, **7**, 205–15.

Branehog, I., Ridell, B., Swolin, B. and Weinfeld, A. (1982), The relation of platelet kinetics to bone marrow megakaryocytes in chronic granulocytic leukaemia. *Scand. J. Haematol.*, **29**, 411–20.

Burkhardt, R., Bartl, R., Beil, E., Denmler, K., Hofmann, E., Irrgang, U., Kronseder, A., Langegger, H., Saar, U., Ulrich, M. and Wiemann, H. (1975), Myelofibrosis–osteomyelosclerosis syndrome. Review of literature and histomorphology. In: *Advances in the Biosciences*, Vol. 16, Pergamon Press, Oxford, pp. 9–56.

Burkhardt, R., Frisch, B. and Bartl, R. (1982), Bone biopsy in haematological disorders. *J. clin. Pathol.*, **35**, 257–84.

Caligaris-Cappio, F. Vigliani, R., Novarino, A., Camussi, G., Campama, D. and Gavosto, F. (1981), Idiopathic myelofibrosis: a possible role for immune-complexes in the pathogenesis of bone marrow fibrosis. *Brit. J. Haematol.*, **49**, 17–21.

Castro-Malaspina, H. and Moore, M. A. S. (1982), Pathophysiological mechanisms operating in the development of myelofibrosis: role of megakaryocytes. *Nouv. Rev. Fr. Hematol.*, **24**, 221–6.

Castro-Malaspina, H., Gay, R. E., Jhanwar, S. C., Hamilton, J. A., Chiarieri, D. R., Meyers, P. A., Gay, S. and Moore, M. A. S. (1982), Characteristics of bone marrow fibroblast colony-forming cells (CFU-F) and their progeny in patients with myeloproliferative disorders. *Blood*, **59**, 1046–54.

Coulombel, L., Kalousek, D. J., Eaves, C. J., Gupta, C. M. and Eaves, A. C. (1983), Long term culture reveals chromosomally normal hematopoietic progenitor cells in patients with Philadelphia chromosome-positive chronic myelogenous leukemia. *New Engl. J. Med.*, **308**, 1493–8.

Crowley, J. P. and Myers, T. J. (1983), Humoral and cellular studies of eosinophils in reactive and myeloproliferative syndromes with marked eosinophilia. *Am. J. clin. Pathol.*, **79**, 301–5.

Dameshek, W. (1951), Some speculations on the myeloproliferative syndromes. *Blood*, **2**, 372–5.

Denburg, J. A., Wilson, W. E. C. and Bienenstock, J. (1982), Basophil production in myeloproliferative disorders: Increases during acute blastic transformation of chronic myeloid leukemia. *Blood*, **60**, 113–20.

Duhamel, G. and Stachowiak, J. (1981), Bone marrow fibrosis in malignant hemopathies and cancers. Histological study of 2,768 biopsies. *Sem. Hop. Paris*, **57**, 111–16.

Ellis, J. T. and Peterson, P. (1979), The bone marrow in polycythemia vera. *Pathol. Ann.*, **14**, 383–403.

Feremans, W., Marcelis, L. and Ardichvili, D. (1983), Chronic neutrophilic leukaemia with enlarged lymph nodes and lysozyme deficiency. *J. clin. Pathol.*, **36**, 324–8.

Fialkow, P. J., Singer, J. W., Adamson, J. W. *et al.*, (1981), Acute non-lymphocytic leukemia: heterogeneity of stem cell origin. *Blood*, **57**, 1068–73.

Fialkow, P. J., Faguet, G. B., Jacobson, R. J., Vaidya, K. and Murphy, S. (1982), Evidence that essential thrombocythemia is a clonal disorder with origin in a multipotent stem cell. *Blood*, **58**, 916–19.

Flaum, M. A., Schooley, R. T., Fauci, A. S. and Gralnick, H. R. (1981), A clinicopathologic correlation of the idiopathic hypereosinophilic syndrome. I. Hematologic manifestations. *Blood*, **58**, 1012–20.

Frisch, B., Bartl, R., Burkhardt, R., Jäger, K. and Pappenberger, R. (1984a), Bone marrow histology in the chronic myeloproliferative disorders: criteria for recognition, classification and prognostic evaluation. A study of 3500 biopsies. *Biblthca haemat.*, **50**, 57–80.

Frisch, B., Bartl, R., Burkhardt, R. and Jäger, K. (1984b), Histologic criteria for classification and differential diagnosis in the chronic myeloproliferative disorders. *Haematologia*, **17**, 209–26.

Gaetani, G. F., Ferraris, A. M., Galiano, S., Giuntini, P., Canepa, L. and d'Urso, M. (1982), Primary thrombocythemia: clonal origin of platelets, erythrocytes, and granulocytes in a Gd^B/Gd Mediterranean subject. *Blood*, **59**, 76–9.

Georgii, A. (1983), Histopathology and clinics in chronic myeloproliferative diseases. *Verh. Dtsch. Ges. Path.*, **67**, 214–34.

Georgii, A., Vykoupil, K. F. and Thiele, J. (1980), Chronic megakaryocytic granulocytic myelosis-CMGM. A subtype of chronic myeloid leukemia. *Virchows Arch. Abt. A Path. Anat.*, **389**, 253–68.

Gilbert, H. S. (1973), The spectrum of myeloproliferative disorders. *Med. Clin. N. Am.*, **57**, 355–93.

Goldman, J. M. and Dao-Pei Lu (1982), New approaches in chronic granulocytic leukemia–origin, prognosis and treatment. *Sem. Haemat.*, **19**, 241–56.

Gomez, G. A., Sokal, J. E. and Ealsh, D. (1982), Prognostic factors at diagnosis of chronic myelocytic leukemia. *Cancer*, **47**, 2470–777.

Gordon, B. R., Coleman, M., Kohen, P. and Day, N. K. (1981), Immunologic abnormalities in myelofibrosis with activation of the complement system. *Blood*, **58**, 904–10.

Harker, L. A., Zimmerman, T. S. (Eds) (1983), Platelet disorders. *Clin. Haemat.*, **12**, No. 1, W. B. Saunders, Eastbourne.

Hasselbach, H. and Berild, D. (1983), Transition of myelofibrosis to polycythaemia vera. *Scand. J. Haematol*, **30**, 161–6.

Hernandez-Nieto, L., Muncunilli, J., Rozman, C., Febregues, M., Feliv, E., Granena, A., Montserrat-Costa, E. and Nomdedev, B. (1978), Secondary myelofibrosis and/or osteosclerosis. An assessment of 4000 biopsies. *Sangre*, **23**, 402–10.

Hickling, R. A. (1937), Chronic non-leukaemic myelosis. *Q. J. Med.*, **6**, 253–75.

Islam, A., Catovsky, D., Goldman, J. M. and Galton, D. A. G. (1981), Histological study of the bone marrow in blast transformation. II. Bone marrow fibre content before and after autografting. *Histopathology*, **5**, 491–8.

Jäger, K., Burkhardt, R., Bartl, R., Frisch, B. and Mahl, G. (1983), Lymphoid infiltrates in chronic myeloproliferative disorders (MPD). *Verh. Dtsch. Ges. Path.*, **67**, 239–42.

Karcher, D. S., Pearson, C. E., Butler, W. M., Hurwitz, M. A. and Cassell, P. F. (1982), Giant lymph node hyperplasia involving the thymus with associated nephrotic syndrome and myelofibrosis. *Am. J. clin. Pathol.*, **77**, 101–4.

Kersey, J. H. (1983), Chronic myelocytic (multipotent-stem-cell) leukemia. *New Engl. J. Med.*, **309**, 851–2.

Koffler, H. P. and Golde, D. W. (1981), Chronic myelogenous leukemia—New concepts. *New Engl. J. Med.*, **304**, 1269–74.

Kurnick, J. E., Mahmood, T., Napoli, N. and Block, M. H. (1980), Extension of myeloid tissue into the lower extremities in polycythemia. *Am. J. clin. Pathol.*, **74**, 427–31.

Laszlo, J. (1975), Myeloproliferative disorders (MPD): myelofibrosis, myelosclerosis, extramedullary hematopoiesis, undifferentiated MPD, and hemorrhagic thrombocythemia. *Sem. Haemat.*, **12**, 409–32.

Laszlo, J., Iland, H., Murphy, S., Peterson, P., Briere, J. and Rosenthal, D. (1983), Essential thrombocythemia: clinical and laboratory characteristics at presentation. *Clin. Res.*, **31**, 535A.

Lucie, N. P. and Young, G. (1983), Marrow cellularity in the diagnosis of polycythaemia. *J. clin. Pathol.*, **36**, 180–3.

Manoharan, A., Catovsky, D., Clein, P., Traub, H. E., Costello, C., O'Brien, M., Boralossa, H. and Galton, D. A. G. (1981), Simultaneous or spontaneous occurrence of lympho- and myeloproliferative disorders: a report of 4 cases. *Brit. J. Haematol.*, **48**, 111–16.

Manoharan, A., Smart, R. C. and Pitney, W. R. (1982), Prognostic factors in myelofibrosis. *Pathology*, **14**, 455–61.

McBrine, P. A., Miller, A., Zimelman, A. P. and Koft, R. S. (1980), Polycythemia vera with myelofibrosis and myeloid metaplasia. Acute hepatic failure following splenectomy. *Am. J. clin. Pathol.*, **74**, 693–6.

McGlave, P. B., Brunning, R. D., Hurd, D. D. and Kim, T. H. (1982), Reversal of severe bone marrow fibrosis and osteosclerosis following allogeneic bone marrow transplantation for chronic granulocytic leukaemia. *Brit. J. Haematol.*, **52**, 189–94.

Moore, M. A. S. (1982), Pathogenesis of MF. In: *Recent Advances in Haematology* (ed. A. V. Hoffbrand), Churchill Livingstone, Edinburgh, pp. 136–9.

Oblon, D. J., Elfenbein, G. J., Braylan, R. C., Jones, J. and Weiner, R. S. (1983), The reversal of myelofibrosis associated with chronic myelogenous leukaemia after allogenic bone marrow transplantation. *Exp. Hemat.*, **11**, 681–5.

Papayannis, A. G. Nikiforakis, E. and Anagnostou-Keramida, D. (1982), Development of chronic lymphocytic leukaemia in a patient with polycythaemia vera. *Scand. J. Haematol.*, **29**, 65–9.

Radley, J. M. and Haller, C. J. (1983), Fate of senescent megakaryocytes in the bone marrow. *Brit. J. Haematol.*, **53**, 277–87.

Spiers, A. S. D. (1979), Annotation. Metamorphosis of chronic granulocytic leukaemia, diagnosis, classification and management.

Thiele, J., Holgado, S., Choritz, H. and Georgii, A. (1983), Density distribution and size of megakaryocytes in inflammatory reactions of the bone marrow (myelitis) and chronic myeloproliferative diseases. *Scand. J. Haematol.*, **31**, 329–41.

Tura, S. and Baccarini, M. (1981), The Italian cooperative study group on chronic myeloid leukaemia. Staging of chronic myeloid leukaemia. *Brit. J. Haematol.*, **47**, 105–19.

Varki, A., Lottenberg, R., Griffith, R. and Reinhard, E. (1983), The syndrome of idiopathic myelofibrosis. A clinicopathologic review with emphasis on the prognostic variables predicting survival. *Medicine*, **62**, 353–71.

Verhest, A. and Monsieur, R. (1983), Philadelphia chromosome-positive thrombocythemia with leukemic transformation. *New Engl. J. Med.*, **308**, 1603.

Vykoupil, K. F., Thiele, J., Stangel, W., Krmpotic, E. and Georgii, A. (1980), Polycythaemia vera. I. Histopathology, ultrastructure and cytogenetics of the bone marrow in comparison with secondary polycythaemia. *Virch. Arch. Abt. A Path. Anat.*, **389**, 307–24.

Williams, W. C. and Weiss, G. B. (1982), Megakaryoblastic transformation of chronic myelogenous leukaemia. *Cancer*, **49**, 921–6.

9 Acute leukaemias and myelodysplasias

In early cases of acute leukaemia, there is a diffuse interstitial distribution of the blasts (without wide paratrabecular seams) while the marrow architecture and fat cells are to some extent preserved. Alternatively, the interstitial infiltration of blasts is accompanied by an exudative or serous marrow atrophy, with partial disappearance of marrow and fat. In these cases the differential diagnosis includes hairy cell leukaemia, early myelofibrosis and aplastic anaemia.

There are, however, two main types of histological picture in the bone marrow in acute leukaemia, namely: (1) hyper-cellular and (2) hypocellular (Figs 9.1 and 9.2, Plate VIIc and d). The hyper-cellular type predominates.

9.1 Hyperplastic type

In this type, the marrow architecture is effaced, only vestiges of normal haematopoiesis remain, fat cells have virtually disappeared, sinusoids are disrupted, and the marrow cavities are occupied by sheets of leukaemic cells presenting a uniform monomorphic picture. In some cases the cells are very densely packed, so that a dry tap on attempts at aspiration may occur e.g. in acute myeloid leukaemia (AML); in others there is a somewhat looser arrangement. This is often seen in acute lymphatic leukaemia (ALL) in which extravasated erythrocytes, and some connective tissue elements, reticulin fibres and macrophages and other cells are interspersed among the leukaemic cells. In other cases, areas of necrotic cells are found, possibly due to rapid growth, and disruption of the blood supply. Though residual haematopoietic precursors are present in both myeloid and lymphoid acute leukaemias, there may be a difference in their derivation. In AML there is presumably a panmyelosis with granulocytes, erythrocytes and megakaryocytes belonging to the same clone. In ALL there is replacement of normal

146

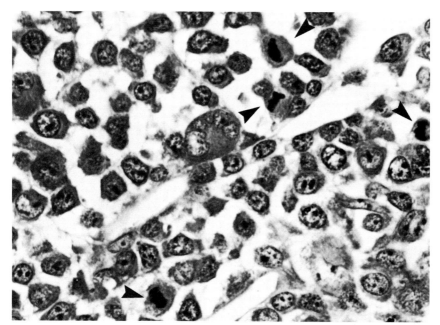

Fig. 9.1 Acute myeloid leukaemia: precise phenotypic characterization requires marker and enzyme studies; note mitotic figures. × 1000, Giemsa.

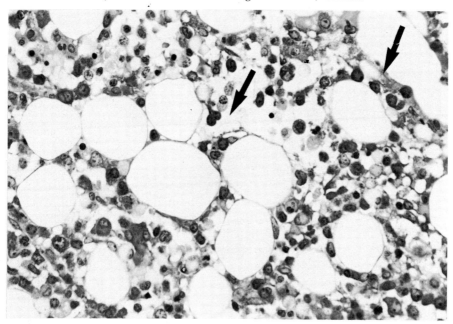

Fig. 9.2 Bone biopsy in case of hypoplastic acute leukaemia; note preservation of fat cells, myeloblasts loosely dispersed in the interstitial spaces; some are indicated by arrows. × 250, Giemsa.

elements and the morphological abnormalities of those left may be due to extraneous causes such as relative folate deficiency. The cytological appearance of the cells indicates the major cell line in the majority of the cases though it is not always possible to distinguish lymphoblasts from myeloblasts on histology. Phenotypic classification of the sub-groups must be accomplished by means of enzymic and other markers on smears of peripheral blood, aspirates of bone marrow or cryostat sections of bone biopsies. Leukaemia of platelet precursors (immature megakaryocytic or megakaryoblastic myelosis) may present with diverse features (Bain *et al.*, 1983; Bevan *et al.*, 1982). In erythroleukaemia, the erythroid cells are megaloblastic with dyserythropoietic characteristics and PAS positive inclusions. There is a concomitant increase in myeloblasts and anomalies in megakaryocytes (Roggli and Saleem, 1982). The degree of fibrosis which accompanies the acute leukaemias varies widely, from mild to marked, and may resemble an acute myelosclerosis (AMF) (see below). In acute leukaemias in adults, progressive fibrosis is thought by some workers to be associated with impending relapse and resolution of the fibrosis with remission.

Collagen fibrosis with osteolytic lesions has also been documented in acute myelomonocytic leukaemia (Delacrétaz *et al.*, 1983).

9.2   Hypoplastic acute leukaemias (hypo-cellular type)

The bone marrow shows a reduction in normal haematopoietic cells, an increase in fat cells between which are narrow bands of immature precursors (Plate VIIc). On closer examination, many of these cells are blasts with a high nucleocytoplasm ratio. When there is little or no progression, this state corresponds to 'smouldering' leukaemia, in which foci of blasts are scattered throughout the marrow, without overgrowing it, for variable periods of time. This situation is more easily recognized in bone biopsies than in smears of aspirates, likewise biopsies are more reliable for detection of early relapse and therefore in planning therapy. Hypoplastic acute leukaemias are rare in children, but a hypoplastic phase may precede typical acute leukaemia (Sills and Stockman, 1981). 'Smouldering' leukaemias are mainly diseases of older people and are included in the myelodysplastic syndromes (see below). Hypercalcaemia may complicate acute leukaemias, due in part to production of an osteoclast stimulating factor similar to that secreted by myeloma cells (Gewirtz *et al.*, 1983). In these cases osteoclastic resorption may be observed in the bone marrow biopsy.

Osteoporosis due to attenuation of the trabecular bone is more frequently seen, while osteomalacia may develop during the course of therapy.

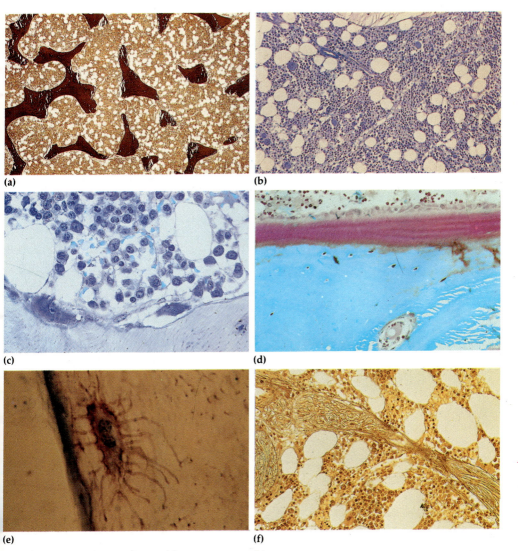

Plate 1 Appearances of normal bone marrow and bone.
(a) Haematopoietic tissue (light brown) fat (white) and trabecular bone (dark brown) within normal limits. × 200, Gomori. (b) High magnification to show haematopoietic tissue. × 500, Giemsa. (c) Trabecular surface with osteoclasts in Howship's lacunae. × 750, Giemsa. (d) Trabecular surface with row of osteoblasts on lamellar osteoid (red) and mineralized bone (blue). × 750, Ladewig. (e) Trabecular surface with osteoid (green line) and osteocyte within its lacuna, and canaliculi connecting with other osteocytes. × 2000, Giemsa. (f) Longitudinal and tangential section through nerve in normal bone marrow. × 500, Gomori.

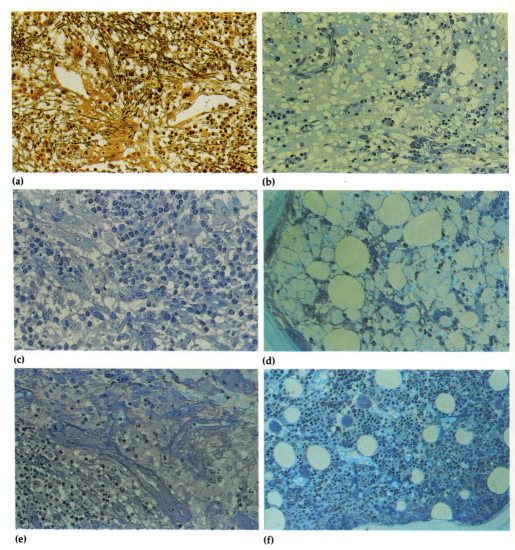

(a)

(b)

(c)

(d)

(e)

(f)

Plate II Non-specific bone marrow reactions.
(a) Sclerosing myelitis. × 750, Gomori. (b) Exudative myelitis. × 750, Giemsa. (c) Granulomatous myelitis. × 750, Giemsa. (d) Foam cells in bone marrow of patient with renal insufficiency. × 750, Giemsa. (e) Bone biopsy of 12 year old child with chronic osteomyelitis. × 750, Giemsa. (f) Leukaemoid reaction in bone marrow of patient with Hodgkin's disease without bone marrow involvement. × 500, Giemsa.

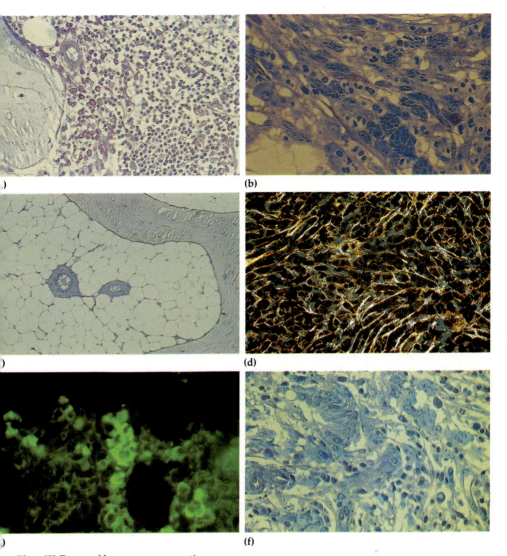

Plate III Types of bone marrow reaction.
(a) Systemic mastocytosis with endosteal and paratrabecular mast cells, lymphocytes and lymphoid cell aggregate. × 500, Giemsa. (b) Macrophages with crystalloid inclusions in systemic mastocytosis; such cells are also frequently seen in CML and megakaryocytic myelosis. × 2000, Giemsa. (c) Complete replacement of haematopoietic tissue by fat cells around arteries with sclerosis of walls. × 200, Giemsa. (d) Case of malignant myelofibrosis viewed in polarized light to illustrate the extent of bone marrow fibrosis. × 2000, Gomori. (e) Case of plasmacytosis in the bone marrow diagnosed as early multiple myeloma by monoclonality of plasma cells, cryostat section, FITC IgM. × 2000. (f) Epithelioid cells in the bone marrow in a case of malignant lymphoma diagnosed as Lennert's lymphoma by lymph node biopsy. × 1500, Giemsa.

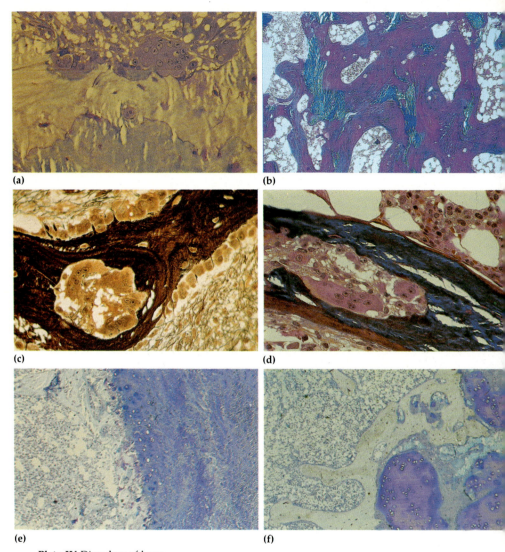

Plate IV Disorders of bone.
(a) Paget's disease of bone, showing mosaic pattern, giant osteoclast, osteoblasts, and paratrabecular fibrosis. × 500, Giemsa. (b) Renal osteodystrophy, osteoid red, mineralized bone blue. × 200, Ladewig. (c) Bone biopsy in case of primary hyperparathyroidism; note excavating osteoclasts within the bone and osteoblasts on its surface, and paratrabecular fibrosis. × 500, Gomori. (d) Renal osteopathy presenting osteolytic lesions similar to those of primary hyperparathyroidism. × 200, Ladewig. (e) Epiphyseal junction in case of osteogenesis imperfecta; note poorly developed cortical and trabecular bone. × 200, Giemsa. (f) Bone biopsy of patient with chondrosarcoma; note cartilaginous masses (red). × 200, Giemsa.

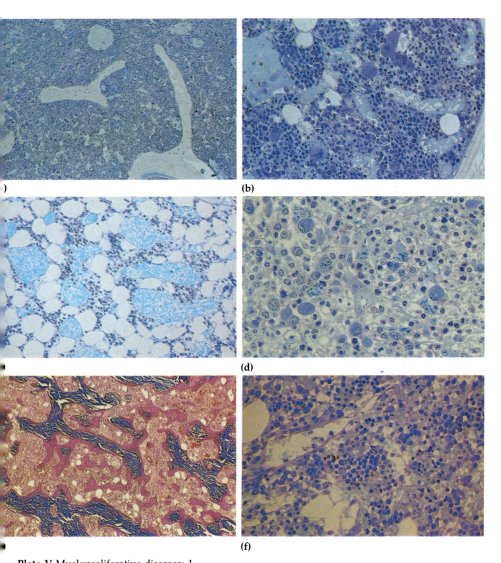

Plate V Myeloproliferative diseases: 1.
(a) PV with trilinear proliferation; hypercellular marrow, absence of fat cells, and reduction in trabecular bone. × 500, Giemsa. (b) PV showing erythroid and megakaryocytic hyperplasia; note dilated sinusoids. × 500, Giemsa. (c) Case of clinical PV, hypocellularity in iliac crest biopsy; note engorged sinusoids. × 500, Giemsa. (d) Transitional phase of megakaryocytic myelosis to myelofibrosis; note mononuclear megakaryocytes and macrophages with crystals. × 500, Giemsa. (e) Osteomyelosclerosis; note osteoid (red), trabecular bone (blue) and fibrosis of the marrow with residual fat cells. × 500 , Ladewig. (f) Case of spherocytosis; to illustrate compensatory erythroid hyperplasia for comparison. × 500, Giemsa.

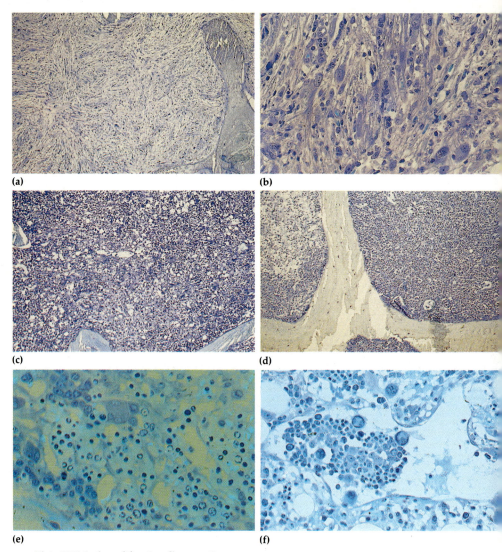

(a) (b)

(c) (d)

(e) (f)

Plate VI Myeloproliferative diseases: 2.
(a) Iliac crest biopsy of 46 year old patient with pancytopenia and splenomegaly and complaint of increasing tiredness of 6 months' duration; note almost acellular fibrosis. × 200, Giemsa. (b) Biopsy taken 2 months later, typical picture of myelofibrosis with numerous megakaryocytes. × 750, Giemsa. (c) A month later the patient developed acute leukaemia and died within a week; section from iliac crest showing residual haematopoietic tissue. × 200, Giemsa. (d) Sheets of blasts from (c), × 200, Giemsa. (e) marked dyserythropoiesis in the bone marrow in megakaryocytic myelosis with incipient fibrosis. × 750, Giemsa. (f) Intravascular haematopoietic tissue in myelofibrosis. × 750, Giemsa

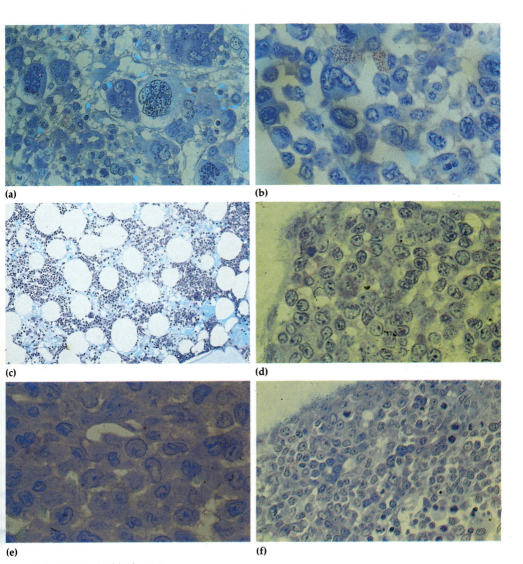

Plate VII Myeloid leukaemias.
(a) Mixed erythro- and megakaryoblastic. × 1500, Giemsa. (b) Myelomonocytic. × 1500, Giemsa. (c) Hypo-cellular undifferentiated. × 500, Giemsa. (d) Myeloblastic. × 1500, Giemsa. (e) Monocytic. × 1500, Giemsa. (f) Promyelocytic. × 750, Giemsa.

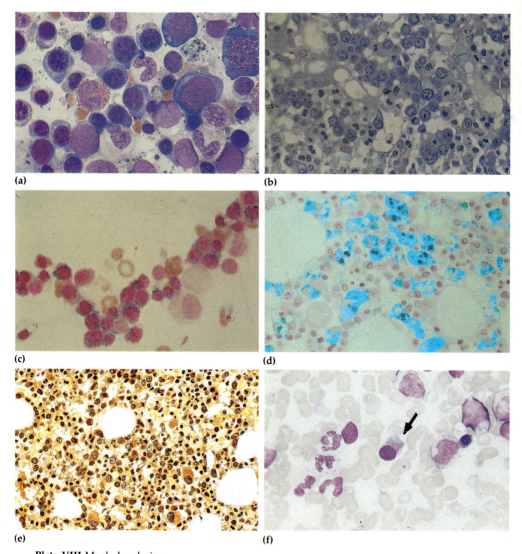

Plate VIII Myelodysplasias.
(a) Smear of aspirate of patient with refractory anaemia showing erythroblasts at all stages of maturation. × 2000, Giemsa. (b) Biopsy section of patient with refractory anaemia, showing clusters of immature precursors. × 800, Giemsa. (c) Numerous ringed sideroblasts from a case of sideroblastic anaemia. × 2000, Giemsa. (d) Massive accumulation of iron in macrophages in a case of refractory anaemia. × 800, Berlin Blue. (e) Biopsy section in myelodysplasia showing increased cellularity and micromegakaryocytes. × 500, Gomori. (f) Smear of bone marrow aspirate in myelodysplasia; micromegakaryocyte indicated by arrow. × 1500, Giemsa.

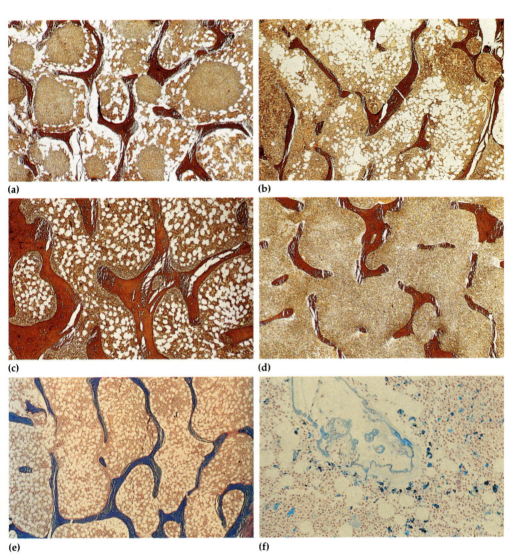

Plate IX Growth patterns of malignant lymphomas in the bone marrow.
(a) CLL, nodular. × 40, Gomori. (b) Hairy cell leukaemia, patchy. × 40, Gomori. (c) Centrocytic, paratrabecular. × 40, Gomori. (d) Immunocytoma, packed marrow. × 40, Gomori. (e) Multiple myeloma, interstitial pattern, with hypo-cellular marrow and marked osteoporosis. × 40, Ladewig. (f) Iron overload in multiple myeloma with endosteal deposition of iron. × 200, Berlin blue.

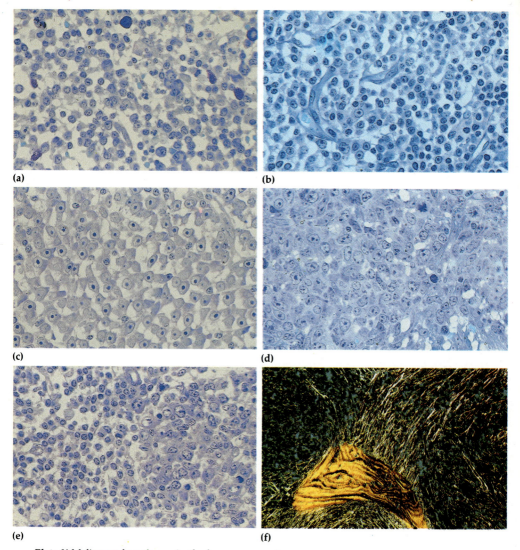

Plate X Malignant lymphoma in the bone marrow.
(a) Polymorphic immunocytoma. × 2000, Giemsa. (b) CLL with nucleolated cells and blasts.
× 2000, Giemsa. (c) ML immunoblastic. × 2000, Giemsa. (d) ML centroblastic. × 2000, Giemsa. (e)
ML centroblastic–centrocytic. × 2000, Giemsa. (f) ML centrocytic in polarized light; fibres radiating
from bone. × 2000, Gomori.

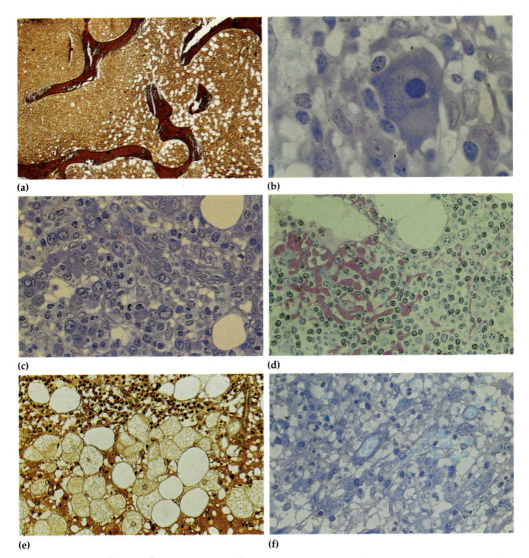

Plate XI Miscellaneous bone marrow reactions.
(a) Partial involvement of the bone marrow by lymphogranulomatous tissue containing Reed–Sternberg and HD cells. × 20, Gomori. (b) Mononuclear HD cell in bone marrow with involvement by HD. × 2000, Gomori. (c) Pleomorphic cell infiltrate in patients with angio-immunoblastic lymphadenopathy (AILD) diagnosed by lymph node biopsy. × 750, Giemsa. (d) AILD in bone marrow showing PAS + interstitial material. × 750, Giemsa. (e) Histiocytes and foam cells in a case of ML immunocytoma in the bone marrow. × 750, Gomori. (f) Histiocytosis. × 800, Giemsa.

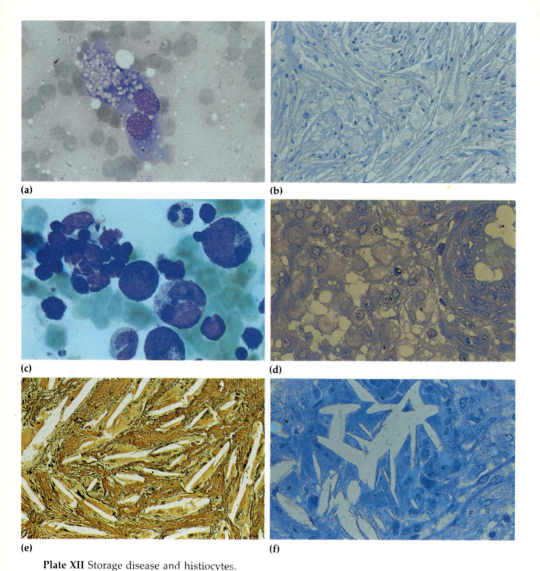

(a)   (b)

(c)   (d)

(e)   (f)

Plate XII Storage disease and histiocytes.
(a) Bone marrow smear from a case of Hand–Schüller–Christian disease. × 2000, Giemsa. (b) Biopsy section from the same child showing the lipid-laden macrophages and fibrosis. × 800, Giemsa. (c) Smear of bone marrow aspirate of child with Farquhar's disease, macrophages with engulfed normoblasts. × 2000, Giemsa. (d) Bone marrow biopsy section showing accumulation of histiocytes in a case of Fabry's disease. × 750, Giemsa. (e) Xanthoma. × 750, Gomori. (f) Cystinosis; in both (e) and (f) the large cholesterol crystals have been dissolved out. × 750, Giemsa.

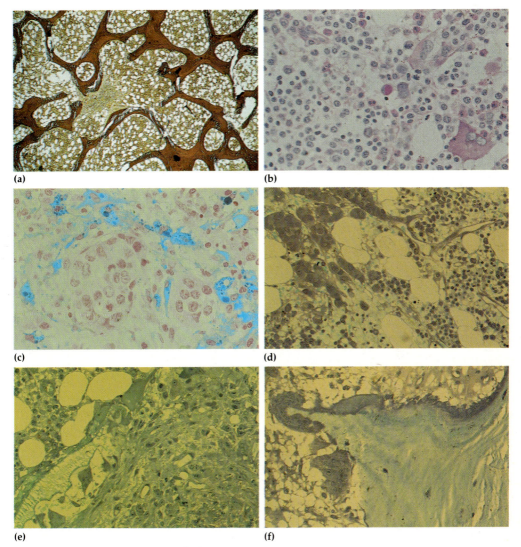

(a)

(b)

(c)

(d)

(e)

(f)

Plate XIII Micrometastases in the bone marrow.
(a) One focus of tumour cells with pronounced reactive fibrosis. × 20, Gomori. (b) Isolated tumour cells in bone marrow identified by PAS reaction. × 750. (c) Small metastases surrounded by iron-containing macrophages. × 750, Berlin blue. (d) Interstitial spread of metastases with marginal angiogenesis. × 750, Giemsa. (e) Osteoclasts resorbing bone in front of advancing metastasis. × 750, Giemsa. (f) Mixed osteoblastic and osteoclastic reaction near metastatic focus. × 750, Giemsa.

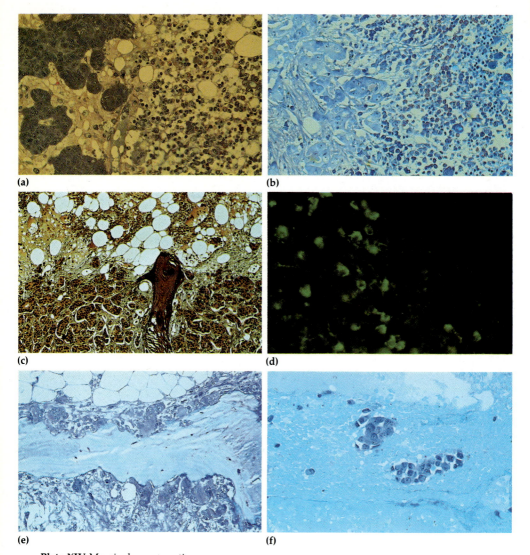

(a)   (b)

(c)   (d)

(e)   (f)

Plate XIV Marginal zone reactions.
(a) Metastases with broad marginal zone containing lymphocytes and plasma cells. × 750, Giemsa. (b) Mixed reaction with strong eosinophilic component to metastases of bronchogenic cancer. × 500, Giemsa. (c) Area of œdema and fibrosis separating metastases of prostatic carcinoma from the residual marrow. × 500, Gomori. (d) Cryostat section, FITC IgG: plasma cells around metastatic focus. × 2000, Giemsa. (e) Osteoclastic resorption near metastases of unknown primary tumour. × 950, Giemsa. (f) Tumour cells in blood clot, together with small negative biopsy. × 2000, Giemsa.

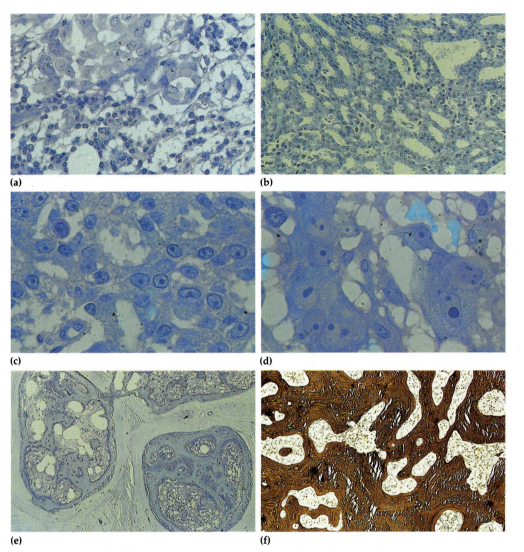

Plate XV Histological variations in metastases of prostatic cancer.
(a) Pale nuclei with fairly abundant cytoplasm and tendency to tubule formation; note lymphocytic reaction. × 750, Giemsa. (b) Smaller, more closely packed cells, cribriform pattern. × 750, Giemsa. (c) Groups of tumour cells from mainly solid type metastasis. × 750, Giemsa. (d) Large cells with prominent nucleoli of anaplastic metastases. × 750, Giemsa. (e) Osteoblastic metastasis; note small groups of tumour cells within loose fibrous tissue, osteoid encroaching on the marrow cavities. × 500, Giemsa. (f) later stage; picture similar to osteomyelosclerosis, few remaining tumour cells within the marrow spaces. × 500, Gomori.

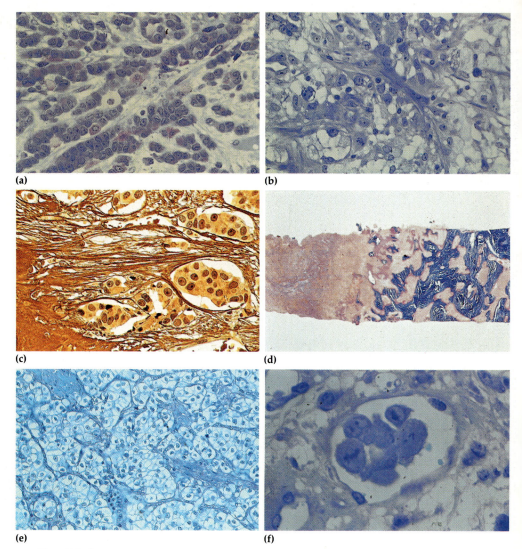

Plate XVI Carcinoma metastases.
(a) Mammary carcinoma tumour cells in 'Indian file' arrangement, with mast cells in close apposition. × 2000, Giemsa. (b) Small groups of cancer cells, capillary proliferation and lipomacrophages. × 750, Giemsa. (c) Scirrhous metastases, clusters of tumour cells encapsulated within fibres attached to the bone. × 200, Gomori. (d) Low power view of carcinomatous osteodysplasia, showing osteolytic lesions. × 20, Ladewig. (e) Metastases of hypernephroma, showing groups of large, clear cells. × 500, Giemsa. (f) Intravascular tumour embolus; note mitotic figure. × 2000, Giemsa.

The preleukaemic erythroid disorders (also called diGuglielmo syndrome) include acute and chronic erythraemic myelosis and erythroleukaemia (in its early stages). The bone marrow is hyper-cellular, with increased erythroid precursors, megakaryoblasts and megakaryocytes, and a decrease in myeloid elements (Fig. 9.3). The erythroblasts vary greatly in size from small to gigantic and multinucleated, they may show numerous mitotic figures, many abnormal, and they have PAS positive cytoplasmic inclusions (Fig. 9.4, Plate VIIa).

9.3   Acute promyelocytic leukaemia

This is considered a variant of acute myeloblastic leukaemia; the marrow is hyper-cellular with broad paratrabecular seams of promyelocytes and myelocytes (Plate VIIf), with variable granulation, and there are relatively few mature granulocytes. Erythroid precursors and megakaryocytes are also reduced.

Another variant is the microgranular form, and here the promyelocytes may have a monocytoid configuration of the nucleus.

9.4   The myelodysplastic syndromes (MDS)

This is a group of disorders presenting with varying degrees of anaemia, leucopenia and thrombocytopenia occurring 'spontaneously', usually in patients over 50 years of age and occasionally evolving into acute leukaemias (Block et al., 1953; Shively, 1980). In the bone marrow, there is increased cellularity, ineffective erythropoiesis (or haematopoiesis) and iron overload. Two types of chronic refractory anaemias were recognized by early workers (see Lewis and Gordon Smith, 1982), namely refractory anaemia with excess of blasts, and refractory anaemia with proliferative dysplasia.

Myelodysplasia may develop at some time after therapy for malignancies in younger people as well (Hoover and Traumeni, 1981; Anderson et al., 1981). The myelodysplastic syndromes have been called the 'grey zone' disorders (Van Slyck et al., 1983), as the literature on the subject is difficult to interpret and contains identity confusion between patients with smouldering leukaemias, preleukaemias and other myelodysplastic states, including chronic myelomonocytic leukaemia and elderly patients with leukaemia. The acquired sideroblastic anaemias have also been included (Bottomley, 1982); and possibly also subacute myeloid leukaemia (Cohen et al., 1979).

Proposals for the classification of these disorders have rested on examination of smears of aspirates (Bennett et al., 1982), and five groups are distinguished. On the other hand Joseph et al. (1982) distinguished

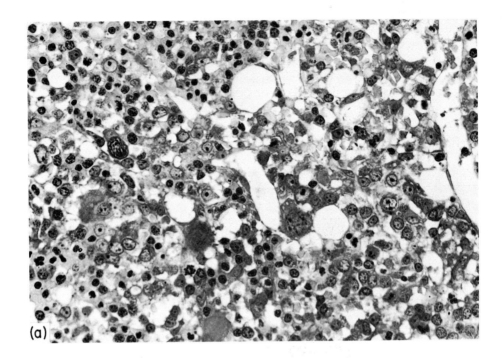

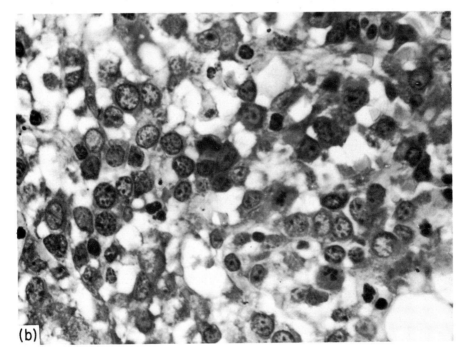

only three major subgroups in the smouldering leukaemias, namely refractory anaemia with excess of blasts (RAEB); chronic myelomonocytic leukaemia (CMML); and chronic erythraemic myelosis (CEM). It should be remembered that material obtained by aspiration differs according to the suction applied and to the ease or the difficulty with which cells are dislodged from the marrow. This in turn depends on the degree of 'packing' of the cells, and on the amount of fibrosis present; an increase in reticular fibres is a feature in many myelodysplastic states and acute myelodysplasia may also occur with myelofibrosis (Sultan *et al.*, 1981). Hence, specific criteria based on biopsy sections as well as on smears of aspirates would decrease the uncertainty and enable more valid comparison of the results obtained. Proposals for the classification of the myelodysplastic states based on bone marrow histology have been suggested (Frisch *et al.*, 1983).

In a comparative study of smears and bone biopsy sections of 40 patients with myelodysplasia, Tricot *et al.* (1984) have shown that the biopsies could *not* be classified according to criteria of the FAB group which was based on smears of aspirates (Bennett *et al.*, 1982); moreover the latter had no prognostic significance, whereas certain parameters derived from the histological sections did. In a recent study of clinical prognostic factors (Coiffier *et al.*, 1983) 193 patients were analysed and the most significant variables (in descending order) were the following: excess of blasts, neutropenia, thrombopenia, circulating blasts, types of erythropoietic insufficiency and decrease of *in vitro* growth. The most significant determinant (the excess of blasts) is far more accurately determined in sections (for the reasons mentioned above) and also because they may be clustered in inaccessible marrow areas within paratrabecular regions, which although not reached by the aspiration needle, would be evident in the biopsy section. The South Western Oncology Study Group (Van Slyck *et al.*, 1983) has defined 'smouldering' acute granulocytic leukaemia as follows: clustering of blasts, presence of micromyeloblasts and a blast differential of between 20% and 40%. Thiele (1983) has described the histopathology of the preleukaemic syndromes and demonstrated that they may precede both acute and chronic myeloid leukaemias.

In smouldering myeloblastic leukaemia, a cell line similar to that in acute leukaemia is present in the bone marrow for months or years: this clone has a certain proliferative advantage and normal haematopoietic tissue is suppressed from the early stages on; the importance in recog-

Fig. 9.3 (a) Chronic erythraemic myelosis; note islands of erythropoiesis with maturation, and few remaining fat cells. × 400, Giemsa; (b) chronic erythraemic myelosis; note fairly monomorphic aspect of the immature cells. × 1000, Giemsa.

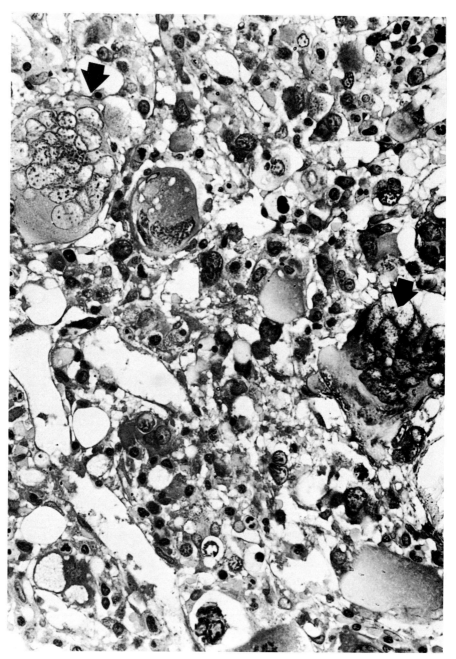

Fig. 9.4 Erythroblastic and megakaryoblastic myelosis, complete effacement of marrow architecture; note giant syncytial masses at arrows, these have haemoglobinized cytoplasm. × 600, Giemsa.

nition of these conditions lies in the fact that attempts may be made to stimulate the leukaemic clone to differentiate, for example, by small doses of cytosine arabinoside.

With these considerations in mind, it might be advisable to redefine the myelodysplastic syndromes on the basis of histological findings. In this case, all patients in whom a diagnosis of overt leukaemia could be made on the peripheral blood smear or on the smears of buffy coat or aspirate, by the presence of Auer rods, or the criteria as given above for 'smouldering' acute granulocytic leukaemia, or patients in whom a diagnosis of myelomonocytic leukaemia or chronic monocytic leukaemia (Bearman *et al.*, 1981) is made, should be excluded from the category of the myelodysplastic states. The presence of Auer rods in myeloid cells in the bone marrow has recently been described in a sub-group of patients with RAEB, who did not differ in any way (including disease course) from those who did not have the Auer rods. Hence, the authors conclude that their presence did not imply overt leukaemia (Seignurin and Audhuy, 1983). As suggested by Pierre *et al.* (1982), these syndromes would then only include (1) the refractory anaemias with or without sideroblasts (Figs 9.5, 9.6) and (2) the refractory anaemias with excess of blasts (Fig. 9.5), with or without monocytosis, but which by definition cannot be classified as leukaemia, and (3) a group which would accommodate patients with refractory cytopenias, who do not fit into either 1 or 2 (Plate VIIIa–d). Under this heading might also come the cases of otherwise unexplained refractory anaemias who later develop one of the chronic myeloproliferative disorders. Severe iron deficiency may cause apparent absence of sideroblasts, even in sideroblastic anaemia. A transient syndrome mimicking myelodysplasia may occur in hypothermia (O'Brien *et al.*, 1982).

In the myelodysplastic syndromes, all three cell lines show morphological abnormalities which reflect their dysplastic maturation (Figs 9.7, 9.8). They represent stem cell disorders and up to 50% of the cases are characterized by chromosomal aberrations (Koffler and Golde, 1980; Second International Workshop on Chromosomes, 1980; Nowell, 1982). In most cases, the bone marrow is hyper-cellular, with increased precursors of all three cell lines with few fat cells and variable disruption of its normal architectural pattern. Alternatively, the marrow may have a patchy appearance, with some preservation of its normal architecture. The infiltration may be diffuse and/or paratrabecular, and more reticulin fibres are often present than in the acute leukaemias. Monocytes, mast cells (Prokocimer and Polliack, 1981; Yoo and Lessin 1982), plasma cells and eosinophils are also frequently prominent. In the first group there is marked accumulation of iron (Plate VIIIc–d) and numerous ringed sideroblasts (which are better seen in smears of aspirates stained for iron),

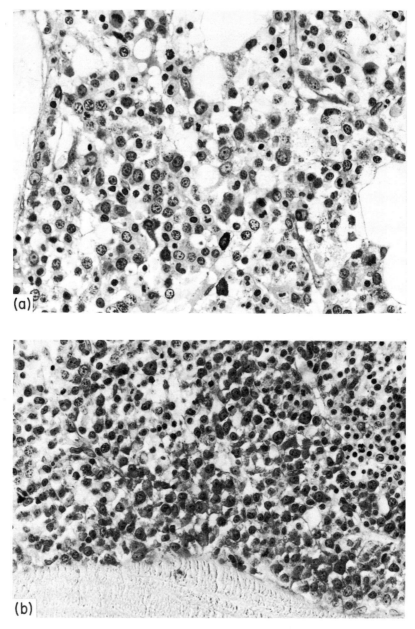

Fig. 9.5 (a) Cellular bone marrow in elderly patient with sideroblastic anaemia; note preponderance of immature cells. × 400, Giemsa; (b) bone marrow biopsy of 65 year old patient with refractory anaemia with excess of blasts (RAEB); note paratrabecular seam of myeloid precursors extending into the marrow cavity. × 400, Giemsa.

a reduction in granulopoiesis, some reticulin fibrosis, interstitial oedema, and lymphoid nodules (in 7% of cases). In the second group marrows are hyper-cellular with markedly dysplastic maturation as well as maturation inhibition, presence of lymphoid nodules (in 40%) and increased megakaryocytes, among them many micro forms (Fig. 9.7; Plate VIIIe–f). In these marrows there are also variable deposits of iron in the stromal cells and sideroblasts, not necessarily ringed. In both groups, focal aggregates of immature precursors are dispersed throughout the marrow. The typical features of dyserythropoiesis (see above) are present to greater or lesser degrees. The myeloid series (especially the neutrophil line) shows hypogranularity or coarse granules, and Pelger–Huet-like nuclear anomalies. Megakaryocytes are increased and vary in size and configuration of their nuclei: characteristic for MDS is the presence of micromegakaryocytes (Wiesneth et al., 1980), as well as mono- and multinucleated forms characterized by 2–5 small round nuclei (Wheeler et al., 1983). The distinction between the smaller megakaryocytes and erythroblasts is not always possible by morphology and may require enzyme or marker studies to appreciate fully the megakaryocyte population in the bone marrow. By definition, the first group has more sideroblasts and the second a greater overall number of immature cells, nevertheless the boundaries between the two groups are not sharp (Juneja et al., 1983). As pointed out recently by Peto et al. (1983), assessment of erythroid expansion in sideroblastic anaemias may be as useful as ferrokinetic studies in predicting risk of iron overload and need for prophylactic therapy.

The 5q-syndrome may also present as refractory or macrocytic anaemia (Tinegate et al., 1983). As described by Mahmood et al. (1979), this syndrome includes macrocytic anaemia, thrombocytosis and non-lobulated megakaryocytes.

Several studies have recently been made to identify prognostic factors in the myelodysplastic syndrome (Thiele et al., 1980; Economopoulos et al., 1981; Kanatakis et al., 1983; Tricot et al., 1984) but there is no agreement on these as yet.

Murray et al. (1983) recently addressed the question of normal pluripotent stem cells being present in the bone marrow of patients with dysmyelopoiesis, which would be able to repopulate the marrow with normal cells after therapy-induced aplasia. They achieved remission after intensive chemotherapy, albeit not of long duration.

Our own experience with bone marrow histology in the myelodysplastic syndromes (Frisch et al., 1983) is briefly outlined below. Conditions included in the differential diagnosis of MDS are given in Table 9.1. All biopsies were initially taken because of unexplained cytopenia(s), when bone marrow disease was suspected but a definite diagnosis could

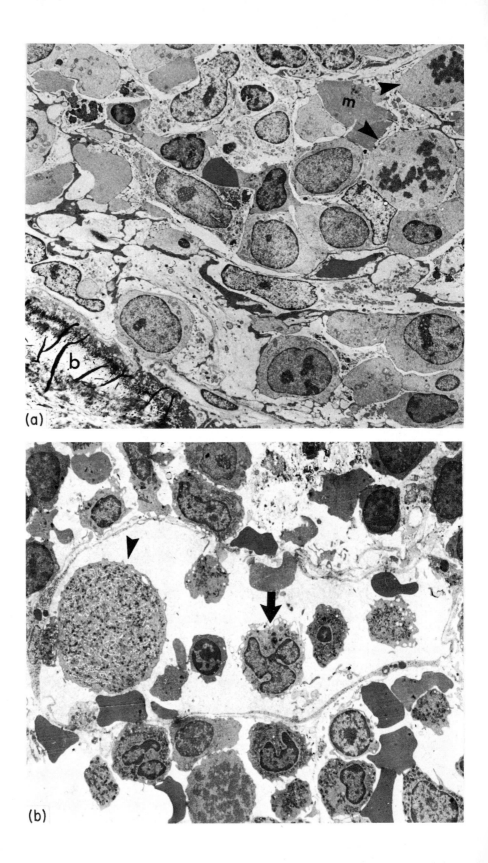

(a)

(b)

Table 9.1 Myelodysplastic syndromes: differential diagnosis of bone marrow histology

Pernicious anaemia	Cytotoxic dysplasias
Malignancies elsewhere	Other acquired hypoplasias
Congenital hypoplasias	Leukaemoid reactions
Rheumatic conditions	Malignant lymphomas
Other chronic disorders	Hodgkin's disease
Haemolytic conditions	Myeloproliferative disorders

not be made from the peripheral blood and other investigations. All biopsies were scored according to their cellularity (Fig. 9.9a) into three groups: hypo-, normo- and hypercellular (Fig. 9.9b, c, d). In all cases there was a more or less pronounced degree of topographic distortion (Fig. 9.10) and a preponderance of early forms of the three cell lines (Fig. 9.11). Moreover invariably there were alterations in the bone marrow stroma as described schematically in Fig. 9.12a and illustrated in Fig. 9.12b,c,d. As already pointed out by Tricot *et al.*, 1984, the bone marrow histology could not be classified according to the criteria of the FAB Group (Bennett *et al.*, 1982). Consequently, the following histological criteria were applied and the biopsies were assigned to one of four categories:

(1) Suspected acute leukosis (hypocellular): decrease in all haematopoietic elements, the residual cells being mainly immature.

(2) Suspected myeloproliferation: increase in megakaryocytes with some atypical forms.

(3) Suspected sideroblastosis: increase in iron in the stromal cells and presence of numerous sideroblasts both ringed and non-ringed.

(4) Marked dysplasia and maturation inhibition: dysplasia and shift to the left.

The correlation between the initial histology and the subsequent course in a large group of patients is given in Table 9.2.

However, there are certain pitfalls in the histological diagnosis of MDS, so that difficulties may be encountered. Four examples of such pitfalls are illustrated as follows:

(1) Site discordance illustrated by a patient who had anaemia, leucopenia and thrombocytopenia and massive sideroblastosis (mostly

---

Fig. 9.6 (a) Electron micrograph in case of sideroblastic anaemia; numerous immature precursors in paratrabecular region; bone (b), mitotic figures (m). × 2000; (b) electron micrograph in case of myelodysplasia; note sinusoid with platelets and piece of megakaryocyte (arrow), monocyte (large arrow), surrounded by mostly immature haematopoietic precursors. × 1800.

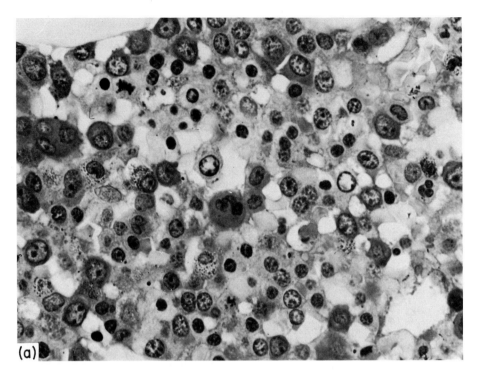

(a)

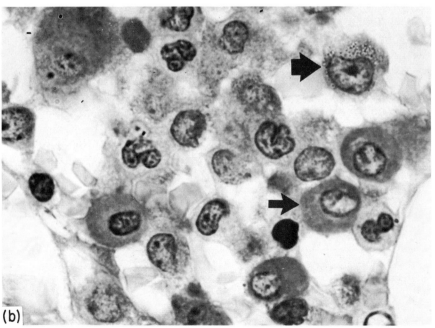

(b)

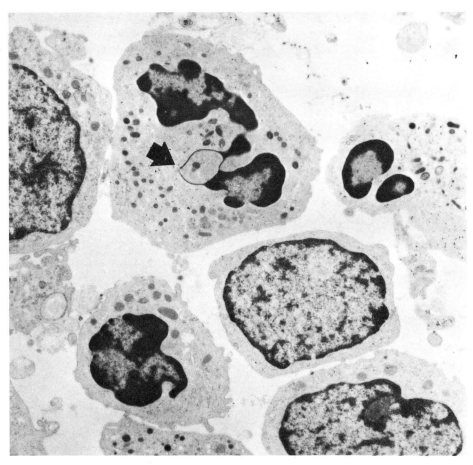

Fig. 9.8 Electron micrograph of bone biopsy of patient with myelodysplastic syndrome; note granulation of myeloid cells, and nuclear loop (arrow). × 6400.

ringed sideroblasts) in smears of the sternal aspirate. Two weeks later acute myelo-monocytic myelosis with almost complete replacement of the bone marrow was found in the histological sections of the iliac crest biopsy.

(2) Temporal variability, as exemplified by a patient who had pancytopenia for several months together with a picture of typical MDS in the bone biopsy sections—a dry tap was obtained on aspirate. This

Fig. 9.7 (a) Myelodysplasia, with dyserythropoiesis, immature and hypogranulated myeloid precursors and micromegakaryocytes. × 600, Giemsa; (b) myelodysplasia; high power to show micromegakaryocytes (small arrow) and promyelocyte (large arrow) for comparison. × 1000, Giemsa.

patient had been on therapy for cardiac problems and a peptic ulcer and was receiving packed red cells. All drugs were discontinued or changed, and a few weeks later his peripheral blood values began to rise and reached near-normal levels and transfusion therapy was stopped.

RANGE OF CELLULARITY IN MDS

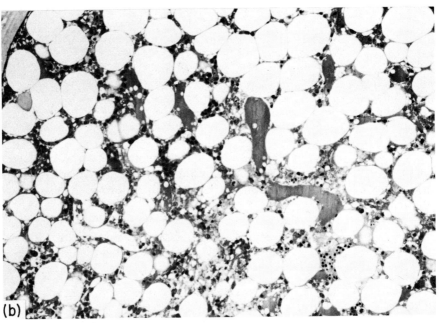

hypocellular	normocellular	hypercellular
< 20 vol %	20 - 50 vol %	> 50 vol %
15 %	25 %	60 %

Fig. 9.9a Diagramatic representation of bone marrow cellularity in MDS.

(b)

Fig. 9.9b Hypocellular type. Giemsa stain, × 100.

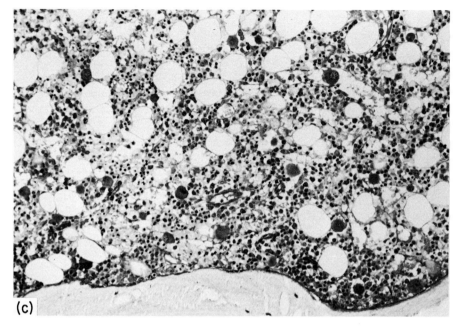

Fig. 9.9c Normocellular type. Giemsa stain, × 100.

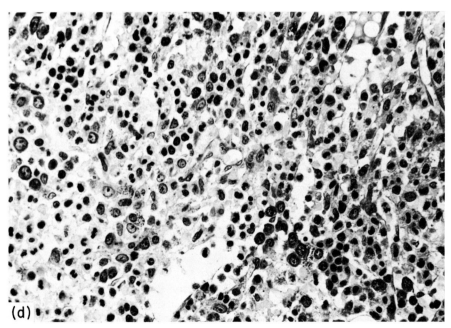

Fig. 9.9d Hypercellular type. Giemsa stain, × 250.

(3) Overlapping of categories as demonstrated by a patient who had pancytopenia with a hypercellular bone marrow and on cytogenetic investigation was found to have some metaphases with a Ph^1 positive chromosome. This patient required maintenance therapy with packed red cells, and four months after the diagnosis of myelodysplasia he died of intercurrent illness, without ever having developed the findings of a typical CML.

Table 9.2 Correlation between initial histology and subsequent course*

Subsequent diagnosis	Suspected acute leukaemia no. 6	Suspected myeloproliferation no. 54	Sideroblastosis no. 62	Dysplastic maturation no. 64
Initial diagnosis unchanged to date	1	33	25	37
Sideroblastic anaemia	—	5	23	1
Myeloproliferation excluded	—	2	8	—
MPD	—	11	—	—
Smouldering leukaemia	5	1	3	11
Acute leukaemia	—	2	3	15

* Sequential biopsies taken within 6–24 month of initial biopsy.
MPD = myeloproliferative disorders.

TOPOGRAPHIC DISTORTION IN MDS

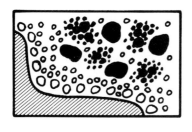
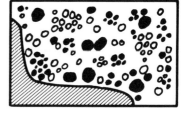

NORMAL   MDS

Fig. 9.10a   Topographic distortion in MDS: Normal (left) shows paratrabecular granulopoiesis, intertrabecular erythroid islands, and parasinusoidal megakaryocytes. MDS (right) shows precursors of the three cell lines dispersed in all marrow regions.

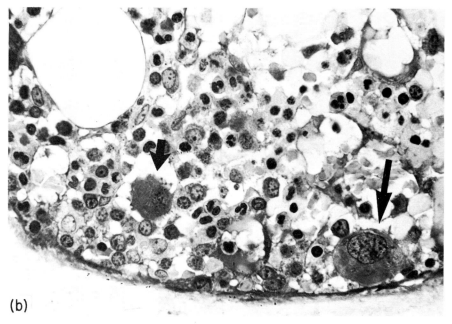

(b)

Fig. 9.10b Bone biopsy section showing paratrabecular megakaryocytes in MDS (arrow). Giemsa stain, × 400.

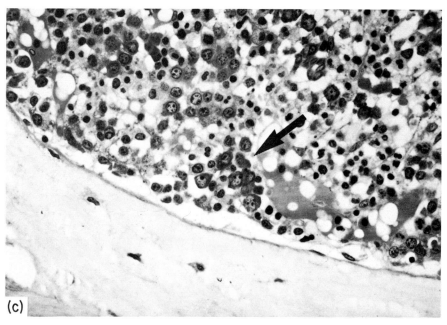

(c)

Fig. 9.10c Bone biopsy section showing paratrabecular erythroid islands in MDS (arrow). Giemsa stain, × 400.

MATURATION INHIBITION IN MDS

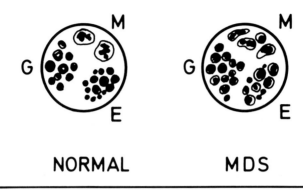

NORMAL   MDS

Fig. 9.11a Diagramatic representation of maturation inhibition in MDS. E = erythropoiesis; G = granulopoiesis; M = megakaryopoiesis.

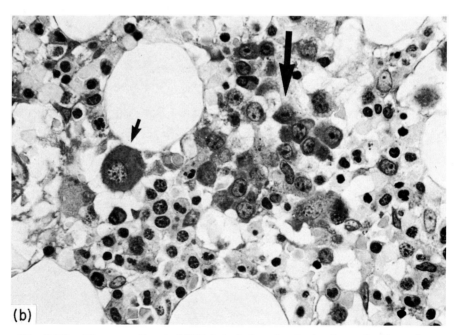

(b)

Fig. 9.11b Biopsy section in MDS: intertrabecular cluster (arrow) of immature precursors and mononuclear megakaryocyte at left (small arrow). Giemsa stain, × 400.

STROMAL REACTIONS IN MDS

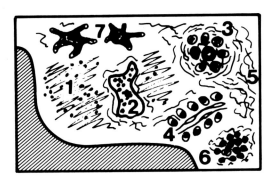

Fig. 9.12a Stromal reactions in MDS. 1. Oedema and extravasated erythrocytes. 2. Ectatic sinusoid with thickened walls. 3. Perivascular infiltration of eosinophils, plasma cells, mast cells. 4. Plasmacytosis around capillaries. 5. Increase in reticulin fibres. 6. Lymphoid cell aggregate. 7. Iron-laden macrophages.

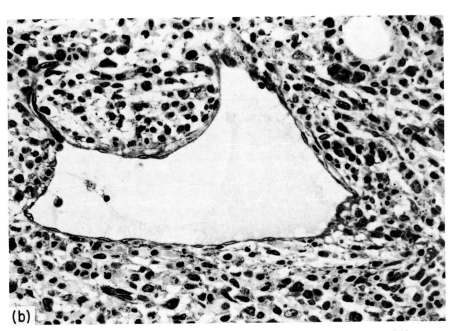

(b)

Fig. 9.12b Example of sclerotic ectatic sinus in MDS. Giemsa stain, × 250.

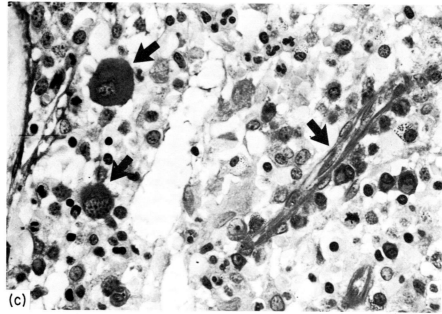

Fig. 9.12c MDS with micro and mononuclear megakaryocytes (arrows, left) and pericapillary plasmacytosis (right), and oedematous marrow stroma. Giemsa stain, × 400.

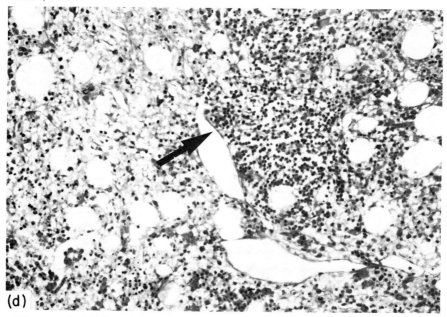

Fig. 9.12d MDS with perivascular lymphoid cell aggregate (arrow). Giemsa stain, × 100.

(4) Is the MDS a basic disorder or is it secondary to another condition? A diagnosis of MDS was made on the basis of peripheral blood findings, smears of sternal aspirate, and bone marrow biopsy sections in a 76 year old patient who presented with anaemia and moderate leucopenia, and thrombocytopenia. Other disorders were excluded. The patient was maintained on three units of packed cells per month. Haematological re-appraisals were carried out at regular intervals. These included peripheral blood films, aspirates and bone biopsies. The diagnosis of MDS (refractory anaemia with excess of blasts) was confirmed at every examination for a period of 18 months when the patient was suddenly hospitalized with acute intractable diarrhoea and abdominal pain. Sigmoidoscopic examination revealed cancer and at laparotomy for palliative surgery, widespread metastatic disease was found. The patient died three days later. The unanswered question remains whether the myelodysplasia in this patient represented a paraneoplastic syndrome and whether this might also be the case in other patients, except that they do not live long enough for the underlying malignancy to be discovered.

It is clear from the foregoing that a diagnosis of MDS is largely made by exclusion, and that MDS may be evoked by both intrinsic and extrinsic causes, as indicated in Fig. 9.13. Moreover it should be borne in mind that intrinsic MDS is a phase in a multi-stage disorder which may or may not

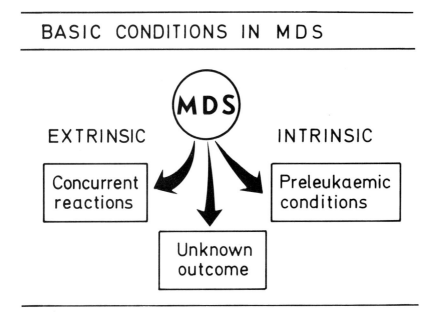

Fig. 9.13   Schematic outline of basic conditions in MDS.

evolve during the life time of the patient (Fig. 9.14). In summary, the following conclusions could be drawn:

(1) Though there is no consistent agreement between aspirate cytology and bone marrow histology, these are complementary and both are required.

(2) Bone marrow histology appears to have some prognostic significance.

(3) The diagnosis of MDS is initially tentative and serial examinations and follow-up are mandatory for periodic re-appraisal.

(4) The diagnosis of MDS can be made only within the framework of a defined clinical setting.

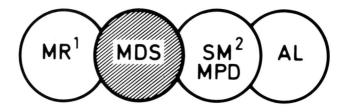

MDS AND ALLIED DISORDERS

1: MR = Myelo –   2: SM = Smouldering
        reactions   leukaemias

Fig. 9.14   Schematic indication of the position of MDS within the myeloproliferative disorders.

The secondary myelodysplastic syndromes

These have been increasingly reported in recent years in patients treated with chemotherapy and/or radiation therapy for Hodgkin's disease and for solid tumours, (Anderson *et al.*, 1981). There appears to be a cumulative risk with the passage of time, that is, more patients are developing myelodysplastic syndromes as several years have passed after completion of their cytotoxic treatment. Various factors are involved. These include:

(1) the type of chemotherapy,
(2) the type of radiation (the incidence after total body irradiation appears to be higher),
(3) intensity and duration of therapy,

(4) the combination and sequence of therapy,

(5) age at time of therapy.

The more widespread use of adjuvant chemotherapy also appears to have increased the incidence of secondary MDS (Bloomfield, 1985). The bone marrow in these syndromes reflects the stage in their development when the biopsy was taken. During the hypoplastic phase there is increased fat, patches of serous atrophy, haematopoiesis is reduced and immature cells predominate; there is oedema, extravasation of erythrocytes, and interstitial infiltration with lymphoid cells, mast and plasma cells and iron-laden macrophages (Fig. 9.15). If and when acute leukaemia develops, this will of course be evident in the biopsy sections (see above).

9.5   PNH (paroxysmal nocturnal haemoglobinuria)

This is now considered to be a clonal stem cell disorder, a primary disease of the bone marrow which affects not only erythroid cells, but also platelets, leucocytes (and even the pluripotent stem cells). PNH can arise from or evolve into other bone marrow diseases, including aplastic anaemia, sideroblastic anaemia, myelofibrosis and acute leukaemia. PNH

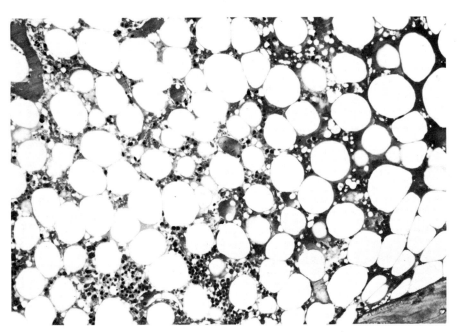

Fig. 9.15   Bone biopsy section of patient with pancytopenia after treatment for lung cancer; note hypoplasia and serous atrophy. Giemsa stain, × 100.

may present with thrombocytopenia, leucopenia or both. The bone marrow may be hyper-plastic, or hypo-plastic and even aplastic, resembling aplastic anaemia.

9.6   Smouldering (or sub-acute) myelomonocytic leukaemia

The bone marrow is hypo- to normocellular or hyper-cellular; the overall architecture is preserved, and there is an interstitial infiltration with monocytic cells which may constitute 20–40% of the nucleated cell population (Fig. 9.16; Plate VIIb). Haematopoietic precursors may be increased or decreased, and there is a slight to moderate increase in reticulin. The mononuclear cells have round to oval, elongated or kidney-shaped nuclei, somewhat like those of the abnormal cells in hairy cell leukaemia. Smouldering myelomonocytic leukaemia is presumed to be a disorderly proliferation of all the marrow cells (Saarni and Linman, 1971).

9.7   Chronic monocytic leukaemia

This has recently been characterized as a separate entity, distinct from myelomonocytic leukaemia, as it affects primarily the monocytic series. There is a pleomorphic cell population of monocytic cells with fairly abundant cytoplasm, larger than hairy cells and with a more prominent nuclear membrane (Bearman et al., 1981).

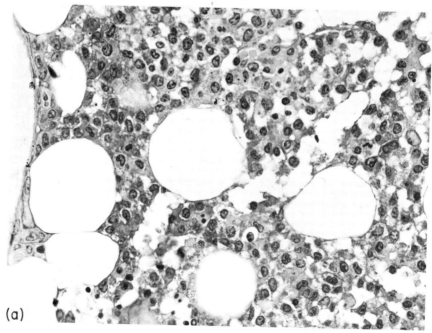

(a)

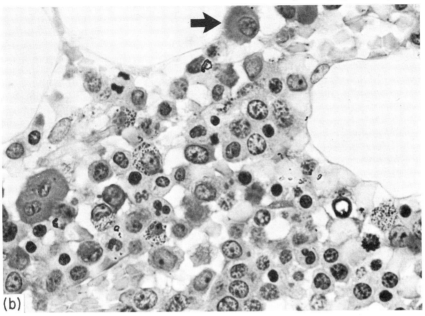

(b)

Fig. 9.16 (a) Myelomonocytic leukaemia; overall bone marrow architecture is preserved but there is an infiltration with monocytoid cells replacing the normal haematopoietic elements, which are dispersed within the infiltration. × 400, Giemsa; (b) myelodysplastic syndrome for comparison, hypercellular marrow, mostly immature precursors, and megakaryocytes (arrow). × 600, Giemsa.

9.8   Acute (malignant) myelofibrosis (AMF)

The clinical criteria of the condition which was originally referred to by Lewis and Szur (1963) as 'malignant myelofibrosis' are peripheral pancytopenia, minimal or no splenomegaly, and a rapid downhill course, with an average duration of disease up to 18 months. The bone marrow histology shows absence of the normal pattern, drastic reduction in haematopoietic precursors, reduction in or absence of fat cells and occupation of the marrow cavities by fibrous tissue (Plate IIId) interspersed with few haematopoietic elements, dysplastic megakaryocytes, and other unidentifiable haematopoietic or reticular cells (Fig. 9.17). This picture may also be seen in some phases of MF, but MF is not characterized by a rapidly progressive fibrosis. However since the initial report by Lewis and Szur, many cases have been reported, not all of whom fit the original criteria (Bergsman and Van Slyck, 1971; Briere *et al.*, 1976; Omar and Jones, 1979; Rupani, 1982). These cases are better referred to as 'acute myelofibrosis' (AMF) and they should be distinguished from the rare syndrome of malignant myelofibrosis. Recent cytogenetic studies sup-

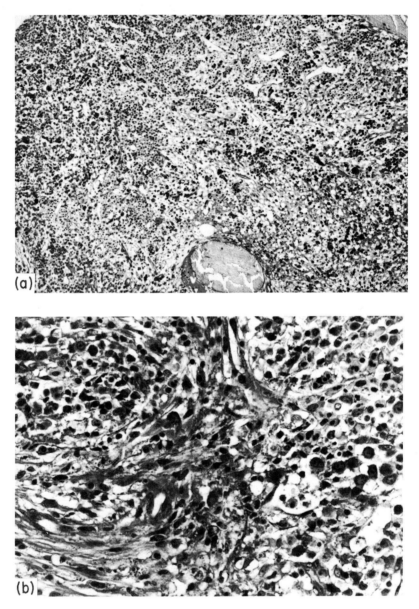

Fig. 9.17 Sections of biopsy in case of acute myelofibrosis: (a) low power view of dense marrow, cellular, with fibrosis. × 100, Giemsa; (b) higher magnification showing fibrosis, capillaries and immature cells. × 400, Giemsa.

port the concept that AMF is a primary malignancy of haematopoietic cells associated with secondary, non-neoplastic fibrosis (Shah *et al.*, 1982; Clare *et al.*, 1982; Mahl *et al.*, 1983). Moreover, if the malignancy is brought under control by intensive chemotherapy, resolution of the fibrosis may be attained (Strebel *et al.*, 1983). A somewhat similar bone marrow histology has also been described as occurring spontaneously, or secondary to cytotoxic therapy, and this appears to be a stem cell disorder. This condition appears to be unresponsive to chemotherapy and rapidly fatal. The bone marrow picture consisted of increased cellularity with dysplastic red and white cell precursors, polymorphic and micromegakaryocytes, unidentifiable blasts and variable infiltration of lymphocytes, plasma and mast cells within a reticulin fibre network. This has been termed acute myelodysplasia with myelofibrosis. A major difference between these cases and AMF is probably the amount of fibrosis; whether they represent a variant of AMF remains to be established. Recognition of 'idiopathic' AMF is important, especially in young people, since chemotherapy is ineffective, but marrow transplantation may offer a cure (Rozman *et al.*, 1982). Acute myelofibrosis may supervene in the course of other haematopoietic disorders (Butler *et al.*, 1982) or itself terminate in acute leukaemia (Tada *et al.*, 1981; Puckett and Cooper, 1981).

9.9   Acute megakaryoblastic leukaemia or myelosis

This entity represents an acute leukaemia of the megakaryocytic cell line analogous to acute myeloblastic or erythroblastic leukaemia, and it may occur together with either or both of these. The bone marrow histology shows a predominant proliferation of megakaryoblasts (Fig. 9.18) which vary in size, are mostly mononuclear and immature and do not produce platelets. Morphologically they resemble the very early erythroblasts of pernicious anaemia. There is little difficulty in recognition of this leukaemia on bone marrow histology, though megakaryoblastic myelosis may present clinically as AMF (Bain *et al.*, 1983); the distinction is made by means of bone marrow histology. Acute megakaryoblastic leukaemia has also been described in infants (Chan *et al.*, 1983). Discrete sclerotic foci, in addition to generalized osteosclerosis, have been reported in acute megakaryoblastic leukaemia (Karasick *et al.*, 1982).

9.10   Acute monoblastic leukaemia

There is complete effacement of the marrow architecture, with replacement of the haematopoietic tissue by a population of polymorphic monoblasts with pleomorphic nuclei (Fig. 9.19). The infiltration is loose

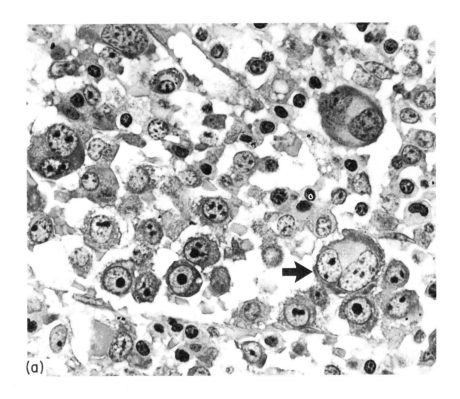

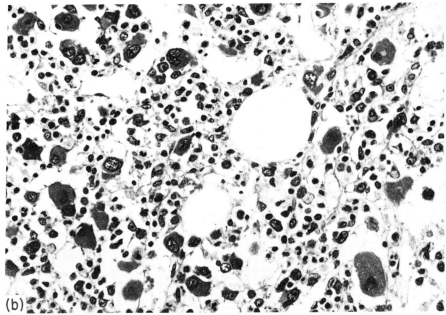

and isolated haematopoietic precursors are dispersed among the monoblasts (Plate VIIe).

9.10.1 Bone marrow appearances after chemotherapy

Post-therapeutic depletion of all haematopoietic elements is seen after aggressive chemotherapy, so that practically only the stroma is left: a reticulin framework, dilated sinusoids, deposition of fibrin in the interstitium, extravasation of red cells, and clusters of plasma cells and sometimes lymphocytes may be prominent in the depleted marrow (see also Wittels, 1980). Histological studies of marrow regeneration have indicated that regenerating haematopoietic tissue requires the presence of fat cells (Islam *et al.* 1980).

References

Alexander, P. (1982), Need for new approaches to the treatment of patients in clinical remission, with special reference to acute myeloid leukaemia. *Brit. J. Cancer*, **46**, 151–9.

Alimena, G., Dallapiccola, B., Gastaldi, R., Mandelli, G., Brandt, L., Mitelman, F. and Nilsson, P. G. (1982), Chromosomal, morphological and clinical correlations in blastic crisis of chronic myeloid leukaemia. A study of 69 cases. *Scand. J. Haematol.*, **28**, 103–17.

Amjad, H., Gezer, S., Inoue, S., Bollinger, R. O., Kaplan, J., Carson, S. and Bishop, C. R. (1980), Acute myelofibrosis terminating in an acute lymphoblastic leukemia. *Cancer*, **46**, 615–18.

Anderson, R. L., Bagby, G. C., Richert-Boe, K., Magenis, R. E. and Koler, R. D. (1981), Therapy related preleukemic syndrome. *Cancer*, **47**, 1867–71.

Bain, B., Manoharan, A., Lampert, I., McKenzie, C. and Catovsky, D. (1983), Lymphoma-like presentation of acute monocytic leukaemia. *J. clin. Pathol.*, **36**, 559–65.

Bartl, R., Frisch, B. and Burkhardt, R. (1982), *Bone Marrow Biopsies Revisited. A New Dimension for Haematologic Malignancies*, Karger, Basel.

Bearman, R. M., Kjeldsberg, C. R., Pangalis, G. A. and Rappaport, H. (1981), Chronic monocytic leukemia in adults. *Cancer*, **48**, 2239–55.

Bennett, J. M., Catovsky, D., Daniel, M. T., Flandrin, G., Galton, D. A. G., Gralnick, H. R. and Sultan, C. (1982), The French–American–British (FAB) Co-Operative Group. Proposals for the classification of the myelodysplastic syndromes. *Br. J. Haematol.*, **51**, 189–99.

Fig. 9.18   (a) Megakaryoblastic myelosis: the megakaryoblasts have round nuclei with single or multiple nucleoli and moderate amounts of cytoplasm; note also numerous binucleate megakaryocytes (arrow) and residual haematopoiesis. × 1000, Giemsa; (b) idiopathic thrombocythaemia for comparison: marrow cellularity increased but not dense; range in size of megakaryocytes, but most are mature. × 400, Gomori.

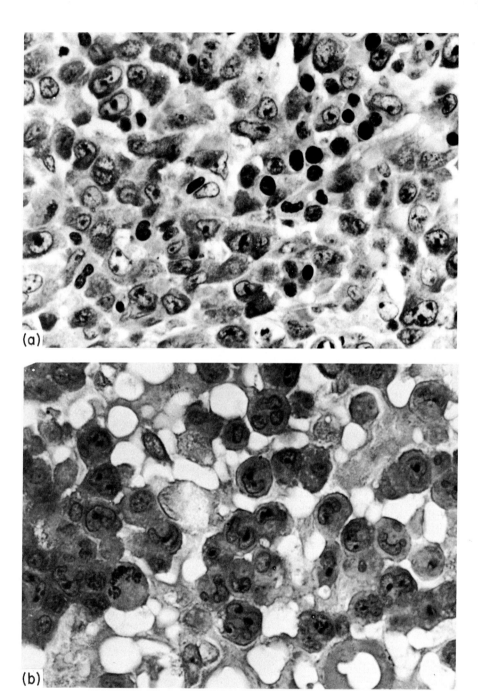

Fig. 9.19 (a) Monoblastic leukaemia, hyper-cellular marrow, erythroblasts in centre. × 1000, Giemsa; (b) monoblastic leukaemia (different case from above); note pleomorphic nuclei with single or several prominent nucleoli. × 1000, Giemsa.

Bergsman, K. L. and Van Slyck, E. J. (1971), Acute myelofibrosis: an accelerated variant of agnogenic metaplasia. *Ann. int. Med.*, **74**, 232–5.

Bevan, D., Rose, M. and Greaves, M. (1982), Leukaemia of platelet precursors: diverse features in four cases. *Brit. J. Haematol.*, **51**, 147–64.

Block, M., Jacobson, L. O. and Bethard, W. F. (1953), Preleukemic acute human leukemia. *J. Am. med. Ass.*, **152**, 1018–28.

Bottomley, S. S. (1982), Sideroblastic anaemia. *Clin. Haematol.*, **11**, 389–409.

Briere, J., Castro-Malaspina, H., Briere, J. F. and Bernard, J. (1976), Les Myelofibroses Aigues ou Subaigues. *Nouv. Rev. Fr. Hemat.*, **16**, 3–22.

Butler, W. M., Taylor, H. G. and Viswanathan, U. (1982), Idiopathic acquired sideroblastic anemia terminating in acute myelosclerosis. *Cancer*, **49**, 2497–99.

Chan, W. C., Byrnes, R. K., Kim, T. H., Varras, A., Schick, C., Green, R. J. and Ragab, A. H. (1983), Acute megakaryoblastic leukemia in early childhood. *Blood*, **62**, 92–8.

Clare, N., Elson, D. and Manhoff, L. (1982), Case reports: Cytogenetic studies of peripheral myeloblasts and bone marrow fibroblasts in acute myelofibrosis. *Am. J. clin. Path.*, **77**, 762–6.

Cohen, J. R., Creger, W. P. and Greenberg, P. L. (1979), Subacute myeloid leukemia. A clinical review. *Am. J. Med.*, **66**, 959–66.

Coiffier, B., Adeleine, P., Viala, J. J., Byron, P. A., Fiere, D., Gentilhomme, O. and Vuvam, H. (1983), Dysmyelopoietic syndromes. A search for prognostic factors in 193 patients. *Cancer*, **52**, 83–90.

Delacrétaz, Fr., Schmidt, P. M., Schmied, P. A. and Saudan, Y. (1983), Acute myelomonocytic leukaemia with collagenous medullary fibrosis and osteosclerotic lesions. *Ann. Pathol.*, **3**, 241–5.

Economopoulos, T., Stathakis, N., Maragoyannis, Z., Gardikas, E. and Dervenoulas, J. (1981), Myelodysplastic syndrome. Clinical and prognostic significance of monocyte count, degree of blastic infiltration, and ring sideroblasts. *Acta Haemat.*, **65**, 97–102.

Frisch, B., Schlag, R., Bartl, R., Kettner, G. and Burkhardt, R. (1983), Histologic characteristics of myelodysplasia. *Verh. Dtsch. Ges. Path.*, **67**, 132–5.

Gewirtz, A. M., Stewart, A. F. Vignery, A. and Hoffman, R. (1983), Hypercalcaemia complicating acute myelogenous leukaemia: a syndrome of multiple aetiologies. *Br. J. Haematol.*, **54**, 133–41.

Hoover, R. and Fraumeni, J. F. (1981), Review of medicinal agents linked to human cancer. *Cancer*, **47**, 1071–80.

Islam, A., Catovsky, D. and Galton, D. A. G. (1980), Histological study of bone marrow regeneration following chemotherapy for acute myeloid leukaemia and chronic granulocytic leukaemia in blast transformation. *Brit. J. Haematol.*, **45**, 535–40.

Joseph, A. S., Cinkotal, K. I., Hunt, L. and Geary, C. G. (1982), Natural history of smouldering leukaemia. *Brit. J. Cancer*, **46**, 160–6.

Juneja, S. K., Imbert, M., Sigaux, F., Houault, H. and Sultan, C. (1983), Prevalence and distribution of ringed sideroblasts in primary myelodysplastic syndromes. *J. clin. Pathol.*, **36**, 566–9.

Kanatakis, S., Chalevelakis, G., Economopoulos, Th., Panani, A., Ferti, A., Vamvasakis, E. and Arapakis, G. (1983), Correlation of haematological electron microscopic and cytogenetic findings in 20 patients with preleukaemia. *Scand. J. Haematol.*, **30**, 89–94.

Karasick, S., Karasick, D. and Schilling, J. (1982), Acute megakaryoblastic leukemia (acute 'malignant' myelofibrosis): an unusual cause of osteosclerosis. *Skeletal Radiol.*, **9**, 45–6.

Koffler, H. P. and Golde, D. W. (1980), Human preleukemia. *Ann. int. Med.*, **93**, 347–53.

Lewis, S. M. and Gordon Smith, E. C. (1982), Aplastic and dysplastic anaemias. In: *Blood and its Disorders*, 2nd edn. (eds R. M. Hardisty and D. J. Weatherall), Blackwell, Oxford, p. 1260.

Lewis, S. M. and Szur, L. (1963), Malignant myelosclerosis. *Brit. med. J.*, **ii**, 472–7.

Mahl, G., Frisch, B., Bartl, R., Burkhardt, R., Jäger, K. and Pappenberger, R. (1983), Acute myelofibrosis: only one extreme of the spectrum of idiopathic myelofibrosis? *Verh. Dtsch. Ges. Path.*, **67**, 272–5.

Mahmood, T., Robinson, W. A., Hamstra, R. D. and Wallner, S. F. (1979), Macrocytic anaemia, thrombocytosis and non-lobulated megakaryocytes the 5q-syndrome, a distinct entity. *Am. J. Med.*, **66**, 946–50.

Murray, C., Cooper, B. and Kitchens, L. W. (1983), Remission of acute myelogenous leukemia in elderly patients with prior refractory dysmyelopoietic anemia. *Cancer*, **52**, 967–70.

Needleman, S. W., Burns, C. P., Dick, F. R. and Armitage, J. O. (1981), Hypoplastic acute leukemia. *Cancer*, **48**, 1410–14.

Nowell, P. C. (1982), Cytogenetics of preleukemia. *Cancer Gen. Cytogen.*, **3**, 265–78.

O'Brien, H., Amess, J. A. L. and Mollin, D. L. (1982), Recurrent thrombocytopenia, erythroid hypoplasia and sideroblastic anaemia associated with hypothermia. *Brit. J. Haematol.*, **51**, 451–6.

Omar, N. and Jones, W. O. (1979), Malignant myelosclerosis (acute myelofibrosis). *Cancer*, **43**, 1211–15.

Peto, T. E. A., Pippard, M. J. and Weatherall, D. J. (1983), Iron overload in mild sideroblastic anaemias. *Lancet*, **1**, 375–8.

Pierre, R., Sultan, C. and Vardiman, J. (1982), *The Myelodysplastic Syndromes*, Hematology Educational Program, American Society of Hematology, pp. 1–5.

Prokocimer, M. and Polliack, A. (1981), Increased bone marrow mast cells in preleukemia and lymphoproliferative disorders. *Am. J. clin. Pathol.*, **75**, 34–8.

Puckett, J. B. and Cooper, M. R. (1981), Acute myelofibrosis evolving into acute myeloblastic leukemia. *Ann. int. Med.*, **94**, 545–6.

Roggli, V. L. and Saleem, A. (1982), Erythroleukemia: a study of 15 cases and literature review. *Cancer*, **49**, 101–8.

Rozman, C., Granena, A., Hernandez-Nieto, M., Vela, E., and Brugues, R. (1982), Bone-marrow transplantation for acute myelofibrosis. *Lancet*, **1**, 618.

Rupani, M. (1982), Acute myelofibrosis. *Am. J. Med.*, **77**, 475–8.

Saarni, M. I. and Linman, J. W. (1971), Myelomonocytic leukemia: disorderly proliferation of all marrow cells. *Cancer*, **27**, 1221–30.

Second International Workshop on Chromosomes in Leukemia: chromosomes in preleukemia. (1980), *Cancer Gen. Cytogen.*, **2**, 108–13.

Seignurin, D. and Audhuy, B. (1983), Auer rods in refractory anemia with excess of blasts: presence and significance. *Am. J. clin. Pathol.*, **80**, 359–62.

Shah, I., Mayeda, K., Koppitch, F., Mahmood, S. and Nemitz, B. (1982), Karyotypic polymorphism in acute myelofibrosis. *Blood*, **60**, 841–50.

Shively, J. A. (1980), Recognition of preleukemia. *Ann. clin. Lab. Sci.*, **10**, 95–9.

Sills, R. H. and Stockman, J. A. (1981), Preleukemic states in children with acute lymphoblastic leukemia. *Cancer*, **48**, 110–12.

Slyck, E. J. Van., Rebuck, J. W., Waddell, C. C. and Janakiraman, N. (1983),

Smouldering acute granulocytic leukemia. Observations on its natural history and morphologic characteristics. *Arch. int. Med.*, **143**, 37–40.

Stavem, P., Rorvik, T. O., Rootwelt, K. and Josefsen, J. O. (1983), Severe iron deficiency causing loss of ring sideroblasts. *Scand. J. Haematol.*, **31**, 389–91.

Strebel, U., Schaffner, A. and Fehr, J. (1983), Die akute Osteomyelofibrose. *Schweiz. Med. Wschr.*, **23**, 844–50.

Sultan, C., Sigaux, F., Imbert, M. and Reyes, F. (1981), Acute myelodysplasia with myelofibrosis: A report of 8 cases. *Brit. J. Haematol.*, **49**, 11–16.

Tada, T., Nitta, M. and Kishimoto, H. (1982), Acute myelofibrosis terminating in erythroleukemia state. *Am. J. clin. Pathol.*, **78**, 102–4.

Thiele, J. (1983), Pathology of preleukaemia. *Verh. Dtsch. Ges. Path.*, **67**, 115–31.

Thiele, J., Vykoupil, K. F. and Georgii, A. (1980), Myeloid dysplasia (MD): a haematological disorder preceding acute and chronic leukaemia. *Virchows Archiv. A. Pathol. Anat. and Hist.*, **389**, 343–68.

Tinegate, H., Gaunt, L. and Hamilton, P. J. (1983), The 5q-syndrome: an under-diagnosed form of macrocytic anaemia. *Brit. J. Haematol.*, **54**, 103–10.

Tricot, G., Wolf-Peeters, C. de., Vlietinck, R. and Verwilghen, R. L. (1984), The importance of bone marrow biopsies in myelodysplastic disorders. *Biblthca haemat.*, **50**, 31–40.

Wheeler, L. A., Hogan, R. P. III., Schwenck, G. R. Jr and Griep, J. A. (1983), Multinucleate megakaryocytes in refractory anemia with excess blasts. *Arch. Pathol. Lab. Med.*, **107**, 277–8.

Wiesneth, M., Pfliefer, H., Kubanek, B. and Heimpel, H. (1980), Micromega-karyocytes in human bone marrow. *Acta Haemat.*, **64**, 65–71.

Wittels, B. (1980), Bone marrow biopsy changes following chemotherapy for acute leukemia. *Am. J. Surg. Pathol.*, **4**, 135–42.

Yoo, D. and Lessin, L. S. (1982), Bone marrow mast cell content in preleukemic syndrome. *Am. J. Med.*, **73**, 539–42.

10 Lymphoproliferative disorders

Bone marrow biopsies are taken to determine the presence or absence of involvement of the marrow in the investigation of patients with known or suspected lymphoproliferative disorders (LPD). Though a considerable range of positive biopsies has been reported in the literature in the past (16–75%), the more recent studies have confirmed the higher incidence and thus have demonstrated the value of bone marrow biopsies in the staging of the malignant lymphomas (see Bartl *et al.*, 1982a, 1984). BMB are now taken routinely to estimate the progression of disease (staging) at initial diagnosis (Table 10.1). Minimal, or even occult bone marrow involvement (Benjamin *et al.*, 1983) has also been described, but the authors did not state the histological method used. In our experience lymphoid cells, even in small amounts, are easily identified in undecalcified plastic embedded sections of biopsies. However with increasing use

Table 10.1 Bone marrow biopsies in lymphoproliferative disease

1. Bone marrow involvement————	initial diagnosis and/or clinical staging
2. Proliferative cell system————	classification
3. Growth pattern————————	sub-grouping
4. Tumour cell burden—————	histological staging in cumulative LPD
5. State of haematopoiesis ———	peripheral blood picture
6. Bone structure———————	hypercalcaemia, alkaline phosphatase increased
7. Sequential biopsy —————	effect of therapy on lymphoproliferation (remission, partial remission, relapse) course of disease effect on haematopoiesis, bone and stroma concurrent diseases amyloidosis consequences of therapy (AML, ALL)
8. Transformation in predominant— cell and proliferative pattern	acceleration of clinical course

180

of BMB as a diagnostic tool, it has become clear that lymphoid cells and nodules may frequently be encountered in the bone marrow as reactions to a variety of non-haematological and haematological conditions as well as forming an integral part of the malignant lymphomas (Table 10.2). Consequently, recognition as benign or malignant is of considerable clinical importance, especially as both the number of lymphocytes and plasma cells, and the occurrence of benign lymphoid nodules increase in the older age groups, while the overall cellularity (haematopoiesis) in the iliac crest, from which bone biopsies are generally taken, tends to decrease. At the same time, the incidence of malignant lymphomas rises. In addition, certain prelymphomatous conditions are now recognized (Lennert *et al.*, 1979). These include persistent and long-term antigenic stimulation which may lead to emergence of a monoclonal growth out of a polyclonal proliferation. For example, immunoproliferative small intestinal disease appears to be an apparently benign and potentially curable disorder initially, but with a malignant terminal stage. Early diagnosis and treatment could possibly avoid this fatal lymphomatous phase. In addition, a deficiency in the number or the function of suppressor T cells may well favour the development of a B cell lymphoma (Lennert *et al.*, 1979).

According to some authors, lymphoid cells may normally comprise up to 20% of the population of nucleated cells in the bone marrow, which itself is an organ of lymphopoiesis and of passage in the migration and the circulation of lymphoid cells (de Sousa, 1981; Pabst *et al.*, 1983). An

Table 10.2 Lymphoproliferations in the bone marrow

Benign
Reactive plasmacytosis
Benign monoclonal gammopathy
Reactive lymphocytosis
Benign lymphoid nodules
Reactive granulomas (with lymphocytic component)

Malignant
Multiple myeloma (MM)
Non-Hodgkin's lymphomas (ML)
Hodgkin's disease (HD)

Equivocal
Certain monoclonal plasmacytoses in stable gammopathies
Lymphocytosis in some rheumatic diseases (e.g. Sjögren's syndrome)
Plasma- and lymphocytosis in heavy chain diseases
Angioimmunoblastic lymphadenopathy (AILD)
Nodular lymphoid hyperplasias
Plasmacytoses with nucleolated plasma cells

---

increase in lymphocytes may be absolute or relative due to a decrease in haematopoiesis (as for example in hypoplastic conditions). The so-called benign lymphoid nodules or benign lymphoid hyperplasia (Hashimoto *et al.*, 1957; Rywlin *et al.*, 1974) may be found in any bone marrow though their occurrence is more frequent in the older age groups, in females, and in certain haematological diseases and other conditions, details of which are given in the appropriate sections.

Four types of benign lymphoid nodules (see Fig. 2.14) have been described (Hashimoto *et al.*, 1957; Rywlin *et al.*, 1974): (1) nodules with germinal centres, 5%; (2) sharply demarcated aggregates, 30%; (3) well defined nodules, 45% and (4) small accumulations of lymphoid cells, 22%. The average size is 0.4 mm (range 0.1–2 mm). They are composed of small lymphocytes, a few plasma cells, histiocytes and capillaries and possibly eosinophils and mast cells within a reticulin fibre network (Fig. 2.14). In 25% of the cases the nodules are multiple, and their localization may be inter- or paratrabecular, or parasinusoidal. Particular care is therefore required before involvement of the bone marrow by malignant lymphoma is diagnosed in an elderly patient. In some cases demonstration of monoclonality may be necessary before a diagnosis is made. And even monoclonality itself may not necessarily prove malignancy. It has recently been demonstrated that reactive lymphoid hyperplasia may show a monoclonal surface immunoglobulin pattern (Levy *et al.*, 1983). The underlying causes for the lymphoid hyperplasia were infectious, autoimmune and immuno-deficiency states. The authors point out that the monoclonality may arise from a clonal but non-neoplastic response to an antigenic stimulus, or that it may be a prelymphomatous state. Long term follow up of the patients is required to document the possible evolution of a neoplastic disease process.

10.1   Classification of the LPD

The assumption is made that the malignant lymphoid cells retain the characteristics of differentiation and maturation (the phenotype) of normal cells, at the level at which the presumed block or maturation arrest and expansion of the clone occurs (Magrath 1981). But this may not always be the case, as some features may be lost because of genetic instability, and others may be altered during the progressive evolution of the malignant cell clones. The Kiel group, as well as Lukes and Collins, utilize morphological and immunological criteria and the similarities between the two sytems of classification of the malignant lymphomas have now been emphasized (Lennert *et al.*, 1983). These authors point out that both systems are flexible enough to be able to accommodate new information, especially on functional capabilities and phenotypic characteristics. A comprehensive evaluation of 564 cases of lymphoproliferative disorders classified according to the International Working Formulation and using immunological criteria showed that the latter could readily be integrated into that classification (Tubbs *et al.*, 1983). Nevertheless, morphology remains the foundation of histopathology and in many cases the distinction between B and T lymphocytes may be made on that basis alone.

It is clear that more and more sub-populations will be detected as the ever increasing batteries of tests are applied to each broad morphological category. Hence the sub-type recognition of LPD in the bone marrow, based on morphological criteria will no doubt be extended with the application of further monoclonal antibodies and other markers.

10.2   Differential diagnosis of LPD in the bone marrow

There are three main areas in which a distinction must be made between benign (reactive) and neoplastic proliferations in the bone marrow.

10.2.1   *Plasmacytosis and multiple myeloma (MM)*

Here the question concerns the differentiation of reactive plasmacytosis in the bone marrow of patients with chronic inflammatory or other diseases, and the plasmacytosis in patients, with benign gammopathy, and with early multiple myeloma. In all three cases, small groups of plasma cells are located near blood vessels, and are dispersed among the haematopoietic and fat cells. In addition, but only in early MM, there are tight clusters of plasma cells in paratrabecular and periarterial regions. These subsequently expand to form the nodules of multiple myelomas as the disease progresses. In rare early cases when the distinction cannot be made on histology alone, immunological investigation on cryostat sections (Falini and Taylor, 1983; Bartl *et al.*, 1984) will identify a monoclonal population of plasma cells (Plate IIIe). With respect to cytology there is no single morphological feature of plasma cells which is found exclusively in the cells of a malignant clone. But a high incidence of certain characteristics may be very suggestive of neoplasia: many cells with large nuclei, prominent nucleoli, multinuclearity, pleomorphism, crystalline or other cytoplasmic or intranuclear inclusions, and nucleocytoplasmic asynchronism (Bartl *et al.*, 1982a). These observations have recently been confirmed by Greipp and Kyle (1983) who also demonstrated that the plasma cell labelling index provides a reliable diagnostic test to differentiate multiple myeloma from other plasmacytoses.

10.2.2   Lymphocytosis, benign lymphoid hyperplasia (BLH) or nodules (BLN) and malignant lymphomas

Increases in lymphocytes (a normal member of the cell population in the bone marrow) may be absolute or relative due to a reduction in haematopoietic elements. Such cases may be difficult to distinguish from early lymphocytic lymphomas with interstitial spread. The same applies to the distinction of BLN from a nodular lymphocytic lymphoma. In both cases immunohistology may be required especially in older age groups in which the incidence of BLN and of lymphomas is higher. Also, as in the lymph nodes, the distinction between benign, reactive, and malignant lymphoid follicles may be facilitated by evaluation of nuclear size, because the mean nuclear diameter and area are significantly greater in the benign than in the malignant conditions (Crocker et al., 1983). Lymphocytosis also occurs in infectious mononucleosis (due to T lymphoblasts), in rheumatic diseases (Humphrey et al., 1982), in infections with cytomegalic virus, in post-transfusion syndrome and in drug hypersensitivity (Gordon et al., 1982). Lymphocytosis may accompany mumps, measles, chicken-pox, infectious hepatitis, toxoplasmosis and other infections (Price, 1983). It must be borne in mind that T cells are normally present in the bone marrow and that there is a functional interaction between T and B cells (both benign and malignant) in the bone marrow (Harris and Bhan, 1983).

10.2.3   Granulomas and Hodgkin's disease (HD)

Infiltrates composed of epithelioid cells, plasma cells, mast cells, histiocytes, lymphoid cells, macrophages and eosinophils, small blood vessels and reticular fibres, in various proportions may occur in numerous conditions. These include: rheumatic diseases, allergies, immune deficiency states and infections due to a variety of agents. In the absence of giant cells in the reactive conditions, and of Reed–Sternberg cells or HD cells in HD, the purely histological distinction between the various entities in the bone marrow is not possible. Moreover, similar infiltrates may be found in angio-immunoblastic lymphadenopathy (AILD), in malignant histiocytosis and systemic mastocytosis. However, in these three conditions the difficulties are usually confined to small bone marrow biopsies and minimal involvement. Otherwise each of the conditions has certain characteristic features: an arborizing, whorl-like arrangement of vessels and deposition of interstitial material in AILD (though not so pronounced in the bone marrow as in the lymph nodes) with preservation of the haematopoietic tissue between the infiltrates; a diffuse spread of histiocytes in the marrow in malignant histiocytosis; and concentric disposition of mastocytes, fibroblasts and lymphocytes around the blood vessels in systemic mastocytosis. For discussion of the inter-relationships within the lymphoproliferative disorders, and for references, see Bartl *et al.* (1984).

10.3   Histology of LPD in the bone marrow

The various forms of the B lymphocyte may be recognized by their morphological characteristics (Robb-Smith and Taylor, 1981). In addition, histological assessment of the bone marrow includes estimation of the relative proportions of the several cell types, which in turn reflect the diverse structural forms of a single neoplastic clone, especially of the B-cell line. Moreover, there is a relationship of morphological diversity to clinical behaviour (Dosoretz *et al.*, 1982). Evaluation of structural patterns and of stromal components are also utilized to support or confirm a diagnosis. Blood vessels in areas involved by lymphoid proliferations may have special features (Freemont, 1983).

The descriptions of the expression of bone marrow involvement given in this chapter are derived from a large series of untreated patients. The distribution of the patients with marrow involvement is given in Table 10.3 and Fig. 10.1. In this book, the Kiel classification is used (Table 10.4)

Table 10.3 Lymphoproliferative disorders in the bone marrow

Histological groups		Cell markers	Frequency %	Bone marrow involvement % in each group
(1729 adult patients)				
LPD of B or T cell lineage				
lymphocytic	LC	BT	16%	99%
lymphoblastic	LB	BTc	2%	45%
centrocytic	CC	B	4%	71%
centroblastic/cytic	CB/CC	B	3%	20%
centroblastic	CB	B	1%	25%
immunocytic	IC	B	15%	85%
immunoblastic	IB	BT	1%	29%
plasmacytic	PC	B	30%	94%
plasmablastic	PB	B	12%	79%
LPD of uncertain cell lineage				
hairy cell leukaemia	HCL	B?	8%	95%
Hodgkin's disease	HD	?	5%	8%
angioimmunoblastic	AILD	?	2%	70%
unclassifiable	UCL	—	2%	—

LPD in the bone marrow
histological groups and frequency

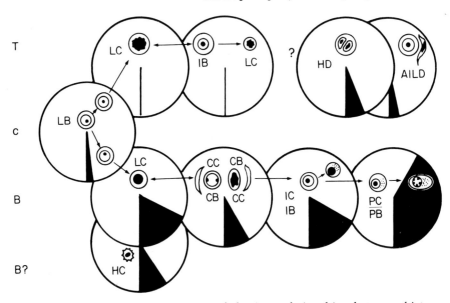

Fig. 10.1 Schematic representation of the interrelationships between histological groups, and the frequency of the LPD in the bone marrow. The size of the black segment indicates the frequency: 100% = all LPD in the bone marrow; T = T cell; B = B cell, c = common; LB = lymphoblastic; LC = lymphocytic; IB = immunoblastic, HD = Hodgkin's disease; AILD = angio-immunoblastic lymphadenopathy; HC = hairy cell; CC = centrocytic; CB = centroblastic; IC = immunocytic; PC = plasmacytic; PB = plasmablastic.

(Lennert, 1981; Lennert *et al.*, 1983). This classification has come into widespread use in Europe (Glimelius *et al.*, 1983; Wright and Isaacson, 1983). Most LPDs with marrow involvement are of B cell lineage (Fig. 10.1). As pointed out by Taylor *et al.* (1979), each B cell neoplasm includes cells in the different stages of the developmental pathway (lymphocytes, follicle centre cells, immunoblasts, and plasma cells), but their relative proportions differ in the various entities. This viewpoint has gained increasing support from immunological studies such as the detection of circulating monoclonal B lymphocytes in the blood of patients with myelomas or lymphomas, and the demonstration of monoclonal cytoplasmic immunoglobulins in leukaemic B lymphocytes from patients with CLL. T cell neoplasms are relatively rare in the bone marrow (Fig. 10.1), less than 1% in our material. Not one of 60 patients with mycosis fungoides had involvement in the bone marrow and it was found in only one patient with Sézary's syndrome. Cases of HCL, HD and AILD as well as of the unclassifiable malignant lymphomas comprise the LPD of

Table 10.4 Modification of the Kiel classification of non-Hodgkin's lymphomas (Lennert *et al.*, 1983)

I. *Low-grade malignancy*
M.L. Lymphocytic
      Chronic lymphocytic leukaemia, B-cell type
      Chronic lymphocytic leukaemia, T-cell type
      Hairy-cell leukaemia (?)
      Mycosis fungoides and Sezary's syndrome
      T-zone lymphoma
M.L. Lymphoplasmacytic/lymphoplasmacytoid (lymphoplasmacytoid
      immunocytoma)
M.L. Plasmacytic (plasmacytoma*)
M.L. Centrocytic
M.L. Centroblastic/centrocytic
      Follicular
      Follicular and diffuse
      Diffuse
      With or without sclerosis

II. *High-grade malignancy*
M.L. Centroblastic
      Primary
      Secondary
M.L. Lymphoblastic
      B-lymphoblastic, Burkitt type and others
      T-lymphoblastic, convoluted-cell type and others
      Unclassified
M.L. Immunoblastic
      With plasmablastic/plasmacytic differentiation (B)
      Without plasmablastic/plasmacytic differentiation (B or T)

* Only extramedullary plasmacytoma.

uncertain cell lineage. When classified according to the predominant cell type, 5 major entities are recognized in the bone marrow: (1) lymphocytic; (2) centrocytic; (3) immunocytic; (4) plasmacytic and (5) hairy cell. Each of these is further classified on the basis of histological and cytological features. Bone marrow involvement in the LPD showed six major types of spread called growth patterns (Fig. 10.2, Table 10.5), but with progressive expansion and replacement of the haematopoietic tissue all patterns merged into the 'packed marrow' type (Plate IXa–e), i.e. complete occupation of the marrow cavities by the neoplastic cells (Fig. 10.2). The amount of infiltration in the biopsy (the tumour cell burden) in the cumulative LPD may be used for histological staging (Bartl *et al.*, 1982a; 1984). Moreover, the numerical quantitation of the infiltration in the biopsy (Fig. 10.2) is important not only for therapy and prognosis, but also for comparison between patients and centres, as these measurements provide an objective basis for the comparison.

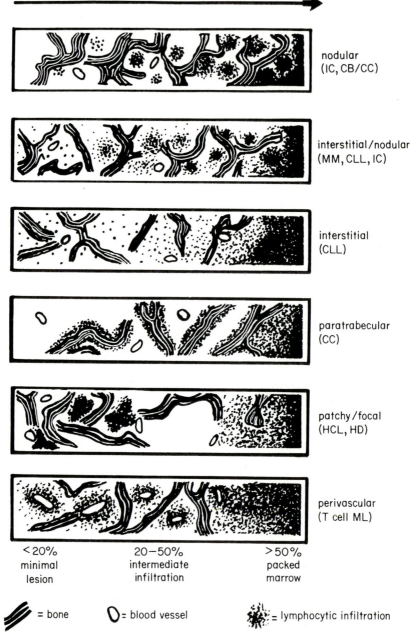

Fig. 10.2 Schematic representation of growth patterns and tumour cell burden (vol %) of lymphoproliferative disorders in the bone marrow.

Table 10.5 Correlation of bone marrow patterns and prognosis in LPD

†	Nod	Nod/Int	Int	Par	Foc	Pac
LC	—	107*	36	—	—	25
IC	74	56	34	—	—	17
PC	50	29	40	—	—	16
CC	—	—	—	29	—	19
CB/CC	50	—	—	—	—	6
Blast	—	—	—	—	—	6
HCL	—	—	—	—	28	18
HD	—	—	—	—	35	29
AILD	—	—	—	—	34	12

* Median survival (months).
The predominant growth pattern in each group is underlined. Nod = nodular, Int = interstitial, Par = paratrabecular, Foc = focal, Pac = packed marrow.
† See Table 10.3 for explanation of abbreviations.

10.4 Malignant lymphoma lymphocytic (LPD of B or T cell origin)

Under this heading are included B 1-CLL, B 2-CLL, T-CLL, P-CLL and Sezary's syndrome (Fig. 10.3). In all these the bone marrow shows variable amounts of infiltration with small lymphocytes with round nuclei (Fig. 10.4) and heavily clumped chromatin demonstrating three growth patterns: (1) interstitial (Fig. 10.5), (2) interstitial/nodular (Fig. 10.5), and (3) packed marrow type. Nodules with follicle centres are present in 25% of the cases. Recent studies have confirmed the more favourable course of nodular as opposed to diffuse lymphomas (Table 10.5) (Damber *et al.*, 1982; Straus *et al.*, 1983; Bartl *et al.*, 1984). There are variable reductions in haematopoietic tissue elements and fat cells. In

Fig. 10.3 Cytological range in the lymphocytic–lymphoblastic spectrum.

Histological groups		Patients, % in each group	Median survivals* (months)
Lymphocytic		283	43
Small, round	(1)	70%	48
Small, notched	(2)	5%	32
Large	(3)	20%	27
Prolymphocytic	(4)	5%	10
Lymphoblastic	(5)	13	6

* from the time of biopsy to death or date of last contact

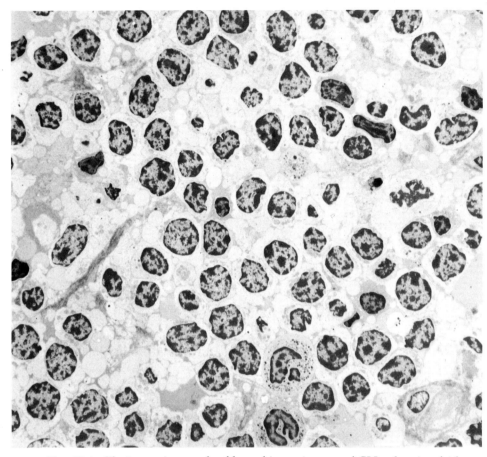

Fig. 10.4 Electron micrograph of bone biopsy in case of CLL, showing fairly round, monomorphic, typical nuclei of the lymphoid cells. × 1000. Compare with Fig. 10.7.

some cases the fat cells are preserved while the haematopoietic precursors are greatly reduced, especially in the vicinity of the infiltrations. In reticulin strains a thin network of fibres is present in the infiltrated areas and accentuated in the perivascular regions. Lymphoid cells are frequently found in the lumina of the sinusoids and around small blood vessels (especially in T-cell lymphomas) (Fig. 10.6). Mast and plasma cells are generally not prominent. There is some variation in size and number of nucleolated cells within the lymphoid cell population (Plate Xb)—a

Fig. 10.5 CLL: (a) early marrow involvement with interstitial spread, haematopoiesis and marrow architecture largely preserved. × 400, Giemsa; (b) nodular growth in the bone marrow. × 60, Giemsa.

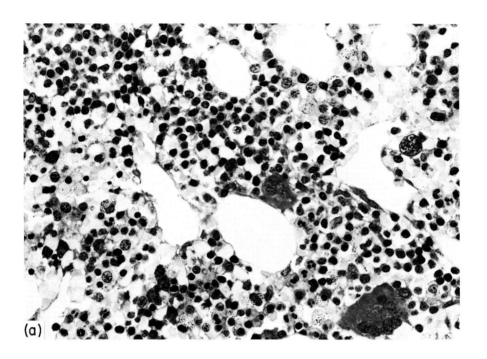

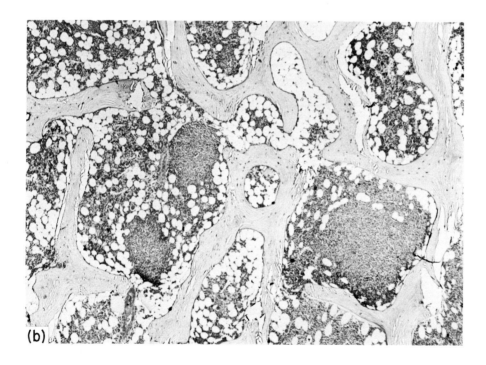

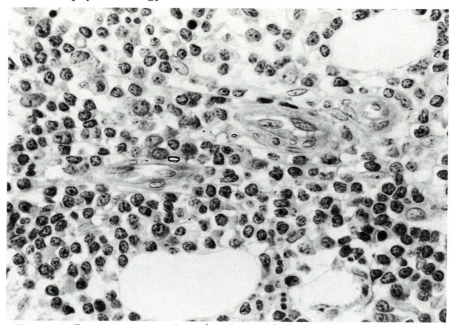

Fig. 10.6 Bone marrow section of patient with T cell lymphatic leukaemia showing perivascular infiltration. × 400, Giemsa.

high proportion indicates P-CLL (prolymphocytic). In these cases the cells have moderate amounts of cytoplasm and a positive acid phosphatase reaction (on imprints, smears or cryostat sections). B2-CLL is characterized by lymphoid cell nuclei with slight indentations or notches (Fig. 10.7), confirmed by marker studies (Ralfkiaer *et al.*, 1983). In cases with T-CLL involvement in the bone marrow the lymphocytes may have round, oval, notched or even convoluted nuclei and a striking perivascular localization. When CLL is complicated by haemolysis, there is erythroid hyperplasia in the bone marrow. Marked osteoclastic activation has been noted in some patients with T cell lymphoma-leukaemia (Grossman *et al.*, 1981) and these patients had hypercalcaemia. CLL with osteolytic bone lesions, hypercalcaemia and a monoclonal protein in the blood has also been described (Redmond *et al.*, 1983).

10.4.1   *Differential diagnosis*

Benign lymphoid hyperplasia and lymphocytic infiltrations due to other causes such as infections (see Table 10.2) must be excluded, as well as

Fig. 10.7 Electron micrographs of bone biopsy of case of CLL: (a) low power × 640, (b) × 2520 to show pleomorphism of the nuclei; complete replacement of marrow. Compare with Fig. 10.4.

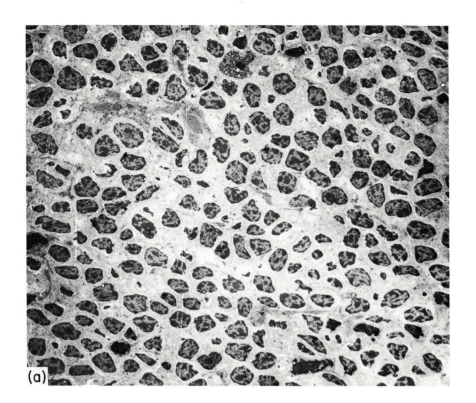

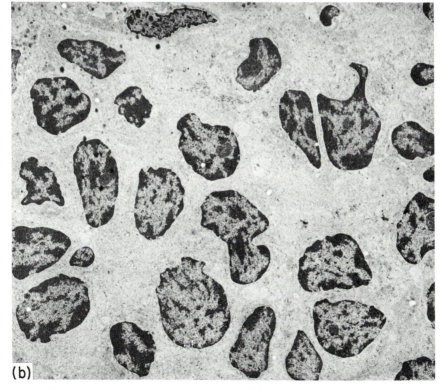

early cases of hairy cell leukaemia, and monocytic leukaemia. CLL may also (rarely) terminate in myeloid leukaemia (Stern *et al.*, 1981).

T-cell lymphomas and leukaemias have now been classified separately (Kadin *et al.*, 1983) and sub-types of T-cell CLL have also been characterized (Huhn *et al.*, 1983). The immunological phenotypes of both the neoplastic B cells and the reactive T cells in the bone marrow in B CLL have been demonstrated by Pizzolo *et al.* (1983). T-cell CLL is classified into two major phenotypic sub-types: T4 and T8. In the latter the leukaemic cells are large and have abundant cytoplasm with azurophilic granules. In contrast to T4, patients with the sub-type T8 present with low lymphocyte counts, little organ or bone marrow involvement and a long clinical course (Brisbane *et al.*, 1983). Some features of LPD of T-cell lineage are given in Table 10.6.

Table 10.6 LPD of T cell lineage in the bone marrow: cytological and histological criteria (facultative)

T-lymphoblastic:
    (1) convoluted nuclei
    (2) paranuclear granules of acid phosphatase activity (on imprints)
    (3) pronounced perivascular infiltrations
T-lymphocytic:
    (1) convoluted nuclei
    (2) azure cytoplasmic granulation (on imprints in Giemsa stain)
    (3) coarse clumps of acid phosphatase activity (on imprints)
    (4) pronounced perivascular infiltrations
    (5) non-nodular growth pattern in the bone marrow
T-immunoblastic:
    (1) no plasmablastic differentiation
    (2) no globular PAS reaction (on imprints)
    (3) polymorphic nuclei

10.5 Malignant lymphoma lymphoblastic

Under this heading are included common ALL, B-ALL, T-ALL and lymphoblastic sarcoma.

Only adult patients will be considered here. In most cases a diffuse packed marrow pattern is found, with few remaining fat cells and only isolated haematopoietic precursors dispersed among the lymphoblasts (Fig. 10.8). In the T-cell variants, there is a pronounced perivascular

Fig. 10.8   Acute lymphoblastic leukaemia: (a) diffuse and fairly dense infiltration in the bone marrow with few remaining haematopoietic cells. The lymphoblasts have a high nucleo-cytoplasmic ratio with narrow cytoplasmic rims. × 400, Giemsa; (b) hypocellular marrow, disruption of architecture; lymphoblasts scattered in oedematous stroma, virtually no remaining haematopoietic cells. × 400, Giemsa.

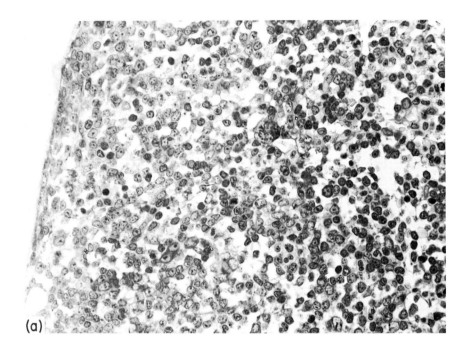

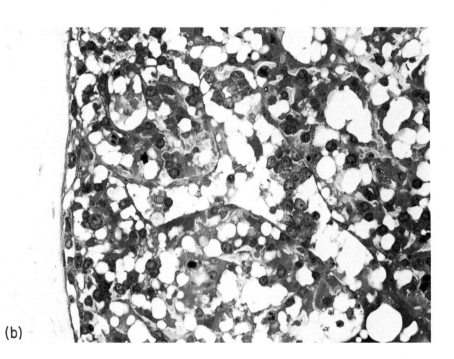

infiltration of lymphoid cells with oval, notched, indented or convoluted nuclei (Fig. 10.9). (Their T-cell origin must be confirmed by studies on imprints, peripheral blood or cryostat sections.) T CLL is rare in the West. Most cases are derived from the helper/inducer subset of T cells and are T4

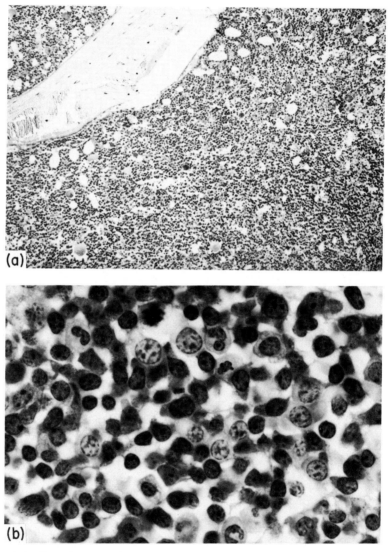

(a)

(b)

Fig. 10.9 Bone biopsy of 16 year old patient with T-cell lymphoblastic lymphoma, established by lymph node biopsy and marker studies: (a) cellular bone marrow. × 100, Giemsa; (b) higher magnification to show diffuse infiltration and the round, oval and occasionally lymphoid cells. × 1000, Giemsa.

positive cells. In bone marrow biopsies there is hypercellularity, with an increase in plasma cells and there are lymphoid aggregates.

A few cases of T CLL have been described which are T8 positive, i.e. of suppressor/cytotoxic cell derivation. In these lymphomas the T cells are large, with abundant cytoplasm, containing azurophilic granules and the nuclei are not convoluted. There is lymphocytosis in the peripheral blood and bone marrow, and this may remain mild for long periods of time. There may be suppression of leucopoiesis so that the peripheral blood may show neutropenia (Brisbane *et al.*, 1983).

Eosinophilia has been observed in patients with a lymphoblastic malignancy (Catovsky *et al.*, 1980) with increases of eosinophilic precursors in the bone marrow. The authors suggested that the hypereosinophilic syndrome in these patients was due to eosinopoietic stimuli produced by the lymphoblasts.

Bone marrow histology before and after chemotherapy for acute lymphoblastic leukaemia is illustrated in Fig. 10.10. Bone marrow findings after transplantation have been studied by Müller-Hermelink and Sale (1983) and Heymer *et al.* (1983).

10.6   Malignant lymphoma centrocytic (synonyms: cleaved cell lymphoma, follicle centre cell lymphoma FCC)

The characteristic picture of bone marrow involvement consists of paratrabecular infiltrations of small to medium-sized lymphoid cells with angulated 'cleaved' nuclei, showing a fairly dense chromatin pattern, and narrow rims of cytoplasm (Figs 10.11, 10.12). The infiltrations are usually enmeshed in a fairly dense reticulin fibre network (Plate Xf), and thus sharply separated from the central haematopoietic tissue. Coarse fibres radiating out from the trabecular surface form a characteristic stromal pattern. The number of blood vessels and cellular stromal elements is higher than in CLL (Table 10.7). Three sub-types may be recognized on the basis of the size and the nuclear morphology of the lymphoid cells: (1) small cleaved, (2) large cleaved, and (3) polymorphous (Figs 10.11 and 10.13).

The small non-cleaved follicle centre cell lymphoma has now been divided into two sub-types, the Burkitt and the non-Burkitt type, and significant biological differences were demonstrated between these variants, including marrow involvement (4.5% in the Burkitt type and 37.5% in the non-Burkitt type) and median survival times (Levine *et al.*, 1983).

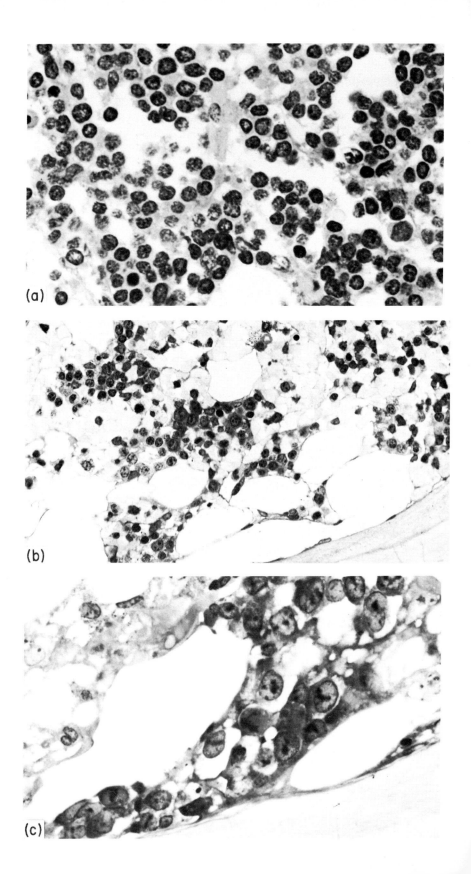

10.6.1   *Differential diagnosis*

The morphological distinction between B2 lymphocytes, small centro-cytes, and T lymphoid cells may be very difficult; the same applies to the differentiation of large centrocytic from monocytic infiltrations. In these cases definite identification is best achieved by enzymic and immunologic methods.

10.7   Malignant lymphoma centroblastic/centrocytic (synonyms: Brill–Symmers' disease, cleaved FCC lymphoma)

Bone marrow involvement is rare in this lymphoma. When found it has a strictly nodular pattern, mostly follicles with germinal centres consisting of centrocytes, centroblasts and lymphocytes, within a network of reticu-lar fibres (Plate Xe, Figs 10.11, 10.14, 10.15). Also present are capillaries

Fig. 10.11 Cytologic range in the centrocytic–centroblastic spectrum.

Histological groups	Patients % in group	Main subtype	Median survival months*
Centrocytic	65		25
Small cleaved	60%	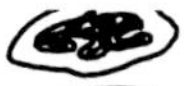	35
Large cleaved	25%	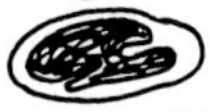	16
Polymorphous	15%	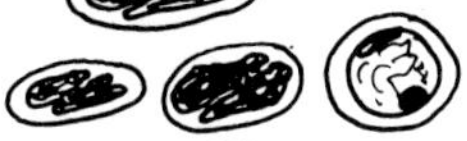	12
Centroblastic/cytic	52	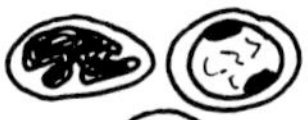	48
Centroblastic	25	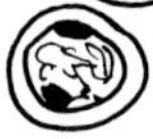	5

* From time of biopsy to date of death or last contact

and histiocytes, while eosinophils, plasma cells and mast cells are found at the margins of the nodules, between which the bone marrow has a normal aspect, both in structure and in cellular composition.

10.7.1   *Differential diagnosis*

When only minimal lesions are found in the bone marrow, their distinc-tion from benign lymphoid hyperplasia or from immunocytoma may not

Fig. 10.10 Acute lymphoblastic leukaemia: (a) before treatment, complete replacement of bone marrow. × 600, Giemsa; (b) biopsy from same patient after chemotherapy, incomplete remission. × 400, Giemsa; (c) high power view of blasts in Fig. (b), bone at lower right. × 1000, Giemsa.

Table 10.7 Quantitative estimation of stromal elements in bone marrows with involvement by LPD

	Norm[0]	LC	LP-oid	LP-tic	PC	CC	CB/CC	HCL	HD	AILD
Arterioles/10 mm²	3	1	1	2	1	2	1	1	12	21
Capillaries/10 mm²	10	2	8	12	5	9	10	25	48	52
Sinusoids/10 mm²	170	30	85	210	70	50	70	215	210	180
Plasma cell/10 mm²	220	25	120	680	210	65	53	160	176	250
Mast cells/10 mm²	20	35	62	234	12	28	21	136	22	12
Histiocytes/10 mm²	52	41	104	126	43	69	90	172	195	148
Trabeculae, vol %	24	22	23	20	19	23	22	24	24	24
OB-index, %**	4	3	3	5	14	8	4	6	7	9
OC-index,/100 mm***	5	4	6	8	31	9	4	8	9	6
Fibres*	—	—	(+)	(+)	(+)	+	+	++	++	+

Histometric evaluation of 30 biopsies in each histologic group, mean values.

[0] Normal individuals, median age of 55 years.

* — = no increase, (+) = thin fibres, + = coarse fibres, ++ = coarse fibrosis.

** Percentage of trabecular surface covered by active osteoblasts.

*** Number of osteoclasts per 100 mm trabecular surface.

See Table 10.3 for explanation of abbreviations. LP-oid = lymphoplasmacytoid; LP-tic = lymphoplasmacytic.

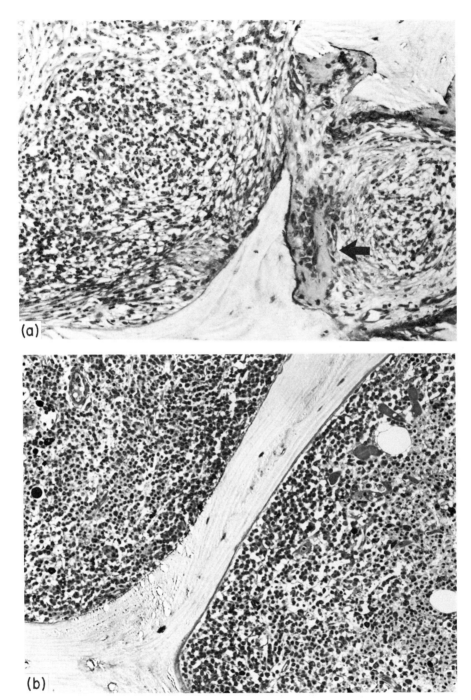

Fig. 10.12 Malignant lymphoma centrocytic: (a) with pronounced osseous remodelling, in particular osteoblastic (arrow); note also accompanying paratrabecular fibrosis; (b) showing wide paratrabecular seams but without increased remodelling and fibrosis; haematopoietic tissue in central marrow areas. Both × 250, Giemsa.

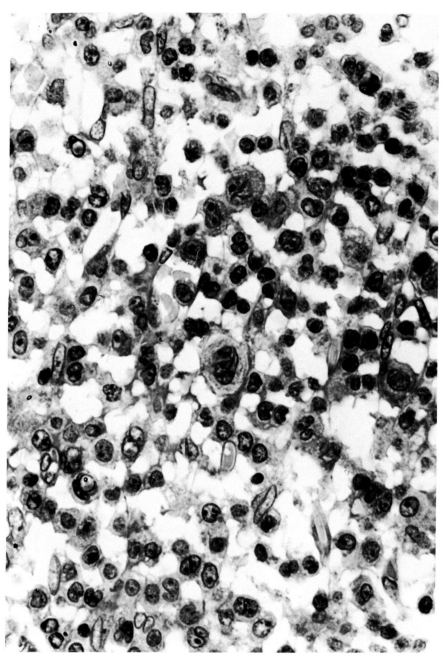

Fig. 10.13 High power view of cytological features of malignant lymphoma centrocytic, pleomorphic sub-type showing somewhat angulated 'cleaved' nuclei with condensed heterochromatin, fairly narrow rims of cytoplasm, and inconspicuous nucleoli. × 1000, Giemsa.

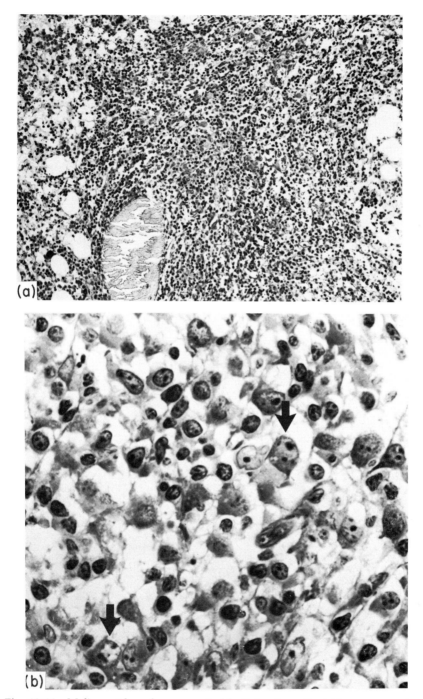

Fig. 10.14 Malignant lymphoma, centroblastic/centrocytic: (a) low power view of bone marrow; note nodular growth pattern. × 100, Giemsa; high power view illustrating centroblasts (arrows) and centrocytes. × 800, Giemsa.

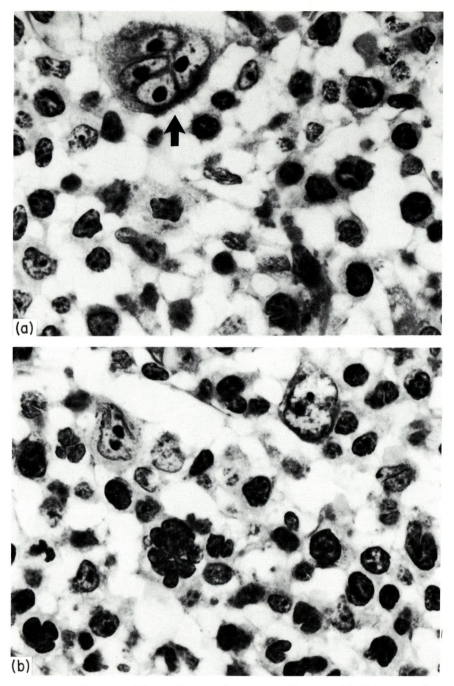

Fig. 10.15 Section of bone biopsy of patient with centroblastic/centrocytic lymphoma: (a) multinucleate cell with large nucleoli (arrow) and polymorphic lymphoid cells. × 1000, Giemsa; (b) centroblasts and convoluted centrocytes. × 1000, Giemsa.

be possible on the basis of histology alone; other investigations are required to confirm or exclude involvement.

Nathwani *et al.* (1983) have reported on the results of a retrospective study of diffuse, mixed cell lymphomas. Two groups were recognized. One had features consistent with follicle centre cell origin and the second group had morphologic features similar to those described for peripheral T cell derived lymphoma. There were significant differences between the two groups: the first lived longer and the second appeared to have a high grade lymphoma.

10.8   Malignant lymphoma centroblastic

The involved marrow shows a packed marrow pattern, and the cells are readily identifiable due to their characteristic nuclear aspect (Plate Xd) and disposition of the nucleoli (Fig. 10.16). Marker studies are generally not required.

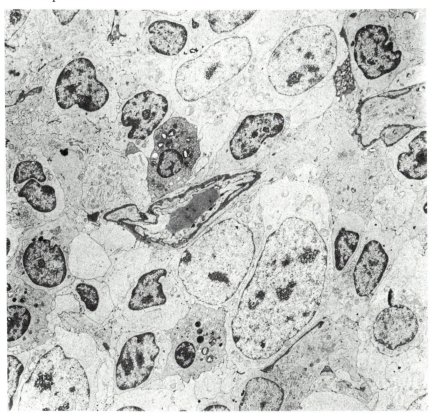

Fig. 10.16   Electron micrograph of bone biopsy, centroblastic lymphoma; only isolated haematopoietic cells left; note blood vessel in centre. × 2000.

10.9 Malignant lymphoma lymphoplasmacytoid, lymphoplasmacytic immunocytoma (Waldenström's macroglobulinaemia)

In this lymphoma the infiltration consists mainly of small lymphocytes with variable numbers of mature plasma cells, lymphoplasmacytoid and lymphoplasmacytic cells (Fig. 10.17), and mast cells in a hypo-cellular to normocellular marrow. Most cases have some lymphoid cells with

Fig. 10.17 Cytological range in the immunocytic–immunoblastic spectrum.

Histological groups	Patients % in group	Main subtype	Median survival months*
Immunocytic	215		46
Lymphoplasmacytoid	49%		75
Lymphoplasmacytic	46%		28
Polymorphous	5%		13
Immunoblastic	30		5

* From time of biopsy to death or date of last contact.

cytoplasmic or nuclear inclusions (PAS positive, called Dutcher bodies). The growth patterns range from nodular to interstitial to packed. As in the lymph nodes, three sub-types (Bartl *et al.*, 1983a), are recognized though these may overlap (Fig. 10.18); the lymphoplasmacytoid, with a

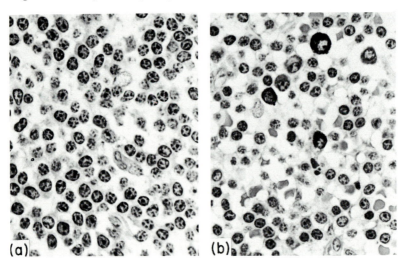
(a)   (b)

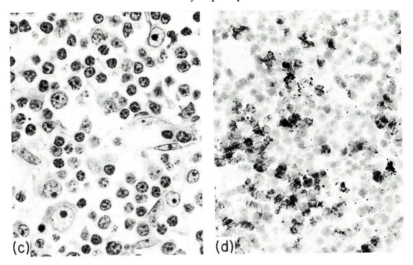

Fig. 10.18 Malignant lymphoma, immunocytic: (a) lymphoplasmacytoid type; (b) lymphoplasmacytic type; (c) pleomorphic type. × 400, Giemsa; (d) T lymphocytes dispersed among B cells in ML immunocytic, pan-T, Papanicolaou stain. × 400.

nodular pattern, the lymphoplasmacytic which shows an interstitial/ nodular pattern and has numerous Marschalko plasma cells and mast cells, and the polymorphous type (Plate Xa), whose cell population consists of lymphocytes, plasma cells, centrocytes, centroblasts (Fig. 10.19), and which usually presents with a packed marrow pattern. The infiltrated areas show a fine reticulin fibrosis. Some haematopoietic precursors are found within the infiltrates as well as occupying the marrow between them. Other stromal features are: hyperplastic and ectatic sinusoids in the lymphoplasmacytic type, with sclerosis of the endothelium and bordered by dense infiltrates of lymphoid cells, and occasional accumulations of histiocytes (Plate XIe). In the paraproteinaemic cases the lumina of the vessels are filled with a homogeneous PAS positive material. Conversion of an immunocytoma to an immunoblastic lymphoma has also been described (Emmerich *et al.*, 1983).

10.9.1 *Differential diagnosis*

In the absence of PAS positive inclusions in the lymphoid cells, the picture may resemble that seen in CLL. However, mast cells are not numerous in the latter. Occasionally CLL with reactive plasmacytosis may present a similar picture. Immunohistology may be used to clarify borderline cases. Evolution into overt malignancy may occur after many

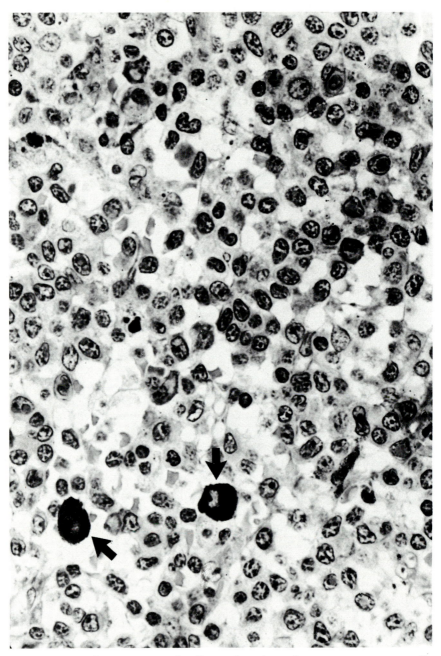

Fig. 10.19 High power view of malignant lymphoma immunocytoma; mast cells (arrows) × 1000, Giemsa.

years of asymptomatic monoclonal macroglobulinaemia (Fine *et al.*, 1982).

10.10   Malignant lymphoma immunoblastic (immunoblastic sarcoma)

Cases in which involvement of the bone marrow occurs usually have a packed marrow type. B-immunoblasts (Plate Xc) are identified by their characteristic round nuclei with prominent nucleoli (Fig. 10.20), in contrast to the polymorphism of the T-immunoblasts (confirmed by immuno-histology on cryostat sections). Immunoblastic sarcoma may also develop in patients with preceding immunocytoma, or multiple myeloma (Falini *et al.*, 1982). Comparative bone marrow and lymph node studies have shown similar histology in most cases (Table 10.8).

Table 10.8 Malignant lymphomas: comparison of lymph node and bone marrow histology

		Lymph node							
		LC	HC	IC	CC	CB/CC	LB	IB	CB
Bone marrow	LC	11*	—	1	1	—	—	—	—
	HC	—	15*	—	—	—	—	—	—
	IC	⑦	—	31*	1	⑧	—	1	—
	CC	—	—	2	8*	2	1	1	—
	CB/CC	—	—	1	—	15*	1	1	—
	LB	—	—	—	—	—	2*	—	—
	IB	—	—	1	—	—	—	2*	—
	CB	—	—	—	—	1	—	—	4*

Mean time interval: congruent cases 10 months, divergent cases 5 months

10.11   Malignant lymphoma plasmacytic (multiple myeloma)

This is divided into two broad groups: plasmacytic primarily mature plasma cells and plasmablastic mainly 'immature' plasma cells (Fig. 10.21). In early cases the plasma cells are dispersed among the haematopoietic and fat cells in addition to small clusters in paratrabecular and peri-arterial regions. Subsequently these plasma cell aggregates expand and coalesce to form 'multiple myelomas' and sheets of plasma cells replacing the normal marrow elements (Figs 10.22, 10.23). All the infiltrated areas have a fibre network which is in most cases fine, but is occasionally coarse. Some lymphocytes are always scattered among the plasma cells, and lymphocytic aggregates are found in 10% of the cases. Usually the residual marrow shows a reduction in haematopoiesis and

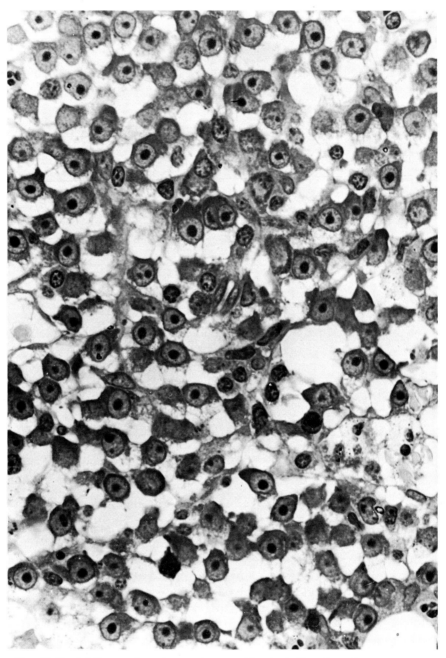

Fig. 10.20 Malignant lymphoma, immunoblastic, infiltration of monomorphic cells with large round nuclei, single prominent nucleoli and moderate amounts of basophilic cytoplasm, no haematopoietic tissue left. × 1000, Giemsa.

Fig. 10.21 Cytological range in the plasmacytic–plasmablastic spectrum.

Histological groups	Patients % in group	Main subtype	Median survival months*
Plasmacytic	546		36
Marschalko	70%	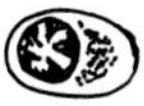	46
Small round	10%	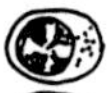	24
Small notched	6%	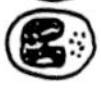	19
Polymorphous	14%	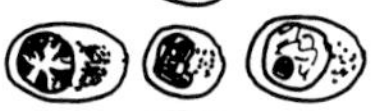	16
Plasmablastic	267	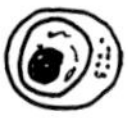	9

* From time of biopsy to death or date of last contact.

maturation arrest of erythropoietic precursors, and an increase in fat cells. Augmented osteoclastic and osteoblastic remodelling are prominent in the majority of cases, and correlate with the amount of plasma cell burden in the biopsy. Few mast cells are found. Four sub-types may be distinguished according to the predominant type of plasma cell present: (1) Marschalko type, (2) small round, (3) small notched, and (4) polymorphous (Fig. 10.24). Patients with the small (micro-type) plasma cells are more likely to have a leukaemic blood picture than the others. Mahmoud *et al.* (1983) have recently demonstrated that there is extension of both myeloid and normal tissue into the appendicular skeleton in some cases of multiple myeloma.

10.12   Malignant lymphoma plasmablastic (multiple myeloma, plasmablastic sarcoma)

The plasmablasts, large polymorphic, often multinucleate plasma cells, usually fill the marrow cavities, thus presenting the packed marrow type (Fig. 10.25). In a few cases a focal sarcomatous pattern is observed. Most cells have moderate to abundant cytoplasm, often with a pronounced perinuclear 'hof'. The nuclei have very prominent nucleoli. Fat cells and residual haematopoiesis are greatly diminished. Mature plasma cells, lymphocytes, and immunoblasts are scattered among the plasmablasts, which are sometimes separated into large nodular aggregates by broad bands of connective tissue fibres. In such areas osteoclastic activity is often prominent. In all cases of multiple myeloma, the plasma cells may have accumulations of secretions within their cytoplasm (rarely also

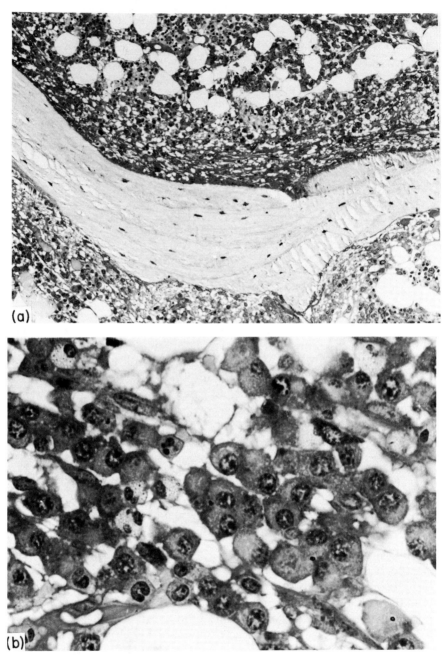

Fig. 10.22 Multiple myeloma: (a) biopsy section illustrating paratrabecular and interstitial infiltration with plasma cells. × 250, Giemsa; (b) high power view of plasma cells. × 1000, Giemsa.

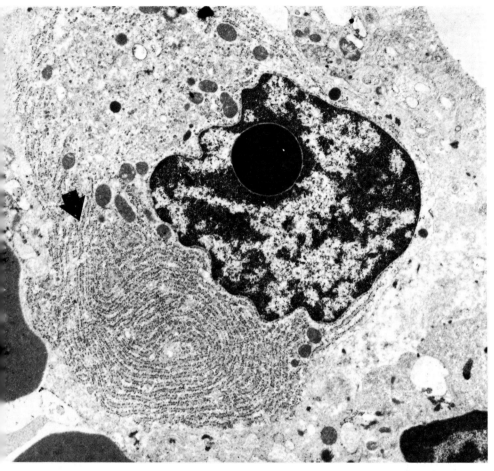

Fig. 10.23   Electron micrograph of plasma cells showing endoplasmic reticulum (arrow) and intranuclear inclusion. × 6400.

within the nuclei). As well as the characteristic Russell bodies these inclusions may have a crystalline or needle-like appearance. In some cases there may be paratrabecular or interstitial infiltrations accompanied by a reduction in haematopoiesis, increase in fat cells or fibrosis. Perivascular amyloidosis may occasionally be found in cases with light chain proteinaemia (about 15% of the patients). In cases of established MM without involvement in the biopsy sections lymphocytosis and an increase in osseous remodelling may be seen.

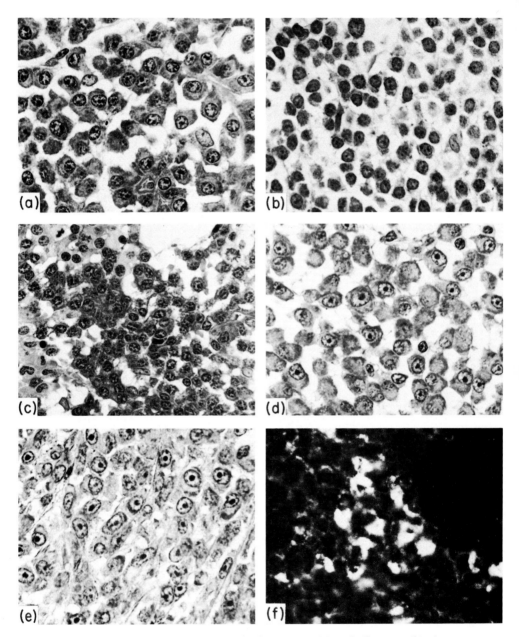

Fig. 10.24 Multiple myeloma: (a) plasmacytic, Marschalko type; (b) plasmacytic, small round type; (c) plasmacytic, small notched type; (d) plasmacytic, polymorphous type; (e) plasmablastic. × 400, Giemsa; (f) early case of MM, IgA, kappa, frozen section, FITC. × 400.

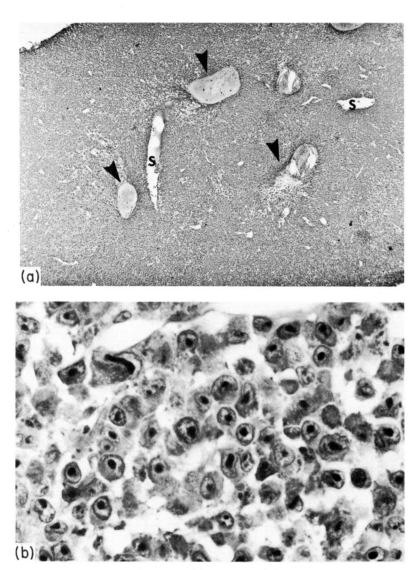

Fig. 10.25 Bone biopsy of 73 year old patient with 3 weeks history of malaise, fever, and transient cerebral disturbances, total protein 85 g/l, albumin 36 g/l, globulin 52 g/l, IgA paraprotein peak, Hb 8.4 g/dl, WBC 13.0×10^9/l, platelets 86×10^9/l, calcium 11.1 mg/dl (2.8 mmol/l): (a) note complete replacement of haematopoietic tissue by monomorphic cell population; trabecular bone (arrows) reduced sinuses (s). $\times$ 40, Giemsa; (b) higher magnification to show the cytological features of the plasmablasts. $\times$ 1000, Giemsa.

10.13   Hairy cell leukaemia

Involvement of the bone marrow is almost invariably present, in the form of a patchy to complete replacement of the normal marrow by hairy cells (Fig. 10.26). They have round to oval to convoluted nuclei, abundant cytoplasm with lateral interdigitating extensions (the hairy processes)

Fig. 10.26 Cytological range in the spectrum of hairy cell leukaemia.

Histological groups	Patients % in group (total = 144)	Predominant cell type	Median survival months*
Ovoid	47%	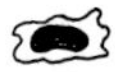	57
Convoluted	37%	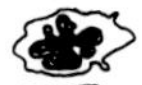	15
Indented	16%	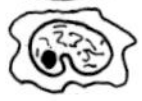	5

* From time of biopsy to death or date of last contact.
Predominant cell, though others also present.

and rod-like cytoplasmic inclusions in about 45% of the cases. The hairy cells are dispersed within a reticular fibre network (Fig. 10.27) which also contains lymphocytes, plasma cells, mast cells, various haematopoietic precursors and extravasated erythrocytes. Numerous small blood vessels, histiocytes and fibroblasts are also intermingled with the hairy cells. At high magnification the hairy cell nuclei display a wide morphologic spectrum with three main configurations (Fig. 10.28), one of which usually predominates in each case: (1) the ovoid in about 47% of the cases, (2) the medium sized and convoluted in about 37%, and (3) the indented in about 16% (Bartl et al., 1983b). Three bone marrow patterns are found: multiple small patches, large confluent areas, and complete replacement. Most evidence to date suggests that hairy cells are of B cell lineage (Su-Ming et al., 1983).

10.13.1   Differential diagnosis

When only moderate involvement is present, centrocytic lymphomas, and myelo-monocytic and monocytic infiltrations may have to be distinguished. However, when undecalcified and plastic embedded bone marrow sections are evaluated at high magnification there are usually no difficulties in recognizing the hairy cells, usually within their characteristic environment.

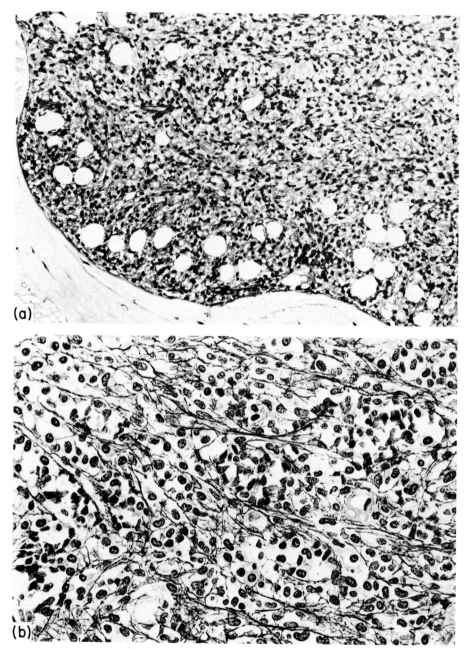

Fig. 10.27 Hairy cell leukaemia: (a) infiltration of rather widely separated cells, within a network of reticulin fibres containing erythrocytes, plasma cells, mast cells and scattered haematopoietic precursor cells. × 250, Giemsa; (b) high power view of part of (a) illustrating the hairy cells within a network of reticular fibres. × 400, Gomori.

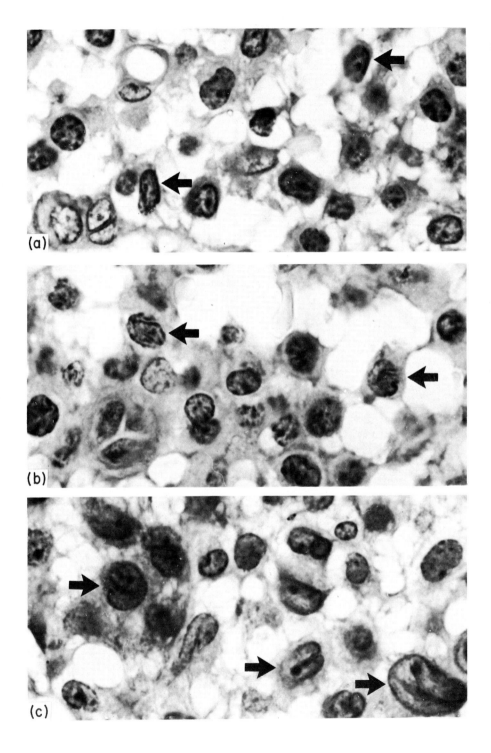

(a)

(b)

(c)

10.14   Hodgkin's disease (HD)

The overall incidence of HD in the bone marrow of patients at initial presentation is 10%. Unlike the lymph nodes there are two main histological types: lymphocytic predominance and lymphocytic depletion (Figs 10.29, 10.30). Bone marrow involvement is extremely rare in stage I and stage II. When correlated with the lymph node histology only 4% of those with nodular sclerosis have bone marrow involvement compared with 22% in the lymphocytic depletion type (Bartl et al., 1982b, 1984).

Fig. 10.29 Cytological range in the spectrum of Hodgkin's disease in the bone marrow

Histological groups	Patients	Cellular composition	Median survival months*
HD low content of lymphocytes	49	†	15
HD high content of lymphocytes	30		55
HD high content of epithelioid cells	5		62

* From time of biopsy to death or date of last contact.
† Order of cells from left to right indicates relative proportions of each type, high to low.

For the initial diagnosis of HD in the bone marrow biopsy, Reed–Sternberg cells within a characteristic stromal environment are mandatory (Lukes, 1971; Myers et al., 1974). However, when HD has already been diagnosed elsewhere, mononuclear Hodgkin's cells within an appropriate setting (Plate XIa–b) are considered evidence of involvement (Jacquillat et al., 1981). The mononuclear HD cell may be accompanied by binuclear HD cells and lacunar cells (Fig. 10.30). These cells are large and pale, their cytoplasm appears extracted, the nuclei may be multi-lobed with small nucleoli. Within the lesions are eosinophils, plasma cells, macrophages, and a greater or lesser degree of fibrosis and lymphocytic infiltration. Capillaries with large prominent nuclei are often quite conspicuous in the lesions. These elements constitute the characteristic environment for the Reed–Sternberg (RS) and mononuclear HD cells. Phagocytes may be abundant in the uninvolved areas between the

Fig. 10.28 High power view of hairy cell sub-types (arrows): (a) ovoid; (b) convoluted; (c) indented; note abundant cytoplasm and long interdigitating processes. × 1000, Giemsa.

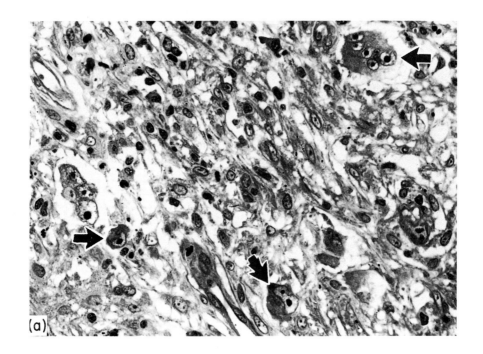

(a)

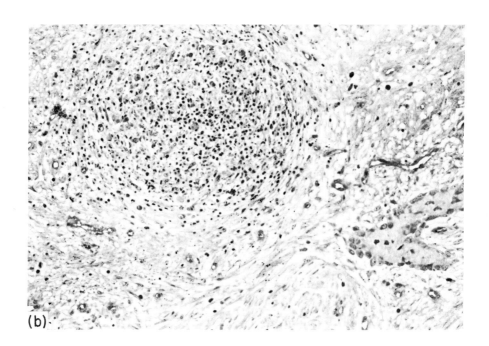

(b)

foci. The suggestion has been made that the RS cells and their precursors are the malignant tissue, while all the other constituents in and around the foci represent the host reaction to antigens on the RS cells, in a graft-versus-host like disease. The lesions in involved biopsies range from small paratrabecular foci to large intertrabecular areas of lymphogranulomatous tissue. There are great variations in fibrosis, in vasculature and in cellular composition of the lesions both in the same biopsy and from patient to patient. It is of interest that certain types of Hodgkin's disease cells in tissue culture stimulate fibroblast growth notably from nodular sclerosing HD (Newcom and O'Rourke, 1982). When there are only small foci, the trabecular structure is usually not affected, but large areas of involvement are usually accompanied by osteosclerosis, osteolysis or osteoporosis of the cancellous bone in their vicinity. Between the foci, the marrow may show an increase in fibres, plasma and mast cells and lymphocytes, in an oedematous stroma, with only remnants of haematopoietic tissue. The variability of the histological findings in HD has led to the speculation that HD is not a single disease, but possibly a number of different disease entities, or that it represents the evolutionary steps of a condition with a very wide spectrum.

Bone marrows of patients with HD may exhibit leukaemoid reactions, or 'tumour myelopathy', or other non-specific changes such as the presence of small epithelioid foci with variable numbers of lymphocytes and plasma cells.

Epithelioid cell granulomas may also be found in the iliac crest biopsies of patients with malignant lymphomas or AILD (diagnosed by lymph node biopsy), with SLE and other immune diseases (see Fig. 4.1), as well as in the absence of a clearcut lymph node histopathology. Two main types have been described, one with lymphocytes and one with plasma cells. In addition, in both types the aggregates contain a mixed population of cells including granulocytes, immunoblasts, plasmablasts, Hodgkin-like cells and micro-'Sternberg–Reed' cells. Multinucleated giant cells may also be present. The significance of these infiltrations is unknown.

10.14.1   Negative bone biopsies in HD

About three quarters of the patients with lymph node documented HD and negative bone marrow biopsies, show some kind of reaction in the

---

Fig. 10.30   (a) Bone marrow involvement in Hodgkin's disease, lymphocytic depletion; Reed–Sternberg and Hodgkin's cells at arrows; note capillaries with prominent endothelia within a fibrous stroma. × 400, Giemsa; (b) non-specific reaction in the bone marrow in HD consisting of epithelioid granuloma; without Reed–Sternberg or Hodgkin's cells. × 250, Giemsa.

bone marrow. This ranges from leukaemoid reactions to epithelioid cell granulomata, foci of fibrous tissue (Fig. 10.30b) and/or lymphocytic nodules (without RS or HD cells). One which is frequently seen is a mixed inflammatory reaction in which there are vascular wall alterations, nucleophagocytosis by histiocytes, infiltrations of lymphocytes, plasma and mast cells especially in perivascular regions; and disturbances of haematopoiesis such as maturation arrest of erythroid precursors and hyperplasia of granulocyte precursors and of megakaryocytes. Alternatively, there may be pronounced hypoplasia of haematopoiesis, increase in fat cells, or exudative reactions, with extensive oedema, reduction in haematopoiesis. In studies of the prognostic significance of these reactions, it was found that hypoplasia, leukaemoid and exudative reactions indicated a poor prognosis, while epithelioid cell granulomas and lymphoid nodules were associated with a more favourable outcome. The negative biopsies of treated patients also showed certain changes: damage to the sinusoidal endothelium, extravasation of red blood cells, oedema, decrease in haematopoiesis. No differences were observed in the negative biopsies of patients treated with chemotherapy or radio-therapy. In some cases the hypo-cellularity persisted for periods of up to 6 months after therapy. Bone marrow changes after chemotherapy with MOPP have also been described by Myers *et al.* (1974).

10.15   Angio-immunoblastic lymphadenopathy (AILD)

Involvement of the bone marrow is thought to occur in about 50% of cases of AILD diagnosed by lymph node histology (Schnaidt *et al.*, 1980). The infiltrates consist of multiple, partly confluent foci having a hetero-geneous cell population which includes immunoblasts, lymphocytes, centrocytes, plasma cells and eosinophils, within a reticulin framework containing arborizing capillaries and interstitial deposits of PAS positive material (Plate XIc–d, Fig. 4.1). The lymphoid proliferation is polyclonal and of B-cell lineage (Ershler *et al.*, 1983). In some patients such manifes-tations are found in the bone marrow in the absence of lym-phadenopathy. In these cases the diagnosis is one of exclusion. Vascular proliferation may be marked, and occur together with fibres in whorl-like arrangements.

10.16   Bone biopsies in acquired immune deficiency syndromes

Aggregates described as 'lymphoid-histiocytic proliferations' have been found in the bone marrows of 38% of cases with AIDS (Guarda and Butler, 1983) and the authors point out that such infiltrates when large could be confused with bone marrow involvement by peripheral T cell lymphoma. The aggregates contain a mixture of lymphocytes of various sizes including transformed cells (Mead and Mason, 1983). We have found lymphoid-histiocytic aggregates in the bone marrow of a patient with AIDS, but these were also accompanied by a very prominent vascular network (Fig. 4.2).

10.17   Lennert's lymphoma (malignant lymphoma, lympho-epithelioid)

Involvement in the bone marrow is characterized by aggregates of epithelioid histiocytes, macrophages, lymphocytes, immunoblasts and possibly eosinophils (Plate IIIf). For discussion of whether Lennert's lymphoma constitutes a separate entity, see Kim et al. (1980). The differential diagnosis has been considered above.

10.17.1   Malignant lymphomas unclassifiable

In a small percentage of cases the infiltrations in the bone marrow cannot be classified, in which case multiparameter enzyme and marker studies must be applied (Warnke et al., 1983; Bain, 1983), if a definite diagnosis is not obtained from examination of a lymph node, or peripheral blood, and when a distinction between lymphoid and other malignancies must be made.

'Malignant lymphomas' of true histiocytic, i.e. macrophage/monocyte, origin have recently been characterized by Isaacson et al. (1983a). The single most reliable criterion was a positive reaction for α_1 anti-trypsin.

10.18   Histological variations of LPD in the bone marrow

Occasionally different cell types are found together in a single biopsy, for example malignant lymphoma or myelodysplasia together with multiple myeloma (Greenberg et al., 1983; Mufti et al., 1983; Kontozoglou and Skinnider, 1983). Concurrent LPD and MPD may also be observed. Conversion to a different cell type (Erickson et al., 1981) or subsequent development of another neoplasia (MPD or other) is occasionally seen if sequential biopsies are taken during the course of the patient's disease. Likewise, coexistence of different patterns (Warnke et al., 1977) or changes from one pattern to another (e.g. nodular to diffuse) or transformation from a cytic to a blastic type may be documented in follow-up biopsies (Hubbard et al., 1982); for example, Richter's syndrome in CLL (Harousseau et al., 1981). In addition, phagocytic histiocytosis may accompany the terminal stages of a lymphoid malignancy, and the question as to whether this is a reactive or malignant histiocytosis has not yet been settled (Manoharan et al., 1981b).

10.19   Heavy chain diseases

The bone marrow may be hyper-cellular, with increases in plasma cells, and/or in lymphocytes, immunoblasts, eosinophils, and occasionally there may be amyloid deposits.

10.19.1   Gamma heavy chain disease

This occurs in the elderly and resembles a malignant lymphoma with lymphadenopathy and hepato-splenomegaly. The bone marrow shows plasmacytosis, lymphocytosis, increases in histiocytes and eosinophils, and usually also lytic bone lesions. No specific histopathological pattern has been observed (Wester *et al.*, 1982).

10.19.2   Alpha heavy chain disease

This occurs in two types.

(1) Mediterranean lymphoma, in which there is an infiltration of the lamina propria of the intestine by lymphocytes, plasma cells and histiocytes and a similar infiltrate may be found in the bone marrow. Three histological categories have been distinguished, and the invasive lymphoma is thought to be of follicle centre cell type (Isaacson *et al.*, 1983b).

(2) Respiratory tract involvement in which the infiltrate occurs in the respiratory tract.

10.19.3   Mu chain disease

This may accompany CLL. Vacuolated plasma cells may be found in the bone marrow in this condition.

Discordance between the expression of malignant lymphomas in lymph nodes and at other sites in the body occurs in a certain number of cases; in one large series investigated by us, it was relatively rare (see Table 10.8).

10.20   Trabecular bone involvement

The presence of an LPD in the bone marrow almost invariably has some effect on the trabecular bone (Plate IX). The most striking and serious complications are generally seen in MM and in centrocytic lymphomas, though osteolytic lesions with or without accompanying hypercalcaemia may occur in any LPD. An early biopsy may give warning of increased osseous remodelling, so that measures may be taken to avoid osteolysis and hypercalcaemia. Frequently, however, the picture may be one of osteopenia or osteoporosis on X-ray.

10.21   Effects of therapy

Of several hundreds of patients examined after treatment, either short or long term, none of those who had involvement in the initial bone biopsy were entirely free of it in subsequent biopsies, even when considerable reduction of the tumour cell burden had been achieved, provided that biopsies of adequate size were examined.

References

Aisenberg, A. C. (1983), Cell lineage in lymphoproliferative disease. *Am. J. Med.*, **74**, 679–85.

Baccarani, M., Cavo. M., Gobbi, M., Laurie, F. and Tura, S. (1982), Staging of chronic lymphocytic leukemia. *Blood*, **6**, 1191–6.

Bain, G. O. (1983), Non-Hodgkin's lymphomas. Analysis of 92 cases using the 'International' classification. *Arch. Pathol. Lab. Med.*, **107**, 64–9.

Bartl, R., Frisch, B. and Burkhardt, R. (1982a). *Bone Marrow Biopsies Revisited. A New Dimension for Haematologic Malignancies*, Karger, Basel.

Bartl, R., Frisch, B., Burkhardt, R., Huhn, D. and Pappenberger, R. (1982b). Assessment of bone marrow histology in Hodgkin's disease: correlation with clinical factors. *Brit. J. Haematol.*, **51**, 345–60.

Bartl, R., Frisch, B., Mahl, G., Burkhardt, R., Fateh-Moghadam, A., Pappenberger, R., Sommerfeld, W. and Hoffmann-Fezer, G. (1983a), Bone marrow histology in Waldenstroem's macroglobulinaemia. Clinical relevance of subtype recognition. *Scand. J. Haematol.*, **31**, 359–75.

Bartl, R., Frisch, B., Hill, W., Burkhardt, R., Sommerfeld, W. and Sund, M. (1983b), Bone marrow histology in hairy cell leukemia: identification of subtypes and their prognostic significance. *Am. J. clin. Pathol.*, **79**, 531–45.

Bartl, R., Frisch, B., Burkhardt, R., Jäger, K., Pappenberger, R. and Hoffmann-Fezer, G. (1984), Lymphoproliferations in the bone marrow: identification and evolution, classification and staging. *J. clin. Path.*, **37**, 233–54.

Benjamin, D., Magrath, I. T., Douglass, E. C. and Corash, L. M. (1983), Derivation of lymphoma cell lines from microscopically normal bone marrow in patients with undifferentiated lymphomas: evidence of occult bone marrow involvement. *Blood*, **61**, 1017–19.

Berg, J. A. (1976), The incidence of multiple primary cancers. I. Development of further cancers in patients with lymphomas, leukemia, and myeloma. *J. natl. Cancer Inst.*, **38**, 741–57.

Bergsagel, D. E. (1982), Plasma cell neoplasms and acute leukaemia. *Clin. Haematol.*, **11**, 221–34.

Berrebi, A., Talmor, M. Vorst, E., Resnitzky, P. and Shtalrid, M. (1983), IgM lambda globular cytoplasmic inclusions in chronic lymphocytic leukaemia resembling immunocytoma. *Scand. J. Haematol.*, **30**, 43–9.

Bluming, A. Z., Cohen, H. G. and Saxon, A. (1979), Angioimmunoblastic lymphadenopathy with dysproteinemia. A pathogenetic link between physiologic lymphoid proliferation and malignant lymphoma. *Am. J. Med.*, **67**, 421–8.

Brisbane, J. U., Berman, L. D., Osband, M. E. and Neiman, R. E. (1983), T8 chronic lymphocytic leukemia: a distinctive disorder related to T8 lymphocytosis. *Am. J. clin. Pathol.*, **80**, 391–6.

Brunning, R. D. and McKenna, R. W. (1979), Bone marrow manifestations of malignant lymphoma and lymphoma-like conditions. In *Pathology Annual, Part 1* (eds S. C. Sommers, and P. P. Rosen), Appleton-Century-Crofts, New York, pp. 1–59.

Carbone, P. P., Kaplan, H. S., Musshoff, K., Smithers, D. W. and Tubiana, M. (1971), Reports of the committee on Hodgkin's disease staging classification. *Cancer Res.*, **31**, 1860–1.

Castellani, R., Bonadonna, G., Spinelli, P., Bajetta, E., Galante, E. and Rilke, F. (1977), Sequential pathologic staging of untreated non-Hodgkin's lymphomas by laparoscopy and laparotomy combined with marrow biopsy. *Cancer*, **40**, 2322–8.

Catovsky, D., Bernasconi, C., Verdonck, P. J., Postma, A., Hows, J., van der Does-van den Berg, A., Rees, J. K. H., Castelli, G., Morra, E. and Galton, D. A. G. (1980), The association of eosinophilia with lymphoblastic leukaemia or lymphoma: a study of seven patients. *Brit. J. Haematol.*, **45**, 523–34.

Catovsky, D., Costello, C., Loukopoulos, D., Fessas, P. R., Foxley, J. M., Traub, N. W., Mills, M. J. and O'Brien, M. (1981), Hairy cell leukemia and myelomatosis: chance association or clinical manifestations of the same B-cell disease spectrum. *Blood*, **57**, 758–63.

Cossman, J., Schnitzer, B. and Deegan, M. J. (1978), Coexistence of two lymphomas with distinctive histologic, ultrastructral, and immunologic features. *Am. J. clin. Pathol.*, **70**, 409–15.

Crocker, J., Jones, E. L. and Curran, J. C. (1983), Study of nuclear sizes in the centres of malignant and benign lymphoid follicles. *J. clin. Pathol.*, **36**, 1332–4.

Damber, L., Lenner, P. and Lundgren, E. (1982), The impact of growth pattern on survival in non-Hodgkin's lymphomas classified according to Lukes and Collins. *Path. Res. Pract.*, **174**, 42–52.

Dosoretz, D. E., Raymond, A. K., Murphy, G. F., Doppke, K. P., Schiller, A. L., Wang, C. C. and Suit, H. D. (1982), Primary lymphoma of bone. The relationship of morphologic diversity to clinical behaviour. *Cancer*, **50**, 1009–14.

Economopoulos, T., Fotopoulos, S., Hatzioannou, J. and Gardikas, C. (1982), 'Prolymphocytoid' cells in chronic lymphocytic leukaemia and their prognostic significance. *Scand. J. Haematol.*, **28**, 238–42.

Emmerich, B., Pemsl, M., Wüst, I., Berdel, W. E., Lechner, S., Thiel, E., Georgii, A., Gössner, W. and Rastetter, J. (1983), Conversion of an IGM secreting immunocytoma in a high grade malignant lymphoma of immunoblastic type. *Blut*, **46**, 81–4.

Erickson, D. J., Cousar, J. B., Flenner, J. M. et al. (1981), Transformation of follicular center cell (FCC) lymphomas (Lukes–Collins classification): progression of small cleaved cell (SCC) type to transformed cell type. *Lab. Invest.*, **44**, 16A.

Ershler, W. B., Moore, A. L., Burns, S. L. and Tindle, B. H. (1983), Immunoblastic lymphadenopathy: failure of, rather than lack of immunoregulation. *J. Med.*, **14**, 81–94.

Falini, B., deSolas, I., Levine, A. M., Parker, J. W., Lukes, R. J. and Taylor, C. R. (1982), Emergence of B-immunoblastic sarcoma in patients with multiple myeloma: a clinicopathologic study of 10 cases. *Blood*, **59**, 923–33.

Falini, B. and Taylor, C. R. (1983), New developments in immunoperoxidase techniques and their application. *Arch. Pathol. Lab. Med.*, **107**, 105–117.

Fine, J. M., Lambin, P., Massari, M. and Leroux, Ph. (1982), Malignant evolution of asymptomatic monoclonal IgM after seven and fifteen years in two siblings of a patient with Waldenström's macroglobulinemia. *Acta Med. Scand.*, **211**, 237–9.

Freemont, A. J. (1983), A possible route for lymphocyte migration into diseased tissues. *J. clin. Pathol.*, **36**, 161–6.

Glimelius, B., Hagberg, H. and Sundström, C. (1983), Morphological classification of non-Hodgkin malignant lymphoma. II. Comparison between Rappaport's classification and the Kiel classification. *Scand. J. Haematol.*, **30**, 13–24.

Gordon, D. S., Jones, B. M., Browning, S. W., Spira, T. J. and Lawrence, D. N. (1982), Persistent polyclonal lymphocytosis of B lymphocytes. *New Engl. J. Med.*, **307**, 232–6.

Greenberg, B. R., MIller, C., Cardiff, R. D., Mackenze, M. R. and Walling, P. (1983), Concurrent development of preleukaemic, lymphoproliferative and plasma cell disorders. *Brit. J. Haematol.*, **53**, 125–33.

Greipp, P. R. and Kyle, R. A. (1983), Clinical, morphological and cell kinetic differences among multiple myeloma, monoclonal gammopathy of undetermined significance and smoldering multiple myeloma. *Blood*, **62**, 166–71.

Grossman, B., Schechter, G. P., Horton, J. E., Pierce, L., Jaffe, E. and Wahl, L. (1981), Hypercalcaemia associated with T-cell lymphomaleukemia. *Am. J. clin. Pathol.*, **75**, 149–55.

Guarda, L. A. and Butler, J. J. (1983), Lymphoma versus AIDS. *Am. J. clin. Pathol.*, **80**, 546.

Harousseau, J. L., Flandrin, G., Tricot, G., Brouet, J. C., Seligmann, M. and Bernard, J. (1981), Malignant lymphoma supervening in chronic lymphocytic leukemia and related disorders. Richter's syndrome: a study of 25 cases. *Cancer*, **48**, 302–8.

Harris, N. L. and Bhan, A. K. (1983), Distribution of T-cell subsets in follicular and diffuse lymphomas of B-cell type. *Am. J. Patol.*, **113**, 172–80.

Hashimoto, M., Masanori, H. and Tsukasa, S. (1957), Lymphoid nodules in human bone marrow. *Acta Pathol. Jap.*, **7**, 33–52.

Heymer, B., Kruger, G., Arnold, R., Schmeiser, T., Friedrich, W., Kubanek, B. and Heimpel, H. (1983), GvH-reaction and morphology of bone marrow after allogenic bone marrow transplantation. *Verh. Dtsch. Ges. Path.*, **67**, 367–71.

Hubbard, S. M., Chabner, B. A., DeVita, V.Tr. Jr, Simon, R., Berard, C., Jones, R. B., Garvin, A. J., Canellos, G. P., Osborne, C. K. and Young, R. C. (1982), Histologic progression in Hodgkin's lymphoma. *Blood*, **59**, 258–64.

Huhn, D., Thiel, R., Rodt, H., Schlimok, G., Theml, H. and Richer, P. (1983), Subtypes of T cell chronic lymphatic leukemia. *Cancer*, **51**, 1434–983.

Humphrey, D. M., Cortez, E. A. and Spiva, D. A. (1982), Immunohistologic studies of cytoplasmic immunoglobulins in rheumatic diseases including two patients with monoclonal patterns and subsequent lymphoma. *Cancer*, **49**, 2049–69.

Hyman, G. A. (1969), Increased incidence of neoplasia in association with chronic lymphocytic leukemia. *Scand. J. Haematol.*, **6**, 98–104.

Isaacson, P., Dennis, M., Wright, J. and Jones, D. B. (1983a), Malignant lymphoma of true histiocytic (monocyte macrophage) origin. *Cancer*, **51**, 80–91.

Isaacson, P., Al-Dewachi, H. S. and Mason, D. Y. (1983b), Middle eastern intestinal lymphoma, a morphological and immunohistochemical study. *J. clin. Pathol.*, **36**, 489–98.

Jacquillat, C., Auclerc, G., Auclerc, M. F., Andrieu, J. M., Weil, M. and Bernard, J. (1981), Hodgkin's disease characteristics and prognosis of forms with initial bone marrow involvement. *Nouv. Presse Med.*, **10**, 95–100.

Kadin, M. E., Kamoun, M. and Lamberg, J. (1981), Erythrophagocytic T$_\gamma$ lymphoma. A clinicopathologic entity resembling malignant histiocytosis. *New Engl. J. Med.*, **304**, 648–53.

Kadin, M. E., Berard, C. W., Nanba, K. and Wakasa, H. (1983), Lymphoproliferative diseases in Japan and Western Countries. *Human Pathol.*, **14**, 745–72.

Kim, H., Nathwani, B. N. and Rappaport, H. (1980), So-called 'Lennert's Lymphoma' is it a clinico-pathological entity? *Cancer*, **45**, 1379–99.

Kontozoglou, T. and Skinnider, L. F. (1983), Concurrent appearance of multiple myeloma with other B-cell lymphoid neoplasms. *Arch. Pathol. Lab. Med.*, **107**, 232–4.

Krause, J. R. (1981), Lymphoproliferative disorders. In: *Bone Marrow Biopsy* (ed. J. R. Krause), Churchill Livingstone, Edinburgh.

Lennert, K. (1981), *Histopathologie der Non-Hodgkin-Lymphome*, Springer-Verlag, Berlin.

Lennert, K., Knecht, H. and Burkert, M. (1979), Prelymphomas. *Verh. Dsch. Ges. Path.*, **63**, 170–96.

Lennert, K. and Burkert, M. (1980), Lymphoplasmacytic/lymphoplasmacytoid lymphoma (LP Immunocytoma). In: *Malignant Lymphoproliferative Diseases* (eds J. G. van den Tweel *et al.*), Martinus Nijhoff, The Hague, pp. 245–7.

Lennert, K., Collins, R. D. and Lukes, R. J. (1983), Concordance of the Kiel and Lukes–Collins classifications of non-Hodgkins lymphomas. *Histopathology*, **7**, 549–59.

Levine, A. M., Pavlova, Z., Pockros, A. W., Parker, J. W., Teitelbaum, A. H., Paganini-Hill, A., Powards, D. R., Lukes, R. J. and Feinstein, D. I. (1983), Small noncleaved follicular center cell (FCC) lymphoma: Burkitt and non-Burkitt variants in the United States. *Cancer*, **52**, 1073–9.

Levy, N., Nelson, J., Mayer, P., Lukes, J. and Parker, J. W. (1983), Reactive lymphoid hyperplasia with single class (monoclonal) surface immunoglobulin. *Am. J. clin. Pathol.*, **80**, 300–8.

Lukes, R. J. (1971), Criteria for involvement of lymph node, bone marrow, spleen and liver in Hodgkin's disease. *Cancer Res.*, **31**, 1733–6.

Lukes, R. J. and Tindle, B. H. (1975), Immunoblastic lymphadenopathy. A hyperimmune entity resembling Hodgkin's disease. *New Engl. J. Med.*, **292**, 1–8.

Magrath, I. T. (1981), Lymphocyte differentiation: an essential basis for the comprehension of lymphoid neoplasia. *J. nat. Cancer Inst.*, **67**, 501–14.

Mahmoud, L. A., Block, M. H., Franks, J. J. and Sayed, N. M. (1983), Marrow biopsy and survival in multiple myeloma. *Am. J. clin. Pathol.*, **80**, 363–9.

Manoharan, A., Catovsky, D., Clein, P., Traub, H. F., Costello, C., O'Brien, M., Boralossa, H. and Galton, D. A. G. (1981a), Simultaneous or spontaneous occurrence of lympho and myeloproliferative disorders: a report of 4 cases. *Brit. J. Haematol.*, **48**, 111–16.

Manoharan, A., Catovsky, D., Lampert, I. A., Al-Mashadhani, Gordon-Smith, E. C. and Galton, D. A. G. (1981b), Histiocytic medullary reticulosis complicating chronic lymphocytic leukaemia: malignant or reactive? *Scand. J. Haematol.*, **26**, 5–13.

Mead, J. H. and Mason, T. E. (1983), Lymphoma versus AIDS. *Am. J. clin. Pathol.*, **80**, 546–7.

Mufti, G. J., Hamblin, T. J., Clein, G. P. and Race, C. (1983), Coexistent myelodysplasia and plasma cell neoplasia. *Brit. J. Haematol.*, **54**, 91–6.

Müller-Hermelink, H. K. and Sale, G. E. (1983), Pathological findings in human bone marrow transplantation. *Verh. Dtsch. Ges. Path.*, **67**, 335–61.

Myers, C. E., Chabner, B. A., Vita, V. T. de and Gralnick, H. R. (1974), Bone marrow involvement in Hodgkin's disease: pathology and response to MOPP chemotherapy. *Blood*, **44**, 197–204.

Nathwani, B. N., Metter, G. E., Gams, R. A., Bartolucci, A. A., Hartsock, R. J., Neiman, R. S., Byrne, G. E., Barcos, M., Kim, H. and Rappaport, H. (1983), Malignant lymphoma, mixed cell type, diffuse. *Blood*, **62**, 200–8.

Newcom, S. R. and O'Rourke, L. (1982), Potentiation of fibroblast growth by nodular sclerosing Hodgkin's disease cell cultures. *Blood*, **60**, 228–37.

Pabst, R., Kaatz, M. and Westermann, J. (1983), In situ labelling of bone marrow lymphocytes with fluorescein isothiocyanate for lymphocyte migration studies in pigs. *Scand. J. Haematol.*, **31**, 267–74.

Pangalis, G. A., Moran, E. M. and Rappaport, H. (1978), Blood and bone marrow findings in angioimmunoblastic lymphadenopathy. *Blood*, **51**, 71–83.

Papayannis, A. G., Nikiforakis, E. and Anagnostou-Keramida, D. (1982), Development of chronic lymphocytic leukaemia in a patient with polycythaemia vera. *Scand. J. Haematol.*, **29**, 65–9.

Paterson, A. D., Kanis, J. A., Cameron, E. C. *et al.* (1983), The use of dichloromethylene diphosphonate for the management of hypercalcaemia in multiple myeloma. *Brit. J. Haematol.*, **54**, 121–32.

Pizzolo, G., Chilosi, M., Ambrosetti, G., Semenzato, L., Fiore-Donati, L. and Perona, G. (1983), Immunohistologic study of bone marrow involvement in B-chronic lymphocytic leukaemia. *Blood*, **62**, 1289–96.

Price, J. (1983), Kawasaki syndrome. *Brit. med. J.*, **288**, 262–3.

Ralfkiaer, E., Geisler, C. Hansen, M. M. and Hou-Jensen, K. (1983), Nuclear clefts in chronic lymphocytic leukaemia. A light microscopic and ultrastructural study of a new prognostic parameter. *Scand. J. Haematol.*, **30**, 5–12.

Redmond, J., Stites, D. P., Beckstead, J. H., George, C. B., Casavant, C. H. and Grandara, D. R. (1983), Chronic lymphocytic leukemia with osteolytic bone lesions, hypercalcemia, and monoclonal protein. *Am. J. clin. Pathol.*, **79**, 616–20.

Robb-Smith, A. H. T. and Taylor, C. R. (1981), *Lymph Node Biopsy*, Heyden, London.

Rywlin, A. M., Ortega, R. S. and Dominguez, G. J. (1974), Lymphoid nodules of bone marrow, normal and abnormal. *Blood*, **43**, 389–400.

Schauer, P. D., Straus, D. J., Bagley, C. M. *et al.* (1981), Angioimmunoblastic lymphadenopathy: clinical spectrum of disease. *Cancer*, **48**, 2493–8.

Schnaidt, U., Vykoupil, K. F., Thiele, J. and Georgii, A. (1980), Angioimmunoblastic lymphadenopathy. Histopathology of bone marrow involvement. *Virchows Arch. (Pathol. Anat.)*, **389**, 369–80.

Skinnider, L. F., Tan, L., Schmidt, J. and Armitage, G. (1982), Chronic lymphocytic leukemia. A review of 745 cases and assessment of clinical staging. *Cancer*, **50**, 2951–5.

Sousa, M. de. (1981), *Lymphocyte Circulation: Experimental and Clinical Aspects*, John Wiley, Chichester.

Spagnolo, D. V., Papadimitriou, J. M., Matz, L. R. and Walters, M. N. I. (1982), Nodular lymphomas with intracellular immunoglobulin inclusions: report of three cases and a review. *Pathology*, **14**, 415–27.

Stern, N., Shemesh, J. and Ramot, B. (1981), Chronic lymphatic leukemia terminating in acute myeloid leukemia: review of the literature. *Cancer*, **47**, 1849–51.

Straus, D. J., Filippa, D. A., Lieberman, P. H., Koziner, B., Thaler, H. T. and Clarkson, B. D. (1983), The non-Hodgkin's lymphomas: a retrospective clinical and pathologic analysis of 499 cases diagnosed between 1958 and 1969. *Cancer,* **51,** 101–9.

Suchman, A. L., Coleman, M., Mouradien, J. A., Wolf, D. J. and Saletan, S. (1981), Aggressive plasma cell myeloma. A terminal phase. *Arch. int. Med.,* **141,** 1315–20.

Su-Ming Hsu, Yan, K. and Jaffe, E. S. (1983), Hairy cell leukaemia: A B cell neoplasm with a unique antigenic phenotype. *Am. J. clin. Pathol.,* **80,** 421–8.

Taylor, C. R., Parker, J. W., Pattengale, P. K. and Lukes, R. J. (1979), Malignant lymphomas: an exercise in immunopathology. In: *Leukemia and non-Hodgkin-lymphoma. Advances in Medical Oncology. Research and Education, Vol VII* (ed. D. G. Crowther), Pergamon Press, Oxford, pp. 125–40.

Tubbs, R. R., Fishleider, A., Weiss, R. A., Sebek, A. and Weick, J. K. (1983), Immunohistologic cellular phenotypes of lymphoproliferative disorders. Comprehensive evaluation of 564 cases including 257 non-Hodgkin's lymphomas classified by the international working formulation. *Am. J. Pathol.,* **113,** 207–21.

Waldenström, J. G. (1982), The benign monoclonal gammapathies: a study of monoclonal antibodies. In: *Advances in Internal Medicine and Pediatrics, Vol. 50* (eds P. Frick *et al.*). Springer Verlag, Berlin, pp. 31–77.

Warner, T. F. C. S. and Krueger, R. G. (1978), Circulating lymphocytes and the spread of myeloma: review of the evidence. *Lancet,* **i,** 1174–6.

Warnke, R. A., Gatter, K. C., Falini, B., Hildreth, P., Woolston, R.-E., Pulford, K., Cordell, J. L., Cohen, B., Wolfe-Peeters, C. de and Mason, D. Y. (1983), Diagnosis of human lymphoma with monoclonal antileukocyte antibodies. *New Eng. J. Med.,* **309,** 1275–81.

Warnke, R. A., Kim, H., Fuks, Z. and Dorfman, R. F. (1977), The coexistence of nodular and diffuse patterns in nodular non-Hodgkin's lymphomas. Significance and clinicopathologic correlation. *Cancer,* **40,** 1229–33.

Wester, S. M., Banks, P. M. and Li, C. Y. (1982), The histopathology of heavy-chain disease. *Am. J. clin. Pathol.,* **78,** 427–36.

Wintrobe, M. M. (1981), *Clinical Hematology,* 8th edn., Lea and Febiger, Philadelphia.

Woda, B. A. and Knowles, D. M. (1979), Nodular lymphocytic lymphoma eventuating into diffuse histocytic lymphoma. Immunoperoxidase demonstration of monoclonality. *Cancer,* **43,** 303–7.

Wright, D. H. (1982), The identification and classification of non-Hodgkin's lymphoma: a review. *Diag. Histopathol.,* **5,** 73–111.

Wright, D. H. and Isaacson, P. G. (1983), *Biopsy Pathology of the Lympho-reticular System,* Chapman and Hall, London.

Zalcberg, J. R., Cornell, F. N., Ireton, H. J. C., McGrath, K. M., McLachlan, R., Woodruff, R. K. and Wiley, J. S. (1982), Chronic lymphatic leukemia developing in a patient with multiple myeloma. Immunologic demonstration of a clonally distinct second malignancy. *Cancer,* **50,** 594–7.

Zucker-Franklin, D., Amorosi, E. L. and Ritz, N. D. (1982), Evolution of Sezary syndrome in the course of hairy cell leukemia. *Blood,* **59,** 1181–90.

11 Reticulo-endothelial mononuclear phagocyte system (macrophages, monocytes)

11.1 Storage diseases

Most storage diseases are inherited, and are the results of enzyme deficiencies, as a consequence of which the incompletely metabolized products of catabolism accumulate in the cells of the reticulo-endothelial system. Many of these products are derived from lipids of the cell membrane.

11.2 Gaucher's disease

Three forms have been described: the infantile, the juvenile, and the adult, based on the time of appearance of the disease, which in turn is connected to the level of enzymic activity retained by the affected cells. The adult type is the most frequent. Gaucher's disease is due to deficiency of the enzyme beta glycocerebrosidase, a lysosomal glucosidase, which splits beta glucosecerebroside (Peters *et al.*, 1977). Large cerebroside-containing macrophages accumulate in the liver, spleen and bone marrow (Fig. 11.1). There may be pigmentation of the skin and in late stages anaemia, leucopenia or thrombocytopenia. The pancytopenia is due to replacement of the normal bone marrow by the Gaucher cells, and possibly to hypersplenism as a consequence of splenomegaly. The accumulation of the Gaucher cells in the bone marrow also leads to destruction of trabecular bone with the appearance of lytic lesions on radiology. The marrow cavities are widened and the cortical bone may be thinned, with a consequent tendency to pathological fractures.

The Gaucher cell is large, and has the appearance of wrinkled silk or paper, due to the elongated rod-shaped structures it contains; the cytoplasm is acid phosphatase positive. At low magnification the marrow

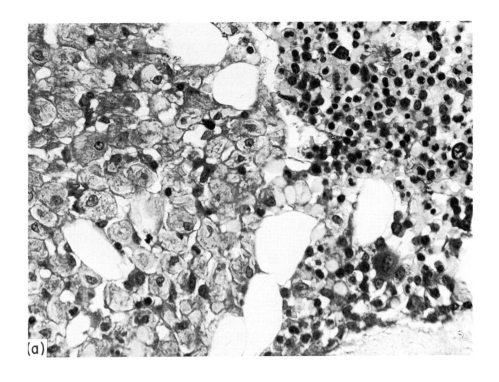

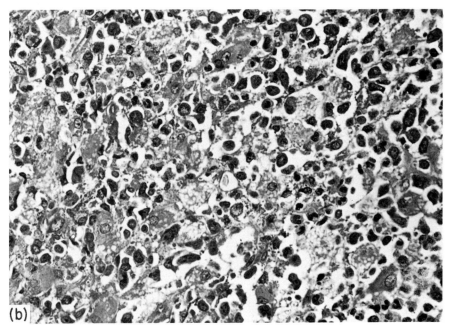

appears hyper-cellular (Fig. 11.1) with loss of fat cells. The Gaucher cells are aggregated in large patches within the marrow cavities or adjacent to the trabeculae which may be attenuated. In the intervening areas there is normal haematopoietic tissue, and between the two, histiocytes in various stages of development to full-blown Gaucher cells will be found. A recent study of immunoglobulin production in Gaucher's disease indicates that there is chronic stimulation of the immune system. At first, this leads to production of polyclonal immunoglobulins and subsequently to the development of monoclonal immunoglobulin and possibly multiple myeloma (Schoenfeld *et al.*, 1982).

11.3   Pseudo-storage or pseudo-Gaucher disease

Cells similar to Gaucher cells in appearance have been observed in the bone marrow in CML, in thalassaemia, after intensive therapy for haematological malignancies (Fig. 11.2), in the CDAs, in tumours (Bhawan *et al.*, 1983) and in other conditions. All have in common a high cellular turnover rate (or destruction), which presumably the macrophage monocyte system cannot cope with, at least temporarily, in some cases (Fig. 11.3).

11.4   Nieman–Pick disease

This most probably represents a heterogeneous group. Most cases occur in infancy and childhood, and the diagnosis is made on clinical grounds. Examination of the bone marrow confirms the diagnosis; there are numerous large foamy cells which have small round eccentric nuclei, and cytoplasm which contains small droplets.

11.5   Fabry's disease

This condition is also called angiokeratoma corporis diffusum universale. It is sex linked (X chromosome) and may be incompletely recessive. There is an inborn error of metabolism of a glycolipid due, according to recent evidence, to the absence of the enzyme alpha galactoside. The result is a storage disease affecting many parenchymal cells (Dawson and Miller, 1983) as well as elements of the mononuclear phagocyte and reticulo-endothelial systems (Plate XIId). The affected cells have a foamy

---

Fig. 11.1   (a) Bone marrow from a case of Gaucher's disease showing aggregate of typical Gaucher cells, left, in various stages of development. × 400, Giemsa; (b) bone marrow from a case of Hand–Schüller–Christian disease; note diffuse infiltration by histiocytes; lymphocytes and plasma cells also present. × 400, Giemsa.

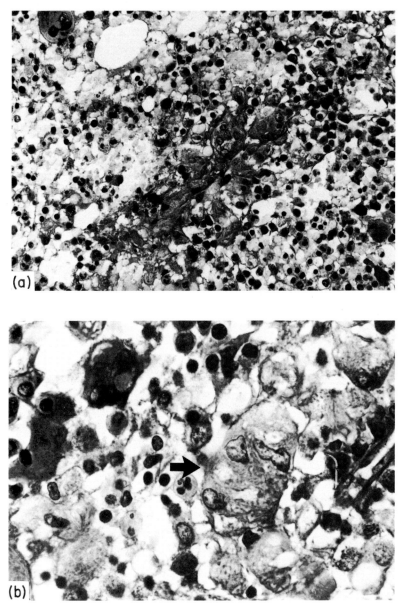

Fig. 11.2 Case of patient with lymphoblastic lymphoma, biopsy taken shortly after intensive chemotherapy; (a) low power view of histiocytes. × 400, Giemsa; (b) histiocytes at high power (arrow). × 1000, Giemsa.

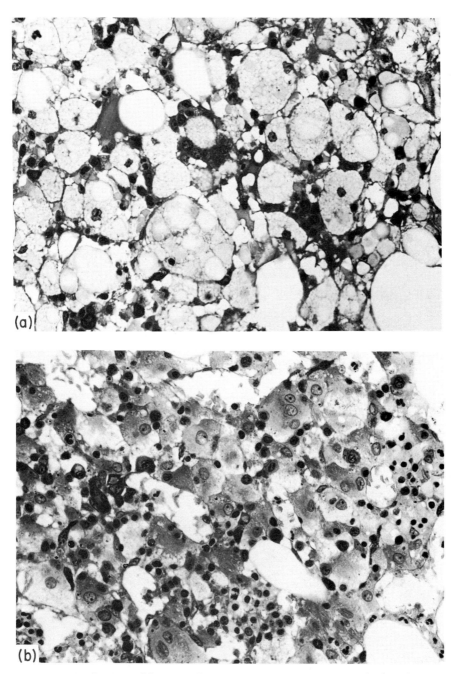

Fig. 11.3 (a) Section of biopsy of patient with prostatic cancer but without metastases in the biopsy, showing aggregate of foam cells. × 400, Giemsa; (b) aggregate of histiocytes in the bone marrow of patient with cytopenia of unclear aetiology, for comparison. × 400, Giemsa.

appearance due to accumulation of metabolic products in the form of laminated whorls.

11.6   Sea-blue histiocytosis

This has been described as an apparently independent condition in which sea-blue coloured inclusions occur in the macrophages in the bone marrow. However, far more frequently such histiocytes are found in the bone marrows of patients with a variety of diseases: thalassaemias, chronic granulomatous disease, CML, megakaryocytic myelosis, polycythaemia vera, histiocytosis, hyperlipoproteinaemia, sickle cell disease, Wolman's disease, sarcoidosis and others. The occurrence of the histiocytes in these disorders is probably due to the overloading of the reticulo-endothelial system, perhaps in the presence of mild (or relative) enzyme deficiency.

11.7   Disorders involving lipid storage

In the hyperlipidaemias (including alpha lipoprotein deficiency and hyper-beta lipoproteinaemia), accumulations of cholesterol or cholesterol esters occur in macrophages in the bone marrow (Plate XIIe–f) as well as in various other organs (Fig. 11.4). Consequently, bone marrow biopsies

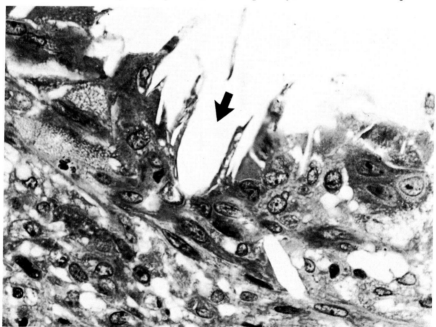

Fig. 11.4   Bone marrow section of patient with xanthomatosis; the cholesterol has been dissolved out of the cells leaving empty spaces (arrow). × 800, Giemsa.

may provide, or confirm, the diagnosis. These macrophages are large, round, multi-loculated, and have small eccentric nuclei. Similar macrophages are also observed in the bone marrow in poorly controlled diabetes, in hypothyroidism, and in dietary hypercholesterolaemia. The mechanism controlling the deposition of cholesterol or its esters is not known.

Cholesterol embolism from atherosclerotic plaques has been observed in the bone marrow in about 20% of proven cases (Pierce et al., 1978).

11.8   Histiocytosis X (Plate XIf; Fig. 11.1)

Included under this heading are eosinophilic granuloma, Hand–Schül-ler–Christian disease and Letterer–Siwe disease, which are thought to be variants of the same underlying disease process. The aetiology is unknown (hence the designation X), though a disorder of immune regulation is considered a strong possibility. Favara et al. (1983) have postulated that histiocytosis X may be a disorder of suppressor T lymphocyte control of autocytotoxic cells (see also Risdall et al., 1983).

11.8.1   Eosinophilic granuloma

This occurs as a benign lesion of bone and consists of single or multiple infiltrates of mononuclear cells (of the reticulo-endothelial system) and eosinophils (Nauert et al., 1983). On electron microscopy the mononuclear cells have the typical Langerhans-type cytoplasmic inclusions (Birbeck granules). Varying degrees of necrosis and foam cells are also present, as well as multinucleated giant cells and fibrosis, especially during the healing phase. Though eosinophilic granulomas of bone have a higher incidence in males and young people, they may also be found as late as the seventh decade of life. Of particular importance is whether the lesions are uni- or multifocal, as the latter indicates a chronic disorder with generalized manifestations.

11.8.2   Hand–Schüller–Christian disease (HSC)

This occurs mainly in children. There is proliferation of histiocytes which accumulate cholesterol esters (Plate XIIa–b). The lesions also contain eosinophils, plasma cells, lymphocytes and fibroblasts. They are found in the bones, as well as in many other organs. There may be exophthalmos and diabetes insipidus if the orbits and hypothalamus are affected. The course may be prolonged, with survival of up to 10 years.

11.8.3   Letterer–Siwe disease

A pathological picture similar to that in HSC and eosinophilic granuloma is seen. However, the histiocytes have distinct cell membranes, and do not give the appearance of a syncytium, which may occur in the former. The cause is unknown, but it is presumed to have an immunological basis; possibly suppressor cell activity is involved.

11.9   Farquhar's disease (lymphohistiocytosis)

A rare familial disease affecting infants and young children. The principal pathological finding is histiocytosis involving lymph nodes, spleen, and bone marrow; in some cases also brain and meninges are affected. The disease is interpreted by some authors as an acute variant of the Letterer–Siwe syndrome. The disease was first described by Farquhar and Claireaux (1952) and later by Marrian and Sanerkin (1963) under the name of familial haemophagocytic reticulosis, because of the phagocytosis of blood cells by the histiocytes (Plate XIIc). They considered the disease to be a variant of histiocytic medullary reticulosis (Berard *et al.*, 1966; Bell *et al.*, 1968). Favara *et al.* (1983) in their review of all the conditions included under the heading histiocytosis X excluded lymphohistioreticulosis with phagocytosis. The disease is rapidly fatal (within a few weeks) but one case which responded to treatment for 7 months has been reported (Lilleyman, 1980).

11.10   Mastocytosis

Systemic mastocytosis (or generalized mastocytosis) is characterized by a proliferation of mast cells in various organs. Though the cutaneous form is the most common, it also occurs without involvement of the skin (Rohner *et al.*, 1982; Horny *et al.*, 1983a, b). The systemic form with urticaria pigmentosa-like lesions has a better prognosis than the second variant, which has been termed malignant mastocytosis. The bone marrow is involved in both types in over 70% of the cases. The histopathology of the bone marrow is typical (Plate IIIa–b): the highly characteristic feature is the presence of the mast cell granulomas. These are preferentially located in the endosteal and the peri-arterial regions. The granulomas consist largely of mast cells, lymphocytes, plasma cells, eosinophilic granulocytes and sea-green histiocytes within a network of reticulin fibres. The trabecular bone is variably affected and shows osteosclerosis, osteopenia and osteolysis. There may be widespread skeletal osteoporosis. The granulomas range from small to large, and have a tendency to a circular or whorl-like configuration. They may be single, but are usually multiple. There may be normal haematopoietic marrow between the granulomas, or this may be reduced with an increase in fat cells. It has recently been demonstrated that the determination of histamine metabolites in the urine (rather than histamine itself) is a specific and sensitive method for the diagnosis of mastocytosis (Keyzer *et al.*, 1983).

Acute leukaemia may supervene on mastocytosis (Fig. 11.5).

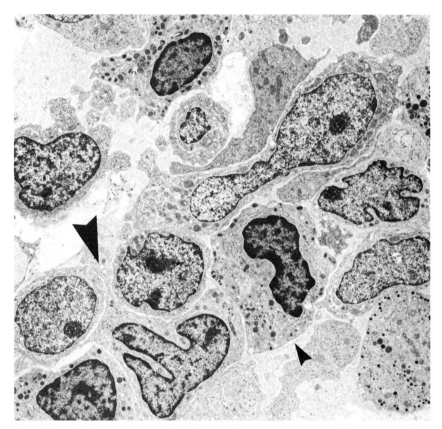

Fig. 11.5 Electron micrograph of bone biopsy of patient with long-standing mastocytosis who developed terminal acute leukaemia; myeloid cells with few granules (small arrow) and leukaemic blasts (large arrow). × 3000.

11.11. Malignant histiocytosis (MH) or histiocytic medullary reticulosis (HMR)

These terms are synonymous and describe a condition characterized by systemic neoplastic proliferation of histologically recognizable histiocytes and their precursors, in the liver, the spleen and bone marrow (Warnke *et al.*, 1975). Lately, however, a virus-associated haemophagocytic syndrome (VAHS) has been recognized which closely resembled HMR or MH both clinically and histologically (Risdall *et al.*, 1979, Editorial, 1983). There is fever, lymphadenopathy, hepato-splenomegaly and pancytopenia. Nevertheless, the disease is presumed to be reactive and at least potentially reversible. Examination of the bone marrow reveals histiocytic hyperplasia with prominent haemophagocytosis (Fig. 11.6). Multinucleated giant cells may also be present and there is disruption of normal architecture, decrease in fat cells, and in haematopoietic tissue.

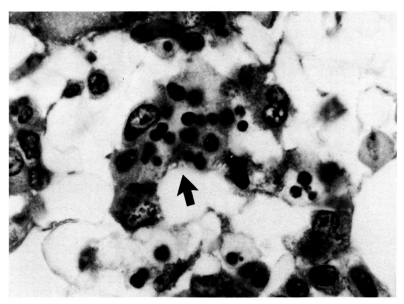

Fig. 11.6   Haemophagocytosis of probable virus association (see text); macrophage containing remnants of numerous nucleated precursors (arrow). × 1200, Giemsa.

Boomsma *et al.* (1983) have shown that angiotensin converting enzyme is present in malignant histiocytes, and that this may be used as an additional parameter for their identification.

Rarely, abnormalities of bone marrow histology simulating histiocytic medullary reticulosis may occur as a concomitant phenomenon in other diseases, for example gastric carcinoma (James *et al.*, 1979); and complicating lymphoproliferative disorders (Manoharan *et al.*, 1981).

The differential diagnosis of histiocytic lesions must also include sinus histiocytosis with massive lymphadenopathy (reviewed by Walker *et al.*, 1981). This is a non-neoplastic, usually self-limited disease, mostly affecting young people, though it may occur at any age. The disease may be accompanied by involvement of the bones, including those of the pelvis. Bone marrow biopsy of a lesion (which appear as lytic foci on X-ray) may show an inflammatory infiltrate consisting of plasma cells, lymphocytes and histiocytes, sometimes with haemophagocytosis.

Kadin *et al.* (1981) have drawn attention to an erythrophagocytic T cell lymphoma with clinical and pathological features resembling malignant histiocytosis. The authors suggested that the tumour cells arose in the spleen, migrated to the lymph nodes and infiltrated other organs, including the bone marrow, as a secondary event. For review of the pathophysiology of the histiocytic disorders see Groopman and Golde (1981); these authors conclude that many of the clinical features, including osteolysis and haemophagocytosis, are mediated by activated macrophages. The cytological and histological distinction between the neoplastic histiocytes of MH (HMR) and the reactive ones of VAHS may be very difficult (if not impossible). Nevertheless, it is clinically very significant as cytotoxic therapy is contra-indicated in VAHS though the viral infection may initiate a condition as rapidly fatal as MH (HMR).

References

Bell, R. J. M., Brafield, A. J. E., Barnes, N. D. and France, N. E. (1968), Familial haemophagocytic reticulosis. *Arch. Dis.Childhood*, **43**, 601–6.

Berard, C. W., Cooper, R. A., Freireich, E. J. and Rabson, A. S. (1966), Disseminated histiocytosis associated with atypical lymphoid cells (lymphohistiocytosis). *Cancer*, **19**, 1429–37.

Bhawan, J., Malhotra, R. and Nail, D. R. (1983), Gaucher-like cells in a granular cell tumor. *Human Pathol.*, **14**, 730–3.

Boomsma, F., Michels, J. J., Prins, E., Abels, J. and Schalekamp, M. A. D. H. (1983), Angiotensin converting enzyme: a tumour marker in malignant histiocytosis. *Brit. med. J.*, **286**, 1106.

Dawson, D. M. and Miller, D. C. (1983), A 47-year-old man with coronary artery disease and variable neurologic abnormalities. *New Engl. J. Med.*, **310**, 106–14.

Editorial (1983), Histiocytic medullary reticulosis. *Lancet*, **1**, 455–6.

Favara, B. E., McCarthy, R. C. and Mierau, G. W. (1983), Histiocytosis X. *Human Pathol.*, **14**, 663–76.

Farquhar, J. W. and Claireaux, A. E. (1952), Familial haemophagocytic reticulosis. *Arch. Dis. Childhood*, **27**, 519–25.

Groopman, J. E. and Golde, D. W. (1981), The histiocytic disorders: a pathophysiologic analysis. *Ann. int. Med.*, **94**, 95–107.

Horny, H. P., Parwaresch, M. R. and Lennert, K. (1983a), Klinisches Bild und Prognose generalisierter Mastozytosen. *Klin. Wochenschr.*, **61**, 785–93.

Horny, H. P., Parwaresch, M. R. and Lennert, K. (1983b), Basophilic leukaemia and generalised mastocytosis. *Verh. Dtsch. Ges. Path.*, **67**, 192–7.

James, L. P., Stass, S. S., Peterson, V. and Schumacher, H. R. (1979), Abnormalities of bone marrow simulating histiocytic medullary reticulosis in a patient with gastric carcinoma. *Am. J. clin. Pathol.*, **71**, 600–2.

Kadin, M. E., Kamoun, M. and Lamberg, J. (1981). Erythrophagocytic T gamma lymphona: a clinicopathologic entity resembling malignant histiocytosis. *New Engl. J. Med.*, **304**, 648–53.

Keyzer, J. J., de Monchy, J. G. R., van Doormal, J. J. and van Voorst Vader, P. C. (1983), Improved diagnosis of mastocytosis by measurement of urinary histamine metabolites. *New Engl. J. Med.*, **309**, 1603–5.

Lilleyman, J. S. (1980), The treatment of familial erythrophagocytic lymphohistiocytosis. *Cancer*, **46**, 468–70.

Manoharan, A., Catovsky, D., Lampert, I. A., Al-Mashadhani, Gordon-Smith, E. C. and Galton, D. A. G. (1981), Histiocytic medullary reticulosis complicating chronic lymphocytic leukaemia: malignant or reactive? *Scand. J. Haematol.*, **26**, 5–13.

Marrian, V. J. and Sanerkin, N. G. (1963), Familial histiocytic reticulosis (familial haemophagocytic reticulosis). *J. clin. Pathol.*, **16**, 65–9.

Nauert, C., Zornoza, J., Ayala, A. and Harle, T. S. (1983), Eosinophilic granuloma of bone: diagnosis and management. *Skeletal Radiol.*, **10**, 227–35.

Peters, S. P., Lee, R. E. and Glew, R. H. (1977), Gaucher's disease, a review. *Medicine*, **56**, 425–42.

Risdall, R. J., McKenna, R. W., Nesbit, M. E., Krivit, W., Balfour, H. H., Simmons, R. L. and Brunning, R. D. (1979), Virus-associated haemophagocytic syndrome: a benign histocytic proliferation distinct from malignant histiocytosis. *Cancer*, **44**, 993–1002.

Risdall, R. J., Dehner, L. P., Duray, P., Krobinsky, N., Robinson, L. and Nesbit, M. E. (1983), Histiocytosis X (Langerhan's cell histiocytosis). *Arch. Pathol. Lab. Med.*, **107**, 59–63.

Rohner, H. G., Bartl, R., Koischwitz, D. and Rodermund, O. E. (1982), Haut-und Knochenbefunde bei der Mastozytose. *Radiologe*, **22**, 545–52.

Pierce, R. J., Wren, M. W. and Consar, J. B. (1978), Cholesterol embolism: diagnosis antemortem by bone marrow biopsy. *Ann. int. Med.*, **89**, 937–8.

Shoenfeld, Y., Gallant, L. A., Shaklai, M., Livni, E., Djaldetti, M. and Pinkhas, J. (1982), Gaucher's disease. A disease with chronic stimulation of the immune system. *Arch. Pathol., Lab. Med.*, **106**, 388–91.

Walker, P. D., Rosai, J. and Dorfman, R. F. (1981), The osseous manifestations of sinus histiocytosis with massive lymphadenopathy. *Am. J. clin. Pathol.*, **75**, 131–9.

Warnke, R. A., Kim, H. and Dorfman, R. F. (1975), Malignant histiocytosis: clinico-pathologic study of 29 cases. *Cancer*, **35**, 215–30.

12 Non-haematological malignancies in the bone marrow

12.1 Metastases and the rate of replication of malignant cells

A tumour cell must divide (or double) 30 times to reach 10^9 cells which is equivalent to a tumour volume of 1 cm^3—the minimal size for clinical detection. Tumour cells dividing once a month would need 30 divisions = 30 months to become clinically detectable. Usually a much longer period has elapsed and the tumours are much larger when the patients seek medical attention. Thus, in almost all patients there has been a considerable time during which metastases could have been formed. This time lag may vary from months to many years—14 as in the case described by Dixon *et al.* (1980); see also Fig. 12.9. Metastases in turn will also require a certain time-lag before becoming clinically evident, and unfortunately there is as yet no reliable test to determine their presence in the early stages of their development (Willis, 1973; Frei, 1974; Weiss, 1976; Springfield, 1982; Finlay *et al.*, 1982; Weiss and Gilbert, 1981). In some cases tumour growth may even be facilitated by cancer therapy.

It is now thought that many primary tumours have the ability to spread as soon as they are established (Adam, 1981; Weiss and Gilbert, 1981), as indicated also by the fact that some remained undetected even at autopsy, though the patients died of widespread metastases (Woods *et al.*, 1980; Steckel and Kagan, 1982). In addition there is a correlation between the site, the size and the properties of the primary tumour and metastasis formation, as for example in cancers of the breast and of the prostate (Kastendieck, 1980; Campbell *et al.*, 1981; Landys, 1982). Moreover, there is some indication that metastatic potential—the tumour cell characteristics—that permit metastases to develop differ in various situations and are amenable to investigation (Carter, 1978; Clarke, 1979). Intravasation (entry of tumour cells into lymphatics or blood vessels) only results in distant metastases if the tumour emboli survive in the bloodstream long enough to be arrested in a blood vessel, to lodge, to grow out into the

243

tissues and to become established at another site. It has long been appreciated that the red, well vascularized, haematopoietic marrow is one of the preferred sites most frequently involved by metastatic cancer after the lungs and the liver (Willis, 1973; Burkhardt *et al.*, 1980; Georgii and Park, 1982). Metastases in bones arise from blood borne tumour emboli arrested in the sinusoids of the red marrow. This sinusoidal system has a large blood flow and a slow perfusion rate. The sinusoids are lined by a discontinuous, often attenuated endothelial layer, lacking tight junctions (Carter, 1982). These conditions are especially favourable for the passage of the tumour cells into the extravascular tissue spaces. Moreover the arrest of the tumour cells and their development into metastases depends on the interaction of the tumour emboli with their environment (Lam *et al.*, 1981; Mundy *et al.*, 1981; Nelson and Nelson, 1981; Woodruff, 1982). The factors involved include: the tumour cell surface properties, the size of the emboli and their homogeneity, the mechanical forces and other aspects of the circulation, the interactions of the tumour cells with host immune cells, with platelets and with other coagulation factors (Donati, 1980; Zacharski *et al.*, 1982), as well as the properties of the endothelium and of the other components of the cell wall (Carr and Underwood, 1974; Hara *et al.*, 1980; Karpatkin and Pearlstein, 1981). When all these aspects are considered, it is not surprising that the red bone marrow provides such a fertile supportive environment for the tumour emboli: the architecture of the marrow vasculature, the megakaryocytes shedding platelets into the sinusoidal lumen, and thus possibly providing platelet derived growth factors, the relatively easy egress from the bloodstream into the tissues, and the provision of other factors which stimulate the metastatic cells by components of the host inflammatory reaction, all of which are present in the bone marrow (Husby *et al.*, 1976; Bassler *et al.*, 1981; Currie, 1981; Rubins, 1983).

12.2   Indications for bone biopsy

In patients with known or suspected malignancies the indications for bone biopsy include the following:

   (1) Part of the initial investigation for staging.
   (2) Because of clinical suspicion of metastases.
   (3) For follow-up and monitoring of therapy.
   (4) Because of anaemia, weakness and fatigue.
   (5) Otherwise unexplained pyrexia.
   (6) Because of hypercalcaemia.
   (7) Raised alkaline phosphatase levels (osseous).

(8) Suspicious areas on X-ray or scan.

(9) When auto-transplantation of bone marrow is contemplated after intensive therapy.

Frequently a cytopenia occurs during the course of treatment and the question arises whether there is therapy-induced hypo- or aplasia or whether there is replacement of the bone marrow by metastases; a bone biopsy will provide the answer in many cases. In addition to these clinical questions, a bone biopsy provides information on the effects of the malignancy on the marrow, the bone, on the reserve capacity of the marrow and on the tumour–host interactions (Joachim, 1976; Burkhardt *et al.*, 1980, 1982; Cohen *et al.*, 1982; Thomas, 1982; Freemont, 1982; Landys, 1982; Rubins, 1983; Carr, 1983; Lang *et al.*, 1983).

In the hypercalcaemia of malignant disease one or more of four mechanisms is involved:

(1) Osteolytic lesions of bone asociated with widespread metastases as in some cases of metastases of carcinomas of breast, thyroid, lung, and in some lymphomas (Plate XIIIe and f).

(2) Osteolysis in the absence of demonstrable osseous metastases, but associated with some carcinomas which elaborate sterols related to vitamin D.

(3) Osteolysis in the absence of demonstrable bony metastases but associated with tumours which appear to secrete a parathyroid-like hormonal substance.

(4) Osteolysis in the absence of demonstrable metastases but in the presence of tumours which secrete some hormonal substance other than PTH or its pro-hormone forms, for example cancers of the lungs, the kidney, uterus, pancreas and colon (Jacobs *et al.*, 1981; Barry *et al.*, 1981; Dady *et al.*, 1981; Galasko, 1982; Burkhardt *et al.*, 1982; Jung *et al.*, 1983; Stewart, 1983).

Thus the production of hypercalcaemia may depend on the involvement of long-range humoral factors produced by the tumour cells, and the direct stimulation of bone resorption (Plate XIIIe and f) by the metastatic deposits in the bones. However, it should be remembered that metastases, especially small ones (Figs 12.1, 12.2, Plate XIIIa, b, c) may be present in the bones in spite of negative X-rays and radionuclide scans as these reflect the sum of the dynamic processes involved—that is both bone formation and bone resorption (Figs 12.3, 12.4, 12.5). In addition, as pointed out by Low (1981), a positive bone scintigraphy is entirely non-specific. Numerous conditions that perturb local bone metabolism will cause a 'hot spot' that represents the localized skeletal response to a fracture, to infection and to humoral stimulation. Moreover, the lytic

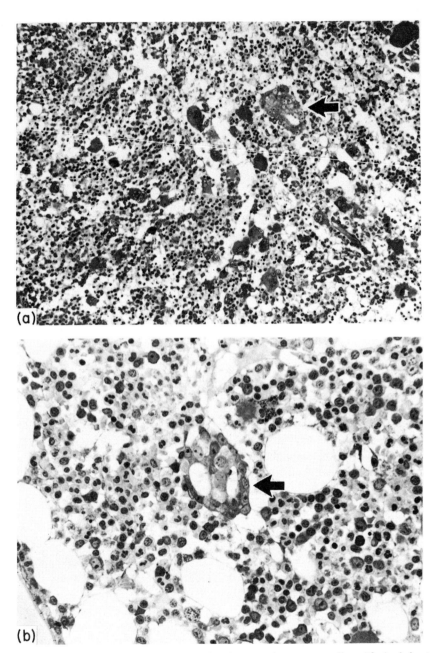

Fig. 12.1 Micrometastases: (a) single cluster of tumour cells with incipient tubular formation (arrow); hyper-cellular marrow; note megakaryocytic hyperplasia. × 250, Giemsa; (b) cluster of tumour cells in sinus, entering interstitial space (at arrow). × 400, Giemsa. Surrounding marrow without obvious reaction. Such micrometastases might easily be overlooked in decalcified and paraffin embedded biopsies, because of the processing and shrinkage.

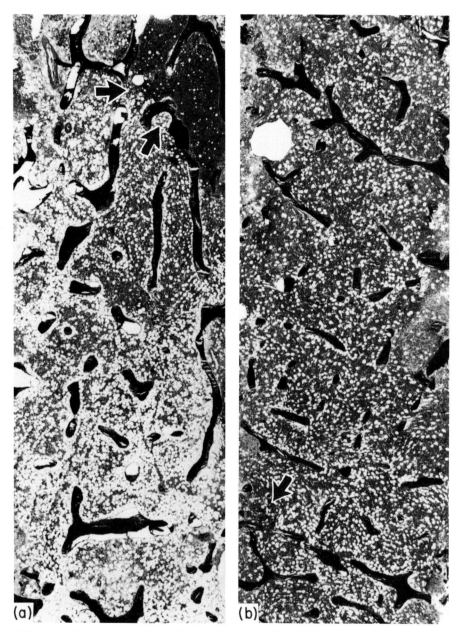

Fig. 12.2 Low power views of biopsy sections of two different biopsies, a and b, to show metastases (arrows). × 10, Gomori. Such metastases would not be detected by other methods.

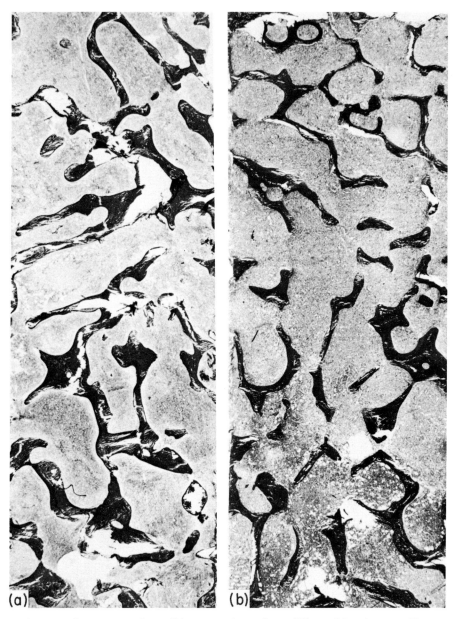

Fig. 12.3 Low power view of biopsy sections of two different biopsies, a and b, to show complete occupation of the marrow cavities by metastases, but with little effect on the trabecular bone. Both × 10, Gomori. Such metastases would give negative X-rays and scans.

component of small metastases as well as early osteolytic foci are not picked up by the X-ray or the scan, and when osseous involvement is detected by iliac crest biopsy, it is fairly safe to assume that in the vast majority of cases this will not be an isolated lesion and the cumulative effect of many such foci throughout the skeleton may well affect the serum calcium levels. This applies especially to tumours such as mammary cancers in which both osseous metastases and hypercalcaemia frequently occur, but no long-range humoral mechanisms have actually been identified (Figs 12.6, 12.7). In these cases the osteolysis is mediated by osteoclast-activating factors (OAF) produced by the neoplastic cells and it may be significantly reduced by therapy with prostaglandin inhibitors and the diphosphonates, or combinations of these two agents.

A raised osseous alkaline phosphatase level is correlated with the presence and activity of osteoblasts, and is frequently observed in prostatic cancer (Fig. 12.8) in men and breast cancer (Fig. 12.9) in women, when a strong osteoblastic reaction has been evoked. In contrast, there is no correlation between the haematological values in the peripheral blood and the size and type of metastases in the bone marrow (Burkhardt *et al.*, 1980).

12.3   Incidence of metastases

In a survey of metastases in autopsy cases, Willis (1973) gave the following incidence for skeletal metastases: cancer of breast and prostate over 75%; thyroid 30–60%; kidney, uterus and bladder up to 50%; lungs up to 40%; neuroblastoma is listed as infrequent, and all others as rare. When all fatal cases are taken together, some series give a figure of 20%, others 30–50% or even more, with careful examination of the bones.

In recent examinations of bone biopsies of 1725 patients with solid tumours (Frisch *et al.*, 1984), the overall involvement found was 35% and the distribution of the metastases according to the primary tumours is given in Table 12.1. The incidence of bone marrow involvement was higher in patients with other indications of dissemination than in those without (Burkhardt *et al.*, 1981). Metastases of occult tumours, and those of prostate, breast and lung comprised 78% of the positive cases, metastases of all other primary tumours together comprised the remaining 22%. Examination of the bone marrow by means of aspirates obtained at primary surgery revealed metastases in 28% of 110 consecutive breast cancer patients (Redding *et al.*, 1983). However, multiple sites were examined. These rates of detection are similar to those reported by other centres where undecalcified bone biopsies are embedded into plastic. Previously published reports of rates of detection differ widely, and most are considerably lower (for references, see Burkhardt *et al.*, 1981). The differences are due to the following factors: (1) the type of the primary tumour, (2) the stage of the disease, (3) the quality of the histological preparation, (4) the size of the biopsy cores. It has previously been shown that an increase in size of the section area available for microscopical examination from 20–30 mm^2 to 30–50 mm^2 increases the yield of positive biopsies by about 10%. Occasionally tumour cells are detected in the blood clot with the biopsy (Plate XIVf).

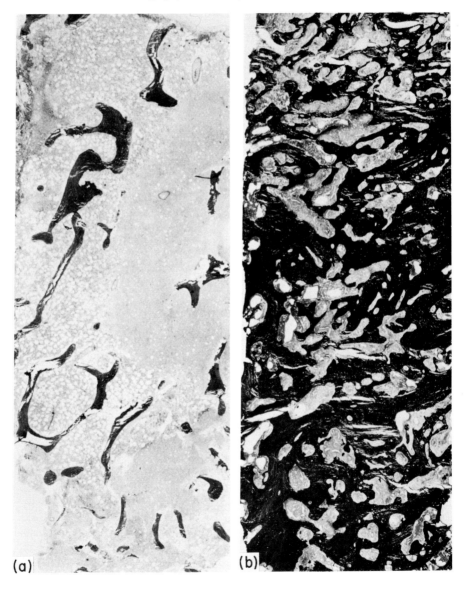

(a)   (b)

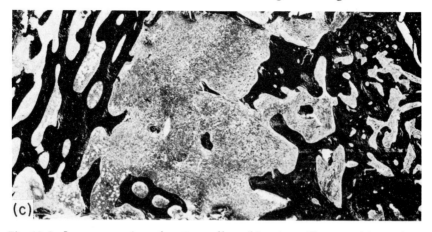

Fig. 12.4   Low power view of sections of bone biopsies to illustrate: (a) osteolytic, (b) osteosclerotic and (c) mixed lytic and sclerotic trabecular bone with metastases. × 10, Gomori.

Table 12.1 Frequency of positive bone marrow biopsies

	No. of patients	No. of positive biopsies	Percentage
Primary tumour			
Breast	504	211	42
Prostate	255	80	32
Lung	389	56	14
Others	294	48	19
Unknown	283	205	72
Biopsy size			
<60 mm^2	1230	357	29
$\geqslant 60$ mm^2	495	243	49
Total	1725	600	35

Bone biopsies in the detection of skeletal metastases have also been investigated by Lang *et al.* (1983) in a meticulous autopsy study of 49 patients who died of breast cancer, and 54 patients who died of broncho-genic carcinoma. They concluded that bilateral posterior iliac crest biop-sies are more effective than single biopsies, and that the length of the biopsy cylinder also has a decisive influence on the rate of detection: 55% in 130 biopsies of less than 25 mm length, and 77% in 46 biopsies over 25 mm in length. Vinceneux *et al.* (1983) reported an incidence of over 50% positive posterior iliac crest biopsies in patients with known primary tumours.

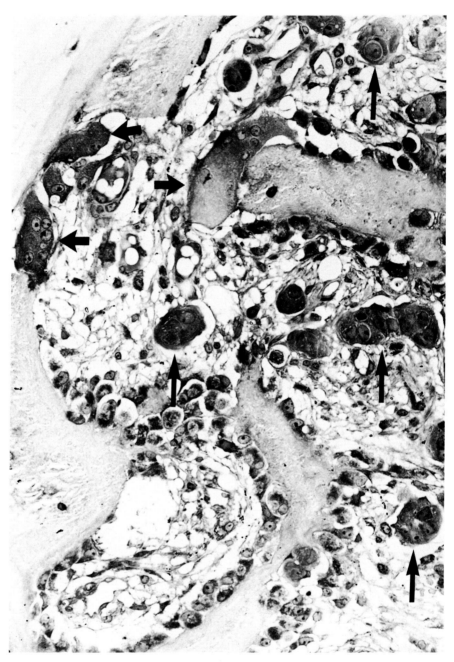

Fig. 12.5 Small groups of tumour cells (long arrows) and mixed osteoclastic (short arrows) and osteoblastic reaction. × 600, Giemsa.

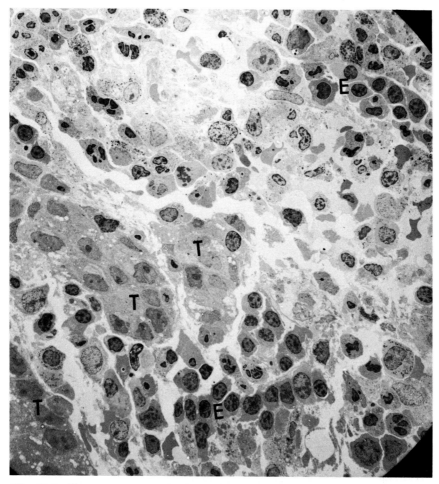

Fig. 12.6   Electron micrograph of bone biopsy of patient with metastases in bone marrow; clusters of tumour cells (T), erythroblasts (E). × 800.

12.4   Histological aspects of metastases

The following histological types are recognized: solid, adenomatous, scirrhous, small cell and mixed; their occurrence in metastases of the various primary tumours is discussed below.

12.4.1   Stroma of the metastases

With the exception of metastatic foci which remain within the vascular system, all metastases are dependent for their successful establishment

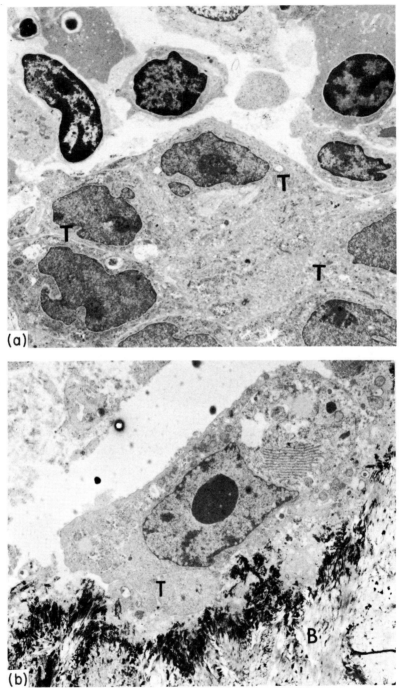

Fig. 12.7 Electron micrographs of bone biopsy of patient with metastatic mammary cancer: (a) group of tumour cells (T) in interstitial space. × 4000; (b) tumour cell (T) on bone in osteolytic lesion. × 6000.

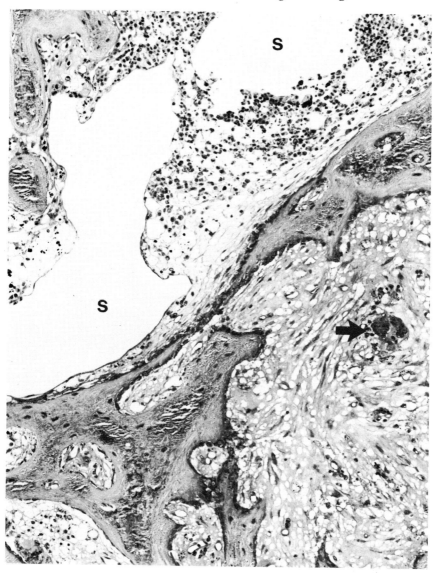

Fig. 12.8   Metastases of prostatic carcinoma (arrow) within acellular marrow, developing fibrosis and osteoblastic new bone formation; two ectatic sinuses (S). × 250, Giemsa.

and continued growth on the stimulation of blood vessels (angiogenesis) from host vessels (Fig. 12.10; Plate XIIId) (Folkman, 1974; Gullino, 1981; Denekamp, 1982). This vascular proliferation is especially prominent at the margins of the invading growths and less so at their centres (Willis,

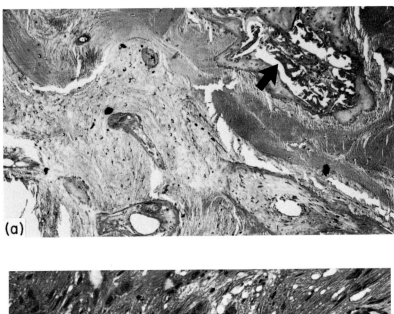

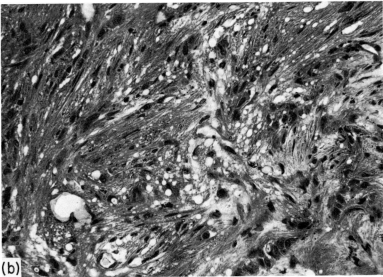

Fig. 12.9 (a) Bone biopsy of patient with bilateral mammary cancer, operated 10 and 11 years previously, no therapy other than mastectomy; the biopsy consisted of sclerotic bone with small marrow cavities filled with connective tissue; only one cavity (arrow) had malignant cells. × 100, Giemsa; (b) bone biopsy section of 48 year old patient (post-mastectomy; no chemotherapy) showing dense connective tissue; tumour cells were only identified in one small area after serial section of the biopsy. × 400, Giemsa.

1973). The structure of these newly formed vessels rarely approaches that of normal veins or arteries; many are irregular channels with scanty perivascular tissue. In some, even the endothelium may be incomplete so that the channels are lined by tumour cells (Peterson, 1979). Others may have pronounced endothelial proliferation (Freemont, 1982). The vascularity of metastases varies greatly—some are richly vascular, others are almost without discernible blood vessels. In some cases the tumour vessels may communicate directly with the arterial blood supply of the host tissues at the periphery of the growths. The adequacy of this peripheral supply is reflected in the proliferation seen at the edges of the tumour, and the inadequacy of that in the deeper areas, by the central necrosis often present. Varying amounts of fibroblasts and fibres (Fig. 12.11) enter with the blood vessels. The proportion of stroma to paren-chyme (the tumour cells) varies greatly from minimal fibrosis accompany-ing the blood vessels, to striking sclerosis that may proceed to total extinction of the tumour in that region (Fig. 12.12). When tumour emboli or cell clusters multiply and expand within the sinusoids the marrow becomes oedematous and almost acellular (Figs 12.13, 12.14). Such areas often extend over several inter-trabecular cavities. The tumour cells themselves may form progressively larger masses, and they may extend along the endothelial surface and line the vascular channels (Fig. 12.13). In these situations large areas of the metastases often become necrotic (Fig. 12.15). The stroma of metastases depends in part on the ability of the tumour cells to differentiate, to produce factors, and to organize them-selves into some sort of structure; this varies even in different parts of the same metastases. It has long been postulated that the host cellular and stromal reactions are elicited by metabolic or secretory products of the tumour cells. Prominent among the substances so far identified are osteoclast and osteoblast (Fig. 12.16), activating factors and angiogenic factors. Other tumour cell products stimulate erythropoiesis, granulopoiesis or thrombopoiesis (Fig. 12.17), and possibly monocytes and lymphocytes. In contrast, inhibitory factors may also be secreted. There is as yet no agreement in the literature concerning the possible function of lymphocytes and other mononuclear cells in host defence mechanisms against neoplasia (Husby et al., 1976; Vose and Moore, 1979; Hartveit, 1981; Daar and Fabre, 1981; Berken, 1982; Key et al., 1982; Haskill et al., 1982; Sokol and Hudson, 1983; Lutz, 1983).

12.5   Bone marrow reactions to metastases

These are found in three situations: (1) within the marrow in the neighbourhood of the metastases, (2) in the marginal area between the metastases and the residual marrow (the interface), and (3) within

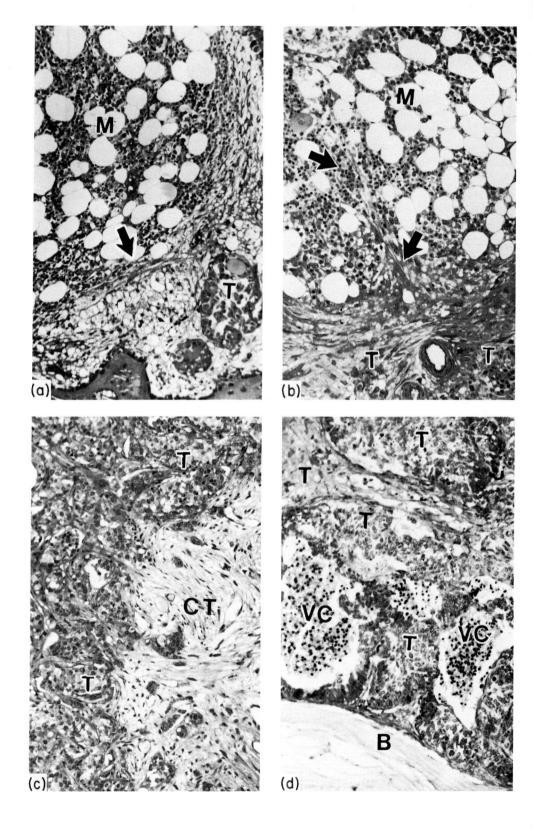

the metastases themselves. These reactions will be considered separately.

12.5.1   *The generalized reaction or tumour myelopathy*

This may be seen in sections containing both metastases and residual bone marrow; in some cases a similar reaction is noted in the bone biopsy in patients with malignancies, but without involvement in the biopsy. The reaction varies greatly from no perceptible morphological change to extensive necrosis of the haematopoietic tissue, or extensive replacement by exudative, almost acellular material. When the marrow is preserved, it may show a decrease in erythropoiesis, an increase in fat cells, plasma cells, iron-containing macrophages and megakaryocytes. Moreover, each of these components may be affected to a different degree.

12.5.2   *The marginal reaction*

This is also highly variable. Rarely, no response occurs at the interface between marrow and tumour cells but usually there is one. This may consist of a zone of fat, fibres, oedema, and degenerating haematopoietic tissue, with various degrees of infiltrations of macrophages (containing haemosiderin), lymphocytes, plasma cells, mast cells, eosinophils, neutrophils, and megakaryocytes (Plate XIVa–d). All these may occur in varying proportions, or any one may predominate. Frequently a zone containing a loose network of fibres enclosing fibroblasts, macrophages, a few fat cells and an assortment of infiltrating cells separates the metastases from the rest of the marrow. In some cases this zone is traversed by blood vessels sprouting from the vessels in the adjacent haematopoietic tissue, and reaching into the metastases, probably in response to angiogenic factors produced by the tumour cells (Plate XIIId).

12.5.3   *The intra-tumour reaction*

An assortment of infiltrating cells may be caught within the metastases as they enlarge, while others enter them together with the blood vessels and the stroma. In this way aggregates of lymphocytes, plasma cells, and macrophages may be formed, and these are then found between the

---

Fig. 12.10   Sections of biopsies with metastatic involvement to show fibrosis and angiogenesis; (a) in marginal reaction (arrow); (b) blood vessels crossing marrow (arrows) towards metastases; (c) connective tissue stroma (CT) and vessels within metastases; (d) large vascular channels (VC) formed by tumour cell masses, T = tumour cells, M = marrow and fat cells, B = bone. × 250, Giemsa.

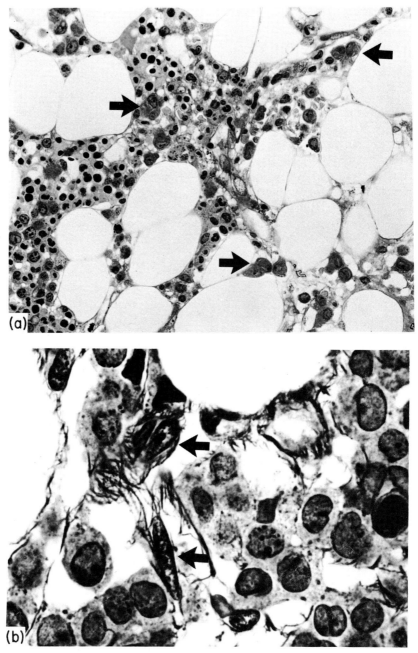

Fig. 12.11 (a) Interstitial spread of metastatic tumour cells (arrows), with incipient fibrosis. × 250, Giemsa; (b) high power view showing reticulin fibres clearly associated with spindle shaped fibroblasts (arrow). × 1000, Gomori.

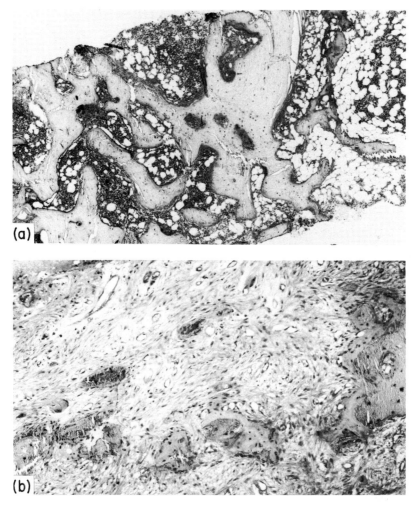

Fig. 12.12 Prostatic carcinoma: (a) bone biopsy showing osteoblastic new bone formation, no metastases in biopsy. × 100, Giemsa; (b) new bone formation, fibrotic marrow, no cancer cells in the biopsy. × 100, Giemsa. Neither patient had received therapy other than resection of prostate.

nodules of tumour cells (Fig. 12.18). Mast cells (as in normal marrow) are often associated with the blood vessels. Macrophages, with or without cellular and nuclear debris, lipomacrophages, foam cells, foreign body giant cells and even granulomata may be found in the vicinity of metastases or even in bone biopsies without evident involvement. The presence of neutrophils in and around metastases may be due to infection, to the accumulation of degeneration and breakdown products, or to

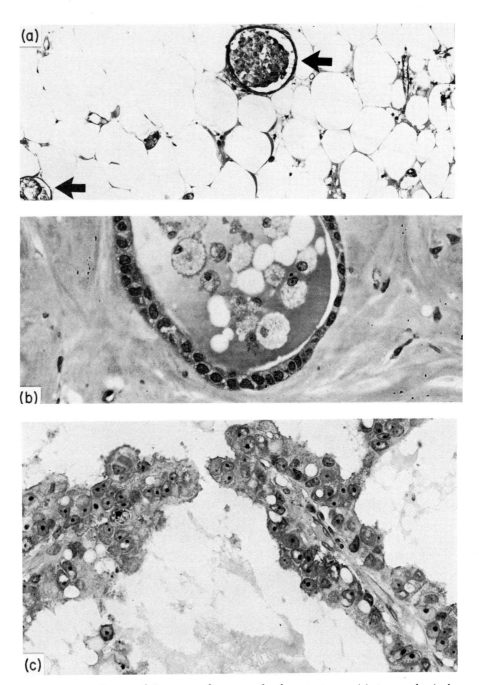

Fig. 12.13 Types of intravascular spread of metastases: (a) two spherical intravascular emboli (arrows) with a hypoplastic marrow. × 250, Giemsa; (b) tumour cells lining dilated sinus in acellular, gelatinous stroma. × 400, Giemsa; (c) vascular channels formed by strands of tumour cells with cores of connective tissue. × 400, Giemsa.

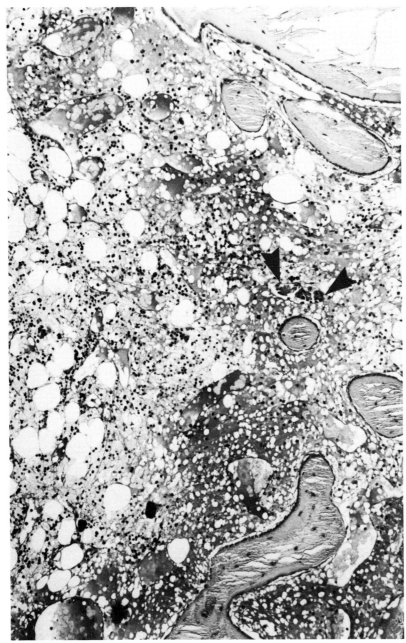

Fig. 12.14 Section of bone biopsy of patient with osteoblastic metastases, clusters of tumour cells (arrows); note oedematous marrow space, no haematopoiesis, only scattered plasma cells, mast cells, lymphoid and stromal elements. × 200, Giemsa.

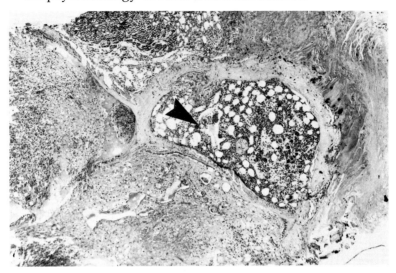

Fig. 12.15 Section of bone biopsy of 80 year old patient with unknown primary tumour; large areas of necrotic metastasis with subcortical preservation of haematopoiesis (arrow), periosteum at right. × 100, Giemsa.

specific factors produced by the tumour cells. Likewise, eosinophilic stimulating factors have also recently been characterized and these account for the eosinophilia sometimes seen in patients with solid tumours. Though the stromal reaction of tumours in its entirety might be considered a reaction of the host to or against the tumour (Joachim, 1976), lymphocytes in particular have been implicated. The participation of lymphoid cells in surveillance against and eradication of neoplasia, has long been postulated, but is still controversial (Drew, 1979). Lymphoid aggregates when found at the margins of, or within the metastases are thought to represent a host defence mechanism. In association with primary tumours, they have been correlated with a more favourable prognosis. Recent work indicates a potential application of activated T lymphocytes in tumour therapy (Rosenberg *et al.*, 1982).

12.6   Trabecular bone in regions of metastases

The presence of the metastases in the marrow has some effect on the trabecular bone in the vast majority of cases (over 95%). Usually both

Fig. 12.16 Illustration of 'activated mesenchyme' near metastases in bone marrow: (a) osteoblasts and osteoclasts (arrows). × 600; (b) elongated fibroblast-like cells, which have red granules in toluidine blue stain, similar to mast cells. × 1000, Giemsa.

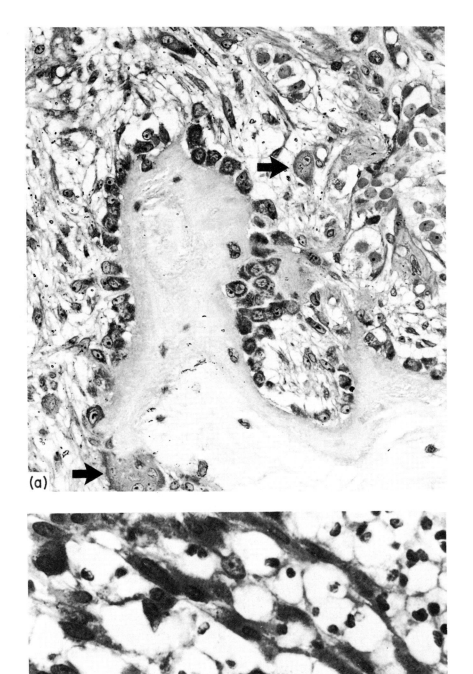
(a)

(b)

osteoblasts and osteoclasts are stimulated, though either may predominate in any one particular case. Rarely the process is purely osteolytic or osteoblastic (Plates XIVe, XVId and XVe–f). Resorption of the cancellous bone in the early stages at least, is accompanied by activation of osteoclasts. Later, when the marrow cavities are entirely occupied by tumour cells which lie directly on the surface of the bone, other mechanisms may also be involved (Mundy *et al.*, 1981; Galasko, 1982). When an

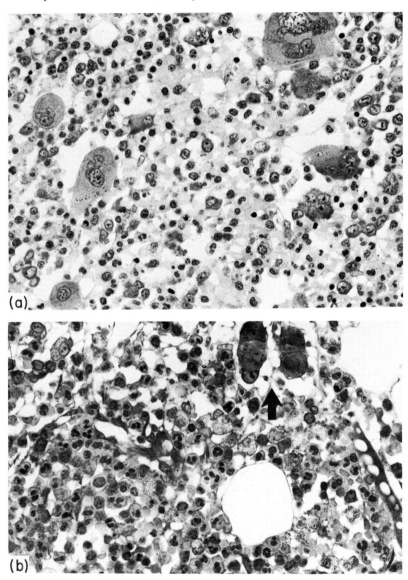

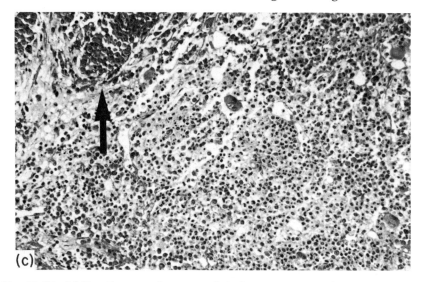

Fig. 12.17 (a) Reactive megakaryocytosis in bone marrow with metastases (not shown); note range in size and nuclear configuration of megakaryocytes. × 250, Giemsa; (b) interstitial spread of small groups of tumour cells. × 400, Giemsa; without optimal histology these could be mistaken for megakaryocytes; (c) granulocytic leukaemoid reaction with metastases (arrow) of pulmonary cancer. × 100, Giemsa.

osteosclerotic reaction is elicited, this may develop from the formation of woven bone, that is mineralization of dense connective tissue stroma, or by the appositional deposition of osteoid on pre-existing trabeculae by osteoblasts, or by osseous sprouts joining up with the trabeculae, which is a combination of the two processes (Burkhardt *et al.*, 1982). However, in all cases the normal trabecular bone structure is destroyed and the bone is thereby weakened, so that pathological fractures may ensue. Early diagnosis is required to prevent them, especially those sub-groups of patients whose tumours have a propensity to settle in the bones (Smalley *et al.*, 1982).

12.7   Prostatic cancer

Cancer of the prostate is now the second most common cancer in Western men. As the life span of the population increases more men are living long enough for prostatic cancer to become clinically significant, to disseminate and thus to increase the contribution made by prostatic cancer to the overall death from malignancies. It has variously been estimated that distant metastases are present at diagnosis in 50–80% of the patients. There are still divergent opinions on the correlation between histology and prognosis, perhaps because the histology of the cells in the primary tumour does not reflect the potential behaviour of the cells at other sites as metastases (Kastendieck, 1980). Another factor is the rate of replication which may be altered in the metastases when the primary tumour is removed. Consequently, though estimates (more or less accurate) may be made of the speed of replication of the primary, these may have little relevance for its metastases (Hill, 1978). Moreover there is some evidence that the variable natural history of prostatic cancer may be related to the

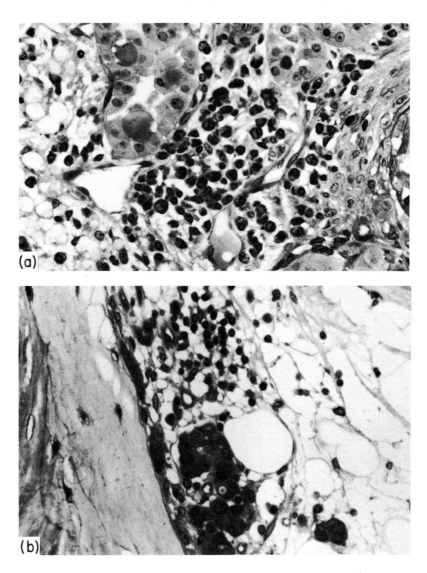

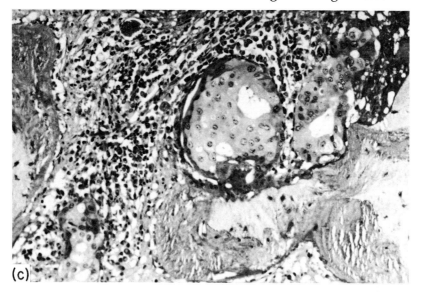

Fig. 12.18 Lymphocytic and plasma cell reaction adjacent to metastatic adeno-carcinoma: (a) of breast. × 600, Giemsa; (b) of colon. × 250, Giemsa; (c) of prostate. × 100, Giemsa.

response of the immune system in the individual patients, and to the hormone responsiveness of the tumour (Pertschuk *et al.*, 1982). From studies recorded in the literature it appears that bony metastases will develop in 75% of the patients with involvement of the pelvic lymph nodes, even if these have been treated by dissection, by external beam radiation or both. Though there is still disagreement concerning the mode of spread and the distribution of osseous metastases, the bones of the pelvic and the lumbar spine are regarded as the most frequent sites for metastases. Both perineural lymphatic spread and dissemination via the vertebral venous plexus have their advocates as possible routes. Willis (1973) maintains that metastatic deposits reach the bones by way of the systemic circulation from secondary deposits in the lungs.

Metastases of prostatic cancer in the bones often appear as lobules separated by bands of connective tissue, which may have some kind of glandular structure or present as solid masses of cells. The alveolar type is usually composed of small to medium sized cells, while the medullary type may consist of large anaplastic cells with large, prominent nucleoli. It should be stressed that the appearance of prostatic cancer cells in the bone marrow varies considerably (Plate XVa–f); nevertheless, all the types appear capable of evoking an osteoblastic reaction. In some cases this is so marked that the tumour cells themselves appear to get swallowed up in it.

In other cases there may be large areas of necrosis when the expansion of the tumour cells has been intravascular. When a considerable portion of the newly formed bone is not mineralized wide osteoid seams result, so that a picture similar to osteomalacia is produced (Smallridge *et al.*, 1981).

12.8   Breast cancer

Breast cancer is today the main cause of death from cancer in women in the US (and many other parts of the world) and about 100 000 new cases are diagnosed each year. Moreover, another important and sobering point is that despite all therapeutic advances and earlier diagnoses the death rate appears to have remained fairly constant over the past several decades (Weiss, 1976; Fox, 1979; Bluming, 1982) and there has been no significant benefit from adjuvant chemotherapy (Smith, 1983). In addition, as pointed out by Willis (1973) and recently confirmed by others (Cho and Choi, 1980) autopsy findings have demonstrated a high incidence of skeletal metastases in patients with mammary cancer who died either in the first or the second five year period irrespective of the immediate cause of death. Such observations raise a number of important issues: (1) correlation between the histological features of the primary tumour and those of the metastases in the bones (see Plates XIIIe and XVIa–d); (2) the effect of the more aggressive treatment schedules on early and late metastatic potential and growth rate; (3) the problem of late recurrences.

With respect to the histopathology of the primary tumour, the natural history of mammary cancer shows that it encompasses a heterogeneous group of diseases, with variable time courses (Henderson and Canellos, 1980). Little if any mention is made of this in many clinical trials, though various studies have indicated an association between histological types (Roses *et al.*, 1982) and probability of recurrence (Fisher *et al.*, 1983). As pointed out by Davies (1983) certain multicentre trials tend to stratify breast tumours only according to lymph node status and ignore the histopathological nature of the primary neoplasm. Nevertheless, a correlation between the histology of the primary tumour and that of its metastases may well provide information for a better understanding of the histological grade and the malignant potential of the primary growth. This is all the more important as some neoplasias may appear histologically malignant, but be relatively benign from the point of view of their biological behaviour (Fox, 1979). Assessment of the results of therapeutic trials (as stressed by Davies (1983)) requires precise classification of the primary tumour, and also of the metastases being treated with a view to eradication.

Similar considerations apply to the hormone dependency of human breast cancer: it is not an all or nothing phenomenon, but a spectrum because of the mixture of receptor positive and receptor negative cells in various proportions in every tumour (Manni, 1983). Therefore clinical trials must also incorporate this sort of information into their experimental design. Finally, there is the question of late recurrences (see Fig. 12.9). These have been documented as occurring from several to over 10 years after removal of a primary tumour (Georgii and Parl, 1982). This necessitates the permanent follow-up at regular intervals of such patients, especially as skeletal metastases may be detected by bone biopsy in the absence of noteworthy changes in the peripheral blood or abnormalities in other tests (Burkhardt *et al.*, 1980; Redding *et al.*, 1983). These 'dormant' metastases appear to be in a kind of equilibrium with the host tissues for variable periods of time. In experimental animals such dormant metastases have been stimulated to grow by perturbation of their environment, i.e. the host tissues, by events such as changes in hormone or immune status, or by surgery (Alexander, 1982).

There are no effective tests available today for the early detection of skeletal metastases other than direct examination of the bone marrow

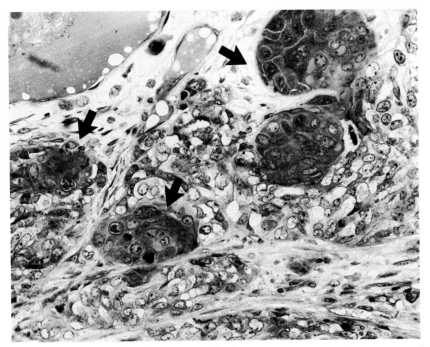

Fig. 12.19 'Combined malignancy' in the bone marrow; nest of squamous cell carcinoma (arrows) within metastases of oat cell carcinoma of lung. × 400, Giemsa.

(Burkhardt *et al.*, 1980; Redding *et al.*, 1983). The relative merits of X-rays and skeletal scintigraphy for early detection of breast carcinoma metastases in bone have been investigated in a large series of patients by Perez *et al.* (1983), and they found that both were unnecessary. Biopsies are considered to be better than serial bone scans to assess response to chemotherapy in breast cancer (Bitran *et al.*, 1980).

12.9   Pulmonary cancer

This accounts for about one third of all cancer deaths in Man. The mortality in women is approximately one quarter that of men but it is increasing (Surgeon General, 1980, 1981). The association between lung cancer and smoking now appears thoroughly documented from clinical, statistical and experimental aspects. In patients with bronchogenic cancer, histological classification of the primary tumour is required before therapy is initiated (Hansen, 1982). The major groups according to the WHO classification are (1) squamous cell carinoma (Fig. 12.19), (2) small cell carcinoma (Fig. 12.20), (3) adenocarcinoma, (4) large cell carcinoma; each of these groups has variants and sub-types. Pulmonary cancer is characterized by early and widespread invasion of the lymphatics, and metastases may occur anywhere, especially in the brain and the bones, even from small and clinically silent primary tumours. Overall about 20% of patients are thought to have positive iliac crest biopsies at diagnosis. In small cell carcinoma, this figure may rise to 30% if bilateral biopsies are taken (Hansen, 1982). An incidence of 17–42% has been reported in anaplastic small cell carcinoma (Hirsch and Hansen, 1980). Studies in large series of patients with the other histological groups have not yet been reported. Cramer *et al.* (1981) have studied the cellular and stromal aspects of metastatic bone disease in patients with lung cancer.

12.10   Metastases of other tumours

12.10.1   Gastro-intestinal tract

About 20% of patients with known gastro-intestinal tumours have skeletal metastases. Recent studies have shown that metastases of colorectal tumours are also far more frequent than previously suspected—in 29% of patients undergoing apparently curative resection occult hepatic

---

Fig. 12.20 Bone biopsy of patient with oat cell carcinoma of lungs: (a) low power to show solid masses of tumour cells and oedematous marrow. × 100, Giemsa; (b) high power illustrating the spindle shaped to oval metastatic cells. × 1000, Giemsa.

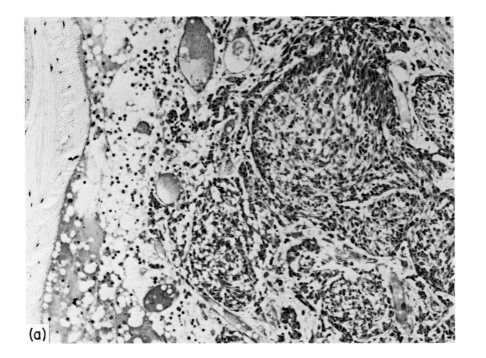

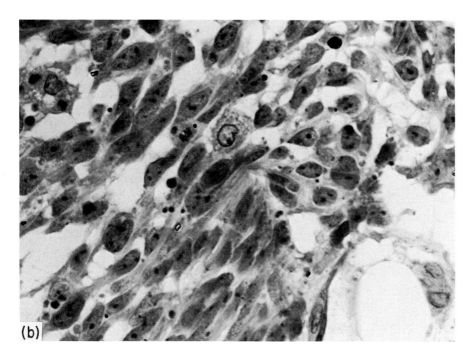

metastases were present at operation and were revealed by computed tomography (Finlay *et al.*, 1982). Such tumours may also metastasize to the bones (Plate XVIf). Carcinoid may produce signet-ring-like cells in metastases (Plate XIIIb).

12.10.2   Renal tumours

Marsden *et al.* (1980) investigated the incidence of metastases of renal tumours in children. They found that these were relatively rare and that males were affected more than females. In adults, metastases of renal carcinoma (hypernephroma) may consist of large, clear cells with a high cytoplasmic to nuclear ratio (Plate XVIe).

12.10.3   Malignant melanoma

Metastases of malignant melanoma may be detected in the bone marrow in a small percentage of the patients. There is no difficulty in recognition if the melanotic granules are present; but when there are no or very few granules, immediate identification may not be possible. However, in the experience of Savage *et al.* (1983) melanoma cells were stained by the Masson Fontana stain even when pigmentation was not observed after routine staining of smears and sections. Cells positive in the Masson Fontana stain did not reveal blue granules (iron) with the Prussian blue method. Though the pleomorphic character of the melanoma cells makes them easy to identify as a rule, in doubtful cases special stains and EM will substantiate the diagnosis.

12.10.4   Neuroblastomas

Secondaries of these tumours may show a rosette-like arrangement of metastatic cells, both in smears and in sections (Abildgaard, 1980; Triche and Askin, 1983).

12.10.5   Medulloblastomas

In some cases, medulloblastomas may metastasize early, and these small cell undifferentiated tumours may then mimic leukaemia (Pollack *et al.*, 1981). Rarely, dissemination to the skeleton occurs before the intracranial mass is evident. Metastases of haemangiopericytomas (a form of angioblastic meningioma) may also be found in the pelvic bones, among others (Anderson and Rovabeck, 1980).

12.10.6   Ovarian and carcinoid tumours

Skeletal deposits of these tumours may consist of signet-ring-like cells, containing strongly PAS positive material.

12.11   Metastases of unknown primary tumours

These are sometimes called ACUP (Adeno-Carcinoma of Unknown Primary). The histological aspect of the metastases may give an indication of their possible source. Metastases of intestinal origin frequently have the histological features of adeno-carcinomas with tubular or acinous structures possibly containing PAS positive material. A medullary arrangement may be observed in metastases of bronchogenic carcinoma.

Solid masses of tumour cells sometimes indicate metastases of prostatic carcinoma (though there is a great histological variation in the metastases of the prostate). A scirrhous type frequently indicates secondaries of mammary carcinoma (Willis, 1973; Nystrom *et al.*, 1979). Metastases of both prostatic and mammary cancer sometimes produce such a strong osteoblastic reaction that the bone in the biopsy resembles that seen in extreme osteosclerosis, with tiny marrow cavities occupied by connective tissue of variable density in which the tumour cells may not be present, or are unrecognizable.

Where morphology is inadequate, there are now many markers available which provide information on the histogenesis of tumours and metastases, for example Factor VIII-related antigen, which indicates a vascular origin (Bell and Flotte, 1982).

A fundamental weakness of modern tumour therapy is that it neglects variation within a given tumour population, both in appearance and in the properties of the cells. Tumour cell diversity is potentially amenable to investigation; one method is correlation of the features of the primary tumour with those of its metastases (Dexter *et al.*, 1981; Weiss *et al.*, 1983). Moreover, such histological diversity characterizes the metastases as well as the primary tumours.

References

Abildgaard, C. F. (1980), Unique features of metastatic neuroblastoma in the bone marrow. *Am. J. clin. Pathol.*, **74**, 363.

Adam. Y. G. (1981). Changing concepts in treating early breast cancer. An overview. *Isr. J. med. Sci.*, **71**, 932–5.

Alexander, P. (1982), Need for new approaches to the treatment of patients in clinical remission, with special reference to acute myeloid leukaemia. *Brit. J. Cancer*, **46**, 151–9.

Anderson, C. and Rovabeck, C. H. (1980), Skeletal metastases of an intra-cranial malignant hemangiopericytoma. *J. Bone Jt Surg.*, **62A**, 145–8.

Barry, W. F., Wells, S. A., Cox, C. E. and Haagensen, D. E. (1981), Clinical and radiographic correlations in breast cancer patients with osseous metastases. *Skeletal Radiol.*, **6**, 27–32.

Bassler, R., Dittmann, A. M. and Dittrich, M. (1981), Mononuclear stromal reactions in mammary carcinoma, with special reference to medullary carcinomas with a lymphoid infiltrate. *Virchows Archiv. (Pathol. Anat.)*, **393**, 75–91.

Bell, D. A. and Flotte, T. J. (1982), Factor VIII related antigen in adenomatoid tumours: implications for histogenesis. *Cancer*, **50**, 932–8.

Berken, A. (1982), Case for adoptive immunotherapy in cancer. *Lancet*, **2**, 1190–2.

Bitran, J. O., Beckerman, C. and Desser, R. K. (1980), The predictive value of serial bone scans in assessing response to chemotherapy in advanced breast cancer. *Cancer*, **45**, 1562–8.

Bluming, A. Z. (1982), Treatment of primary breast cancer without mastectomy. Review of the literature. *Am. J. Med.*, **72**, 820–8.

Burkhardt, R., Frisch, B. and Kettner, G. (1980), The clinical study of micro-metastatic cancer by bone biopsy. *Bull. Cancer*, **67**, 291–305.

Burkhardt, R., Frisch, B., Bartl, R., Kettner, G., Schlag, R. and Hill, W. (1981), Detection of haematologic and non-haematologic cancer by bone biopsy. *Cancer Detect. Prev.*, **4**, 619–27.

Burkhardt, R., Frisch, B., Schlag, R. and Sommerfeld, W. (1982), Carcinomatous osteodysplasia. *Skeletal Radiol.*, **8**, 169–78.

Campbell, F. C., Blamey, R. W., Elston, C. W., Nicholson, R. I., Griffiths, K. and Haybittle, J. L. (1981), Oestrogen-receptor status and sites of metastasis in breast cancer. *Brit. J. Cancer*, **44**, 456–9.

Carr, D. F. (1983), Is staging of cancer of value? *Cancer*, **51**, 2503–5.

Carr, I. and Underwood, J. C. E. (1974), The ultrastructure of the local cellular reaction to neoplasia. *International Review of Cytology* (eds G. H. Bourne and J. F. Danielli), Vol. 37, Academic Press, New York, pp. 329–47.

Carter, R. L. (1978), Metastatic potential of malignant tumours. *Invest. Cell. Pathol.*, **1**, 275–86.

Carter, R. L. (1982), Some aspects of the metastatic process. *J. Clin. Pathol.*, **35**, 1041–9.

Cho, San You and Choi, Hong Yul (1980), Causes of death and metastatic patterns in patients with mammary cancer. *Am. J. clin. Pathol.*, **73**, 232–4.

Clarke, R. L. (1979), Systemic cancer and the metastatic process. *Cancer*, **43**, 790–7.

Cohen, Y., Zidan, J. and McShan, D. (1982), Bone marrow biopsy in solid cancer. *Acta Haemat.*, **68**, 14–19.

Cramer, S. F., Fried, L. and Carter, K. J. (1981), The cellular basis of metastatic bone disease in patients with lung cancer. *Cancer*, **48**, 2649–60.

Currie, G. A. (1981), Platelet-derived growth-factor requirements for in vitro proliferation of normal and malignant mesenchymal cells. *Brit. J. Cancer*, **43**, 335–43.

Daar, A. S. and Fabre, J. W. (1981), Demonstration with monoclonal antibodies of an unusual mononuclear cell infiltrate and loss of normal epithelial membrane antigens in human breast carcinomas. *Lancet*, **2**, 434–7.

Dady, P. J., Powles, T. J., Dowsett, M., Easty, G., Williams, J. and Neville, A. M. (1981), In vitro osteolytic activity of human breast carcinoma tissue and prognosis. *Brit. J. Cancer*, **43**, 222–5.

Davies, J. D. (1983), Nodal status or breast tumour classification? *Lancet*, **2**, 741.

Denekamp, J. (1982), Endothelial cell proliferation as a novel approach to targeting tumour therapy. *Brit. J. Cancer*, **45**, 136–9.

Dexter, D. L., Spremulli, E. N., Fligiel, Z., Barbosa, J. A., Vogel, R., VanVoorhees, A. and Calabresi, P. (1981), Heterogeneity of cancer cells from a single human colon carcinoma. *Am. J. Med.*, **71**, 949–56.

Dixon, D., Reeve, T. S. and Taylor, T. K. F. (1980), Bony metastases from carcinoma of the thyroid gland. *J. Bone. Jt Surg.*, **62B**, 262.

Donati, M. B. (1980), Annotation: malignancy and haemostasis. *Brit. J. Haematol.*, **44**, 173–82.

Drew, S. I. (1979), Immunological surveillance against neoplasia: an immunological quandary. *Human Pathol.*, **10**, 5–14.

Finlay, I. G., Meek, D. R., Gray, H. W., Duncan, J. G., and McArdle, C. S. (1982), Incidence and detection of occult hepatic metastases in colorectal carcinoma. *Brit. med. J.*, **284**, 803–5.

Fisher, E. R., Redmond, C., Fisher, B. and Participating NSABP Investigators (1983), Pathologic findings from the National Surgical Adjuvant Breast Project. VIII. Relationship of chemotherapeutic responsiveness to tumor differentiation. *Cancer*, **51**, 181–91.

Folkman, J. (1974), Tumour angiogenic factor. *Cancer Res.*, **34**, 2109–13.

Fornasier, V. L. and Paley, D. (1983), Leiomyosarcoma in bone: primary or secondary? A case report and review of the literature. *Skeletal Radiol.*, **10**, 147–53.

Fox, M. S. (1979), On the diagnosis and treatment of breast cancer. *J. Am. med. Assoc.*, **241**, 489–94.

Freemont, A. J. (1982), The small blood vessels in areas of lymphocytic infiltration around malignant neoplasms. *Brit. J. Cancer*, **46**, 282–8.

Frei, E. (1974), Rationale for combined therapy. *Cancer*, **40**, 569–73.

Frisch, B., Bartl, R., Mahl, G., Burkhardt, R. (1984), Scope and value of bone marrow biopsies in metastatic cancer. *Invasion Metastasis 4*; Suppl. **1**, 12–30.

Galasko, C. S. B (1982), Mechanisms of lytic and blastic metastatic disease of bone. *Clin. Orthop. Rel. Res.*, **169**, 20–7.

Georgii, A. and Parl, F. F. (1982), Introduction to the topic metastasis. *Verh. Dtsch. Krebs. Ges.*, **3**, 317–20.

Gullino, P. M. (1981), Angiogenesis and neoplasia. *New Engl. J. Med.*, **305**, 884–5.

Hansen, H. H. (1982), Staging of small cell anaplastic carcinoma of the lung. *Recent Advances in Clinical Oncology* (eds C. J. Williams and J. M. A. Whitehouse), Churchill Livingstone, Edinburgh, pp. 285–93.

Hara, Y., Steiner, M. and Baldini, G. (1980), Platelets as a source of growth-promoting factor(s) of tumor cells. *Cancer Res.*, **40**, 1212–16.

Hartveit, F. (1981), Mast cells and metachromasia in human breast cancer: their occurrence, significance and consequence: a preliminary report. *J. Pathol.*, **134**, 7–11.

Haskill, S., Koren, H., Becker, S., Fowler, W. and Walton, L. (1982), Mononuclear-cell infiltration in ovarian cancer. III. Suppressor-cell and ADCC activity of macrophages from ascitic and solid ovarian tumours. *Brit. J. Cancer*, **45**, 747–53.

Henderson, I. C. and Canellos, G. P. (1980), Cancer of the breast. *New Engl. J. Med.*, **302**, 78–90.

Hill, B. T. (1978), The management of human 'solid tumors'. Some observations on the irrelevance of traditional cell cycle kinetics and the value of certain recent concepts. *Cell Biol. intern. Rep.*, **2**, 215–30.

Hirsch, F. R. and Hansen, H. H. (1980), Bone marrow involvement in small cell anaplastic carcinoma of the lung: prognostic and therapeutic aspects. *Cancer,* **46,** 206–11.

Husby, G., Hoagland, P. M., Strickland, R. C. and Williams, R. C. (1976), Tissue T and B cell infiltration of primary and metastatic cancer. *J. clin. Invest.,* **57,** 1471–82.

Ioachim, H. L. (1976), The stromal reactions of tumors: an expression of immune surveillance. *J. nat. Cancer Inst.,* **57,** 465–75.

Jacobs, T. P., Siris, E. S., Bilezikian, J. P., Baquiran, D. C., Shane, E. and Canfield, R. T. (1981), Hypercalcemia of malignancy: treatment with intravenous dichloromethylene diphosphonate. *Ann. int. Med.,* **94,** 312–16.

Jung, A., Chantraine, A., Donath, A. *et al.* (1983), Use of dichloromethylene diphosphate in metastatic bone disease. *New Engl. J. Med.,* **308,** 1499–1501.

Karpatkin, S. and Pearlstein, E. (1981), Role of platelets in tumor cell metastases. *Ann. int. Med.,* **95,** 635–41.

Kastendieck, H. (1980), Prostatic carcinoma. Aspects of pathology, prognosis and therapy. *J. Cancer Res. clin. Oncol.,* **96,** 131–56.

Key, M. Talmadge, J. E. and Fidler, I. J. (1982), Lack of correlation between the progressive growth of spontaneous metastases and their content of infiltrating macrophages. *J. Reticuloendothelial Soc.,* **32,** 387–96.

Killop, J. H. and McDougall, I. R. (1980), The role of skeletal scanning in clinical oncology. *Brit. med. J.,* **281,** 407–9.

Lam, W. C., Delikanty, E. J., Orr, F. W., Wass, J., Varani, J. and Ward, P. A. (1981), The chemotactic response of tumor cells. A model for cancer metastasis. *Am. J. Pathol,* **104,** 69–76.

Landys, K. (1982), Prognostic value of bone marrow biopsy in breast cancer. *Cancer,* **49,** 513–18.

Lang, W., Stauch, G., Soudah, B. and Georgii, A. (1983), The effectiveness of bone marrow punctures for staging carcinomas of breast and lung. *Verh. Dtsch. Ges. Path.,* **67,** 463–5.

Low, J. C. (1981), The radionuclide scan in bone metastases. In *Bone Metastases* (eds L. Weiss and H. A. Gilbert), G. K. Hall Medical Publishers, Boston, Mass., pp. 231–44.

Lutz, D. (1983), Immunotherapy of cancer: a critical review. *Int. J. clin. Pharmac. Therapy Toxicol.,* **21,** 118–29.

Manni, A. (1983), Hormone receptors and breast cancer. *New Eng. J. Med.,* **309,** 1383–4.

Marsden, H. B., Lennox, E. L., Lawler, W. and Kinnier-Wilson, L. M. (1980), Bone metastases in childhood renal tumours. *Brit. J. Cancer,* **41,** 875–9.

Mundy, G. R., DeMartino, S. and Rowe, D. W. (1981), Collagen and collagen-derived fragments are chemotactic for tumor cells. *J. clin. Invest.,* **68,** 1102–5.

Nelson, M. and Nelson, S. D. (1981), Inflammation and tumour growth. II. Tumour growth at sites of inflammation. *Am. J. Pathol.,* **104,** 125–31.

Nystrom, J. S., Weiner, J. M., Wolf, R. M. *et al.* (1979), Identifying the primary site in metastatic cancer of unknown origin. *J. Am. med. Assoc.,* **241,** 381–3.

Perez, D. J., Powles, T. J., Milan, J., Gazet, J. C., Ford, H. T., McCready, V. R., MacDonald, J. S. and Coombes, R. C. (1983), Detection of breast carcinoma metastases in bone: relative merits of X-rays and skeletal scintigraphy. *Lancet,* **2,** 613–16.

Pertschuk, L. P., Rosenthal, H. E., Macchia, R. J., Eisenberg, K. Byer, Feldman, J. G., Wax, S. H., Kim, D. S., Whitmore, W. F., Abrahams, J. I., Gaetjens, E.,

Wise, G. I., Herr, H. W., Karr, J. P., Murphy, G. P. and Sandberg, A. A. (1982), Correlation of histochemical and biochemical analyses of androgen binding in prostatic cancer. Relation to therapeutic response. *Cancer*, **49**, 984–93.

Peterson, H. I. (1979), *Tumour Blood Circulation*, C. R. C. Press, Boca Raton, Florida.

Pollak, E. R., Miller, H. J. and Vye, M. V. (1981), Medulloblastoma presenting as leukemia. *Am. J. clin. Pathol.*, **76**, 98–103.

Redding, W. H., Monaghan, P., Imrie, S. F., Ormerod, M. G., Gazet, J. C., Coombes, R. C., Clink, H. M., Dearnaley, D. P., Sloane, J. P., Powles, T. J. and Neville, A. M. (1983), Detection of micrometastases in patients with primary breast cancer. *Lancet*, **2**, 1271–4.

Rosenberg, S. A., Grimm, E. A., Lotze, M. T. and Mazumder, A. (1982), The growth of human lymphocytes in T cell growth factor: potential applications to tumor immunotherapy. In: *Lymphokines, Vol. 7* (eds E. Pick and S. Mizel), Academic Press, New York.

Roses, D. F., Bell, D. A., Flotte, Th.J., Taylor, R., Ratech, H. and Dubin, J. (1982), Pathologic predictors of recurrence in State I (TINOMA) breast cancer. *Am. J. clin. Pathol.*, **78**, 817–20.

Rubins, J. M. (1983), The role of myelofibrosis in malignant leukoerythroblastosis. *Cancer*, **51**, 308–11.

Savage, R. A., Lucas, F. V. and Hoffman, G. C. (1983), Melanoma in marrow aspirates. *Am. J. clin. Pathol.*, **79**, 268–9.

Smalley, R. V., Scogna, D. Mayer, and Malmud, L. S. (1982), Advanced breast cancer with bone-only metastases. A chemotherapeutically responsive pattern of metastases. *Am. J. clin. Oncol.*, **5**, 161–6.

Smallridge, R. C., Wray, H. L. and Schaaf, M. (1981), Hypocalcemia with osteoblastic metastases in a patient with prostatic Ca. A cause of secondary hyperparathyroidism. *Am. J. Med.*, **71**, 184–8.

Smith, I. E. (1983), Adjuvant chemotherapy for early breast cancer. *Brit. med. J.*, **287**, 379–80.

Sokol, R. J. and Hudson, G. (1983), Disordered function of mononuclear phagocytes in malignant disease. *J. clin Pathol.*, **36**, 316–23.

Springfield, D. S. (1982), Mechanisms of metastasis. *Clin. Orthoped. Rel. Res.*, **169**, 15–19.

Steckel, R. J. and Kagan, A. R. (1982), Evaluation of the unknown primary neoplasm. *Radiol. Clin. N. Amer.*, **20**, 601–5.

Stewart, A. F. (1983), Therapy of malignancy-associated hypercalcemia. *Am. J. Med.*, **74**, 475–80.

Surgeon General (1980), The health consequences of smoking for women: a report. Rockville, Md: Department of Health and Human Services, 1980; 375–8.

Surgeon General (1981), The health consequences of smoking—cancer: a report. Rockville, Md: Department of Health and Human Services; vi (DHSS publication no. (PHS)82-50179).

Thomas, E. D. (1982), The role of marrow transplantation in the eradication of malignant disease. *Cancer*, **49**, 1963–9.

Triche, T. J. and Askin, F. B. (1983), Neuroblastoma and the differential diagnosis of small-, round-, blue-cell tumors. *Human Pathol.*, **14**, 569–95.

Vinceneux, Ph., Cramer, E., Grossin, M. and Kahn, M. F. (1983), Diagnosis of bone metastases. Value of fluoroscopy-guided puncture and systematic aspiration biopsy. *Presse Med.*, **12**, 873–6.

Vose, B. M. and Moore, M. (1979), Suppressor cell activity of lymphocytes infiltrating human lung and breast tumours. *Int. J. Cancer*, **24**, 579–85.

Weiss, L. (1976), *Fundamental Aspects of Metastasis*, North Holland Publishing, Amsterdam.

Weiss, L. and Gilbert, H. A. (ed) (1981) *Bone Metastasis*, G. K. Hall Medical Publishers, Boston.

Weiss, L., Holmes, J. C. and Ward, P. M. (1983), Do metastases arise from pre-existing subpopulations of cancer cells? *Brit. J. Cancer*, **47**, 81–9.

Willis, R. A. (1973), *The Spread of Tumours in the Human Body*, Butterworths, London.

Woodruff, M. (1982), Interaction of cancer and host. *Brit. J. Cancer*, **46**, 313–22.

Woods, R. L., Fox, R. M., Tattersall, M. H. N., Levi, J. A. and Brodie, G. N. (1980), Metastatic adenocarcinomas of unknown primary site. A randomized study of two combination-chemotherapy regimens. *New Engl. J. Med.*, **303**, 87–9.

Zacharski, L. R., Rickles, F. R., Henderson, W. C., Martin, J. F., Forman, W. B., Van Eeckhout, J. P., Cornell, C. J. and Forcier, R. J. (1982), Platelets and malignancy. Rationale and experimental design for the V A cooperative study of RA-233 in the treatment of cancer. *Am. J. clin. Oncol.*, **5**, 593–609.

Appendix: methods

A.1 Biopsy: manual trephines

Several types of trephine needle have been developed. To obtain material the procedure is the same whether the Jamshidi needle (Jamshidi and Swaim, 1971), is used, or one of its modifications, such as that designed by Islam (1982), or a disposable needle with either standard or wide bore (11 or 8 gauge). Examples of optimal biopsies obtained with various types of needles are illustrated in Fig. 1.1.

The patient lies on one side, with legs flexed and knees drawn up (Fig. A.1). The posterior superior iliac spinous process is located by palpation along the iliac crest from front to back, and when found, the spot is marked, e.g. by gentle pressure with the end of a thin wooden applicator.

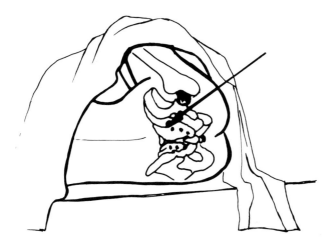

Fig. A.1 Schematic representation of posterior aspect of the bones of the pelvis; arrow points to superior spinous process of the ilium, most commonly used site for biopsies taken with manual trephines.

The skin is cleaned and sterilized with 70% ethanol or 5% chlorhexidine (diluted 1 in 10 in ethanol), and then infiltrated with local anaesthetic (e.g. 2% lignocaine), after which a small area of the periosteum over the posterior iliac spine is also infiltrated. The usual quantity of solution required is about 5 ml though in some cases up to 10 ml may be needed. The skin is again wiped and sterilized and a small 2–3 mm incision is made through which the biopsy needle with the stylet in place is introduced. The direction of the needle is almost horizontal, pointing towards the anterior superior spinous process of the ileum. On reaching the periosteum, pressure is exerted (which may have to be quite considerable) until the stylet is felt to penetrate through the cortex (signalled by a slight 'give' and decrease in resistance), the stylet is then withdrawn, and the needle advanced slowly by means of clockwise–anticlockwise rotary motions until sufficient depth is reached. Depending on the thickness of the layer between skin and periosteum, a biopsy of adequate length will have been obtained when about two-thirds of the needle has been introduced. In patients with a considerable panniculus adiposus, it may be necessary to advance the needle almost up to the handle. In cases in which more material is required (i.e. when double biopsies are recommended, as in staging of Hodgkin's disease) the following procedure is carried out: proceed as outlined above for obtaining a single biopsy, and after an adequate depth has been reached, withdraw to the edge of the marrow, change the angle of direction of the needle slightly, and advance it once more into the marrow space. Alternatively (and usually more effectively) a second biopsy is taken from another spot on the anaesthesized area of the periosteum after complete withdrawal and removal of the first biopsy from the needle (Fig. A.2). Subsequently, the skin is wiped clean; the edges of the incision are approximated, a pressure dressing is applied and firmly taped down with adhesive tape. The patient is checked after 15–30 min in case of bleeding from the site (which is extremely rare). The dressing is left in place for 48 h and the patient advised not to wet it during this time. Biopsies may be taken in this way on ambulatory patients who can often resume normal activity after the biopsy site has been checked after 30 min. However, if the patient has severe anaemia, thrombocytopenia, or any kind of abnormality of coagulation, or bleeding tendency, bone biopsy should only be done after the usual precautions taken before any surgical procedure in such patients. Thrombocytopenia itself is not a contra-indication in hospitalized patients. Bone biopsies have frequently been taken in patients with platelet counts of about $10–20 \times 10^9/l$ without any untoward effects. Bleeding is more likely to occur in patients with polycythaemia vera or idiopathic thrombocythaemia; in which case manual pressure should be applied for 5–10 min.

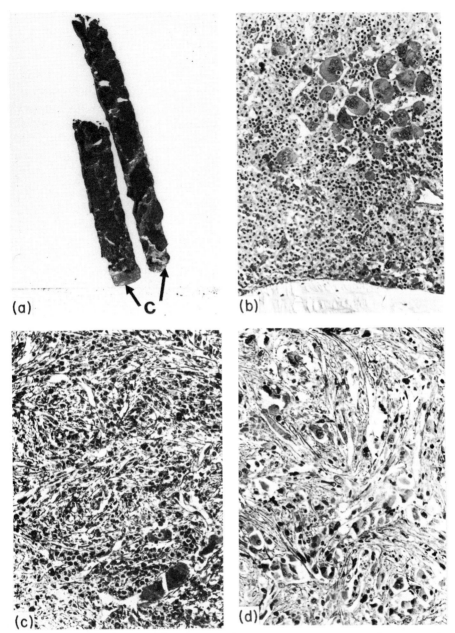

Fig. A.2 Bone biopsy of patient with prostatic carcinoma and suspected metastases: (a) two cores taken by manual trephine from adjacent spots: cortices at bottom (c); note dense cellularity due to myelofibrosis, hyper-cellular phase with extreme megakaryocytic hyperplasia. × 4, toluidine blue; (b) group of polymorphic megakaryocytes. × 100, Giemsa; (c) area of cellularity with incipient fibrosis. × 150, Giemsa; (d) advanced fibrosis with dysplastic haematopoiesis. × 150, Giemsa. The sections were taken from different areas of the same biopsy; illustrating the presence of a myeloproliferative disorder.

A.1.1   Very obese individuals

If difficulty is encountered in locating the superior posterior iliac spinous process, the biopsy may also be taken from the anterior iliac crest. However, the cortex is more difficult to penetrate at this site with a manual trephine.

A.2   Electric drill

With an electric drill (Burkhardt, 1971) biopsies are taken exclusively from the anterior iliac crest. The patient lies on his or her back and one side is slightly elevated by a hard support under the pelvis. After cleansing and disinfection, the skin is infiltrated with local anaesthetic (as described above) followed by infiltration of the anterior, medial and lateral aspects of the anterior iliac crest. A small incision is then made, about 3 cm above the anterior superior iliac spinous process, parallel to the lateral margin. The sub-cutaneous tissue is gently separated with a scalpel until the periosteum is reached, the scalpel is withdrawn, a funnel is introduced through the incision and firmly positioned on the periosteum of the anterior ilium, and the periosteal tissue within the opening of the funnel is scraped off the surface of the bone and removed by a swab. The drill is then applied through the funnel which permits penetration to a depth of about 20 mm; this takes about 10 s of drilling. The drill is withdrawn while still rotating and the biopsy core is then extracted by means of special guided tongs. Two or three haemostatic pellets are inserted, the wound is closed by a single clip or suture, a pressure dressing applied and taped down by adhesive tape. Twenty-four hours' bed rest followed by 24 hours' home rest is advocated, if the patient is not hospitalized. Analgesics may be required for post-operative pain. A few days later the clip or suture is removed at the out-patients' clinic.

A.3   The transilial wide bore needle

This needle (Bordier, 1964) is designed to obtain 'transfixing', or cortex to cortex, iliac crest biopsies. These are taken from the anterior ilium horizontally below the iliac crest. After preparation and anaesthesia of the skin as described above, at a spot about 2 cm below and behind the anterior superior spinous process of the ilium, on its lateral aspect, an incision of approximately 2 cm is made, an area of periosteum larger than the diameter of the biopsy needle is anaesthesized and the needle is inserted through the incision. Both lateral and medial cortices are obtained by this method, which is widely used in nephrology and whenever quantitative measurements of both trabecular and cortical bone are undertaken.

A.4   Processing of biopsy cores

The smaller biopsies are gently pushed out of the needle (according to the manufacturer's directions) on to a glass slide and several imprints made by touching it gently with another glass slide. The biopsy is then immediately placed into fixative. Biopsies with a diameter of 3 mm or more may be longitudinally halved (Bartl et al., 1978) with the aid of an especially designed plastic device (Figs. A.3, A.4). The cut surface is then used for imprints and both halves immediately placed into fixative. If frozen sections are to be made, only one half is fixed and the second is frozen for cutting in a cryostat, after a small piece has been removed for immediate fixation in the appropriate fixative if electron microscopy is also to be done. Both imprints and frozen sections may be used for cytochemistry (Catovsky et al., 1981), as well as for enzyme and antigen–antibody reactions (Harris et al., 1982; Falini et al., 1983; Banks et al., 1983) in addition to routine stains (Fig. A.5). Additional methods may be found in the references provided at the end of this chapter.

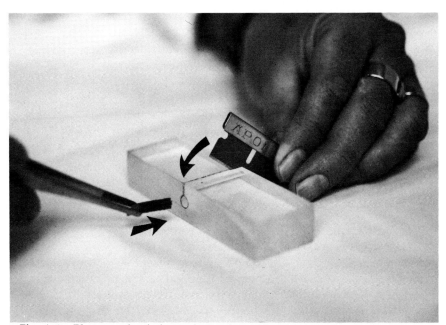

Fig. A.3 Photograph of plastic device for cutting biopsies longitudinally. The bone biopsy (held in forceps at left) is inserted into the plastic holder (at arrow) and cut with the razor blade through the slit in the top of the plastic holder.

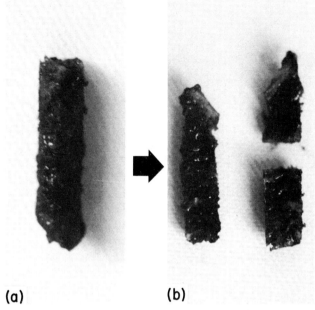

(a)   **(b)**

Fig. A.4   (a) Whole bone biopsy (electric drill); (b) longitudinally halved and cut biopsy pieces.

A.5   Method for plastic embedding of undecalcified bone biopsies

A.5.1   *Fixation*

The solution is made up of formaldehyde 35–40%: 50 ml; absolute methanol: 96 ml; glucose phosphate buffer pH 7.4: 4 ml; the stock formaldehyde is previously neutralized by the addition of 50 g/l $CaCO_3$. To make the buffer add together $Na_2HPO_4.(2H_2O)$: 48.0 g; KH_2PO_4: 8.7 g; glucose (mol. wt. 198.17): 154.0 g; distilled water to 5 litre. This buffer may be sterilized by filtration through a 0.22 μm millipore filter. Store in the refrigerator at 4°C.

Glass containers, capacity 20–25 ml with screw caps are used in fixation, dehydration, infiltration and embedding.

The biopsies are immediately placed into the fixation solution in a glass container and fixed for 16–24 h, with shaking or rotation for the first 2–3 h or longer if possible on a roller mixer. Tissues that have previously been fixed in 10% formalin for longer periods of time (i.e. more than 24 h) should be washed in distilled water for *c* 2 h on the mixer and then transferred to the fixation solution as above. Tissues fixed in 4% or 10% formalin, or 10% neutral buffered formalin, may all be processed into plastic after washing in this way. Tissues fixed in the B-5 fixative, com-

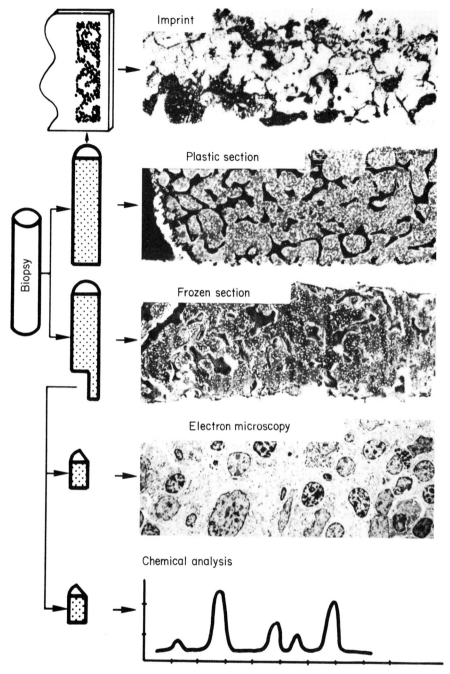

Fig. A.5 Technical possibilities for analysis of bone and bone marrow; from top down: imprints for morphology, cytochemistry and enzymes; plastic sections for histology; frozen sections for enzymes, markers, monoclonal antibodies; electron microscopy and related techniques; chemical analyses EDAX (energy dispersive analysis of X-rays). Reproduced with permission from Frisch and Bartl (1984).

monly used in the United States for bone biopsies, can also be processed into plastic. Tissues which have already been blocked in paraffin may be de-paraffinized and re-hydrated and embedded into plastic. After rinsing in water the same schedule is used as for fresh biopsies.

A.5.2   Dehydration

Transfer the biopsies directly from the fixation solution to absolute methanol, and change the methanol after 30 min, 1 h, 2 h, 4 h and 6 h. A minimum dehydration time of 6–12 h with 6 changes of absolute methanol is required for needle biopsies 2 mm wide. Larger biopsies require longer dehydration, i.e. 16–24 h with at least 6 changes of absolute methanol. Dehydration should be carried out with gentle agitation on a roller as above, if possible, for at least the first 2–3 h. Biopsies longer than the diameter of the vial should be cut into 2 or more segments with a sharp razor blade before infiltration. Biopsies that cannot be completely processed right away (due to weekends, holidays, etc.) should be fixed and dehydrated and left in methanol, as this is less deleterious than prolonged fixation.

A.5.3   Infiltration

The infiltration mixture is made up of 3 ingredients: methylmethacrylate 180 ml, Plastoid N 25 ml, and benzoyl peroxide 3.5 g. First destabilize the methylmethacrylate by passage through a chromatography column filled with basic aluminium oxide to a height of 15–20 cm; passage through two such columns in turn is recommended. The benzoyl peroxide is then placed in an open glass dish and dried in an oven at 37°C for about 30 min before use. The three ingredients are then mixed in the required proportions and the infiltration mixture is kept in a dark loosely stoppered bottle in the refrigerator between changes. It is very important to keep the bottles containing the infiltration mixtures—either fresh or stored—very loosely stoppered, because of the evaporation of components of the mixture. It is best to make up only the estimated required amount and to use fresh each time, though the infiltration mixture may be kept in the refrigerator for periods of up to 2–3 weeks.

After draining off the last absolute methanol the infiltration mixture is poured into the container to reach a level just above the biopsy. The container is left open and placed in a dessicator (Bell jar) connected via a mercury manometer to a vacuum pump (Fig. A.6). The dessicator has a layer of 'Siccapent' (to absorb moisture) at the bottom with a perforated porcelain plate over it, and the glass vials (containing the biopsies and the infiltration fluid) are placed on this plate. The jar is closed (the apposed

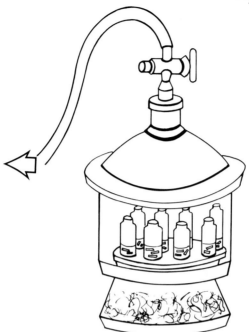

Fig. A.6   Bell jar with rubber tubing leading to vacuum pump. Inside are the glass containers containing the bone biopsies in liquid infiltration medium.

surfaces of lid and jar should first be smeared with vaseline to facilitate opening) and the air is pumped out to a negative pressure of 15–20 mm Hg. The entire infiltration procedure should be carried out with the dessicator in a hood at room temperature. After 30 min air is let into the dessicator, it is opened, the glass container is removed, the infiltration mixture is poured off into an old bottle and replaced by fresh infiltration fluid again just to cover the biopsies (it is very important not to pour the used methacrylate into the sink, as this plastic will eventually harden, therefore use an old bottle and discard when full). The open glass container is replaced in the dessicator, which is closed and the air pumped out as before to a negative pressure of 15–20 mm Hg. This procedure is carried out at the following time intervals to give a total infiltration time of 5–6 h (or more for larger specimens).

(1) Leave for 30 min (the first infiltration after absolute methanol); change.
(2) Leave for 30 min; change.
(3) Leave for 1 h; change.
(4) Leave for 1 h; change and fill.
(5) Leave for 2 (or more) h.

At the last change (No. 4 above) the container is filled with the infiltration mixture to approximately 1 cm from the top. The specimen identification number is written with a lead pencil onto a thin strip of paper which is inserted into the container and this will be fixed into the plastic block when it hardens. The biopsy core is gently pushed as far as possible to one side at the bottom of the vial, so that it lies horizontally and flat and close to the bottom of the container. After a minimum period of 2 h (overnight if the biopsies are large) in the dessicator under negative pressure, the container is removed and closed very tightly with the screw cap and placed in a water bath at 45°C for 1 h to initiate polymerization; and then transferred to a water bath at approximately 34–38°C overnight for hardening. Alternatively, the container may be put into a water bath at 45°C and left overnight; the plastic will have hardened by the morning. The level of the water in both baths should reach to just above the level of the fluid in the container, but no higher—this is to prevent both air and water from penetrating into the container. After the overnight incubation the plastic will generally have hardened; if the top of the block in the container is still soft or even fluid it may be returned to the 45° oven for an hour or so. But if the block is large enough and there is still some fluid plastic at the top this may be poured off (not into the sink, as it will harden later). The container is then placed in the refrigerator (or the freezer compartment) for 15–30 min, after which it is taken out and the glass is shattered with a hammer, the shards are removed, and the block is ready for cutting.

A.5.4   Sections

To facilitate sectioning and mounting, it is advisable to remove that part of the plastic which does not contain the biopsy core: the block is gripped in a vice (as used in workshops) and the plastic is sawn first vertically to a depth of about 5 mm and then horizontally with a small hand saw, leaving a half circle of plastic with the biopsy inside it (Fig. A.7). The block is then trimmed and sections cut at 1–5 μm in a heavy duty microtome (such as Jung's autocut with a tungsten-tipped knife—Jung, Heidelberg); 3 μm is the thickness generally used. A soft brush is used to moisten the surface of the block with 30% alcohol between sections. Each section is grasped at its edge with a pair of tweezers as it comes off the knife, and placed into a petri dish filled with distilled water. Each section is then separately mounted as follows: the section is picked up with tweezers from the distilled water and placed (as flat as possible) onto a gelatinized slide, and several drops of 90% alcohol are dropped onto it. After a few seconds the section will soften and it can then be stretched and the folds smoothed out with a soft brush. The section is brushed gently to avoid

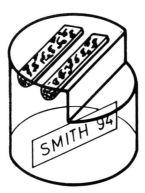

Fig. A.7 Schematic representation of plastic block; note name tag embedded within the plastic, and the top half not containing the biopsy sawn off, and top surface trimmed and ready for cutting.

tearing it, until flat and dry. (This technique requires some practice, but once acquired, mounting is accomplished quite rapidly and even large sections will be flat and free of folds.) The section is covered with a small piece of PVC or a piece of filter paper, so that slides may be stacked one on top of the other and then placed in an oven at 50°C for about 2 h (or longer, even overnight) under a weight, such as a paper-weight. In exceptional cases, 30–60 min will suffice.

Before staining, the methylmethacrylate is dissolved from the sections as follows. The slides are taken from the oven, the PVC slips removed, and the slides are placed sequentially into: benzene (benzol) I, 20 min; benzene II, 10 min; absolute methanol, 1–2 min; 96% methanol, 2 min; 80% methanol, 2 min; methanol–ammonia solution*, 10 min; distilled water, 10 min. Acetone may be used instead of benzene. The slides are then ready for staining and most stains used in routine histopathology can be used; these include Giemsa, haematoxylin and eosin, Van Giesson's, stains for iron, for reticulin, the PAS reaction for glycoproteins. Different time schedules are required according to the thickness of the sections and it is best for each laboratory to determine these for itself.

A.5.5   Materials used for infiltration process

Methylmethacrylate (e.g. Merck Cat. No. 800 590), benzoyl peroxide (e.g. Merck Schuchardt Cat. No. 801 611), Plastoid N (Burnus Gess., Darmstadt, Germany), Siccapent (Merck, Cat. No. 747-8033).

---

* 70% methanol, 100 ml; 25% ammonia, 10 ml.

A.6   Procedure for cleaning and coating glass slides

A.6.1   Covering of slides with chromalalaun gelatin

Put the slides into 4% sodium hydroxide and leave for 24 h. Rinse very well in warm running tap water (c 40°C) for 1 min. Put into 2% hydrochloric acid for 5 min. Rinse again very well in warm running tap water for 1 min, and place the slides into a slide rack. Dip into gelatin solution (heated to 50°C)—see below. Dry the slides in the slide rack at room temperature or under an electric light bulb, or in a warm oven, but keep covered to prevent contamination.

A.6.2   Gelatin solution

Dissolve 6.75 g gelatin in 1500 ml distilled water at 60°C; cool to 50°C and add 58 ml of a 4% potassium chromium (III) sulphate solution; add several crystals of thymol and 4 drops of Plastoid N.

The gelatin solution is stable at room temperature for about 10–14 days, and longer in the refrigerator; gelatinized slides can be kept for 2 days or longer, if put into boxes and kept in the refrigerator.

A.6.3   Toluidine blue stain

This is used for rapid diagnostic evaluation. Dissolve the methylmethacrylate as described above. Then stain in Toluidine blue 0.1% in distilled water, at c 50°C for 5–20 min, dip in water, blot gently, dry in air for 1–5 min, dip into xylol, cover with mounting medium and cover-glass.

A.6.4   Giemsa stain—for cytological details

Remove the methacrylate and put the slides into distilled water for 10 min.

Wash in distilled water: 10 min. Put into Giemsa solution pH 6.7 at 50°C: 45 min. Put into Giemsa solution pH 6.6 at 40°C: 25 min. Dip in distilled water and dry the slides immediately by gentle blotting with filter paper, dip into xylol, cover with a mounting medium and cover glass.

A.6.5   Phosphate buffer pH 6.7, 0.066 mol/l

0.066 mol/l disodium hydrogen phosphate (Na_2HPO_4): 43.4 ml
0.066 mol/l potassium dihydrogen phosphate (KH_2PO_4): 56.6 ml

A.6.6   Phosphate buffer 6.6, 0.066 mol/l

0.066 mol/l disodium hydrogen phosphate (Na$_2$HPO$_4$): 36 ml
0.066 mol/l potassium dihydrogen phosphate (KH$_2$PO$_4$): 64 ml

A.6.7   Giemsa pH 6.7 (prepare fresh before use)

Distilled water: 49 ml
Phosphate buffer pH 6.7: 1 ml
Giemsa solution*: 0.2 ml

A.6.8   Giemsa solution pH 6.6

Distilled water: 49 ml
Phosphate buffer pH 6.6: 1 ml
Giemsa solution*: 0.2 ml

The times for staining are calculated for 3 μm section thickness; thinner sections need more time.

A.6.9   PAS reaction for glycoproteins

Dissolve the methacrylate and put the slides into distilled water for 10 min:
Place in periodic acid at 56°: 30 min
Rinse in running tap water: 2 min
Wash in distilled water.
Put into Schiff's reagent (filter before use): 60 min at room temperature.
Rinse in running tap water: 20 min.
Wash in distilled water: 1 min.
Stain nuclei with Nuclear blue P. Mayer: 35 min.
Rinse in running tap water: 10 min.
Wash in distilled water.
Dry the slides with filter paper, dip briefly into xylol, cover with mounting medium and cover glass.

A.7   Solutions

A.7.1   Periodic acid

Add 4.0 g of potassium metaperiodate (KIO$_4$) to 950 ml of distilled water; warm, until it is dissolved.

* E.g. Merck No. 9204.

After cooling, add 50 ml 2N H_2SO_4.
Keep the solution at room temperature.

A.7.2   Schiff's reagent

Dissolve 5 g para-rosaniline (base) for microscopy in 150 ml 1N HCl. Dissolve 5 g potassium disulphite cryst. in 850 ml distilled water. Mix the two solutions together and keep in darkness for 24 h, then extract with activated charcoal and filter until the solution is clear.

Keep the solution in the refrigerator. It is stable for c 14 days.

A.7.3   Nuclear blue P. Mayer

Dissolve 1.0 g haematoxylin in 1 l of distilled water; add exact 0.2 g sodium iodate and 50 g potassium aluminium sulphate. Dissolve by shaking (the solution becomes blue-violet in colour). Add 50 g chloral hydrate and 1 g citric acid (the colour changes to red-violet). The solution is stable for c 3–4 months. Filter the solution before using.

A.8   Iron reaction—for haemosiderin

Remove the methacrylate and transfer the slides from distilled water into a freshly prepared and filtered 2% potassium ferrocyanide solution for 5 min (iron solution I). Then place the slices into a freshly prepared and filtered acidified ferrocyanide solution for 25 min (iron solution II) at room temperature. Wash with distilled water: 1 min. Stain the nuclei with Nuclear Fast Red: 1–2 h. Rinse in cold running tap water: 5 min. Wash in distilled water: 5 min. Dry between filter paper. Dip into xylol. Cover with mounting medium and cover glass. The times for the reaction and staining are calculated for 3 μm section thickness.

A.8.1   Iron solution I

Potassium ferrocyanide: 2 g; distilled water: 100 ml.

A.8.2   Iron solution II

Potassium ferrocyanide: 1 g; distilled water: 50 ml; 0.2N hydrochloric acid: 50 ml.

A.8.3   Nuclear fast red

Aluminium sulphate: 5 g; distilled water: 100 ml; dissolve by boiling; Nuclear fast red: 0.1 g. Filter the solution after cooling.

A.9   Ladewig staining of undecalcified slides (for mineralized bone and osteoid)

Remove the methacrylate and put the slides into distilled water for 10 min.

Stain with haematoxylin (Weigert) at room temperature for 1–2 h.

Rinse the slides in cold running tap water: 10 min.

Wash with distilled water: 1 min.

Put into 5% tungstophosphoric acid: 3 min.

Wash with distilled water: 1 min.

Lay the slides flat on a staining rack and drop the Ladewig solution onto the sections through a folded filter paper. Leave for 30–35 min.

Wash in distilled water: 30 s.

Differentiate in 96% methanol: 30 s.

Wash in distilled water: 30 s.

Dry with filter paper, dip into xylol and cover with mounting medium and cover glass.

A.9.1   Ladewig solution

Aniline blue, water soluble: 0.5 g; Gold orange: 2.0 g; distilled water: 100 ml; add glacial acetic acid: 8 ml.

Mix ingredients and boil the solution. Filter after cooling; add 1.0 g fuchsin acid (rubin S), heat to boiling point, and then cool; filter when cool. Prepare the solution in the fume cupboard. Use gloves and mask. Fuchsin acid is carcinogenic!

The times for staining are calculated for 3 μm section thickness.

A.10   Goldner staining of undecalcified slides (for connective tissue, mineralized bone and osteoid)

Remove the methacrylate and put the slides into distilled water for 10 min.

Stain with haematoxylin (Weigert) at room temperature: 1–2 h. Rinse the slides in cold running tap water: 10 min. Wash with distilled water: 1 min. Put into fuchsin acid solution: 5 min. Wash briefly with acetic acid: 10 s. Differentiate in tungstophosphoric acid Orange G; 1 min. Wash briefly with 1% acetic acid: 10 s. Lightgreen yellowish: 20–25 min. Wash briefly with 1% acetic acid: c 10 s.

Wash with distilled water for 10 s, dry with paper, dip into xylol and cover with mounting medium and cover glass.

A.10.1   Fuchsin acid solution

Ponceau xylidine: 1.0 g; fuchsin acid: 0.5 g; distilled water: 100 ml; glacial acetic acid: 0.2 ml.

A.10.2   Tungstophosphoric acid—Orange G

Tungstophosphoric acid: 4.0 g; distilled water: 100 ml; Orange G: 2.0 g.

A.10.3   Lightgreen solution

Lightgreen yellowish: 0.2 g; distilled water: 100 ml; glacial acetic acid: 0.2 ml.

A.11   Gomori's silver impregnation (for reticulin fibres)

Remove the methacrylate and put the slides into distilled water for 10 min. Decalcify the sections in 3% acidic acid: 5 min. Wash in distilled water (2 ×): 1 min in each.

A.12   Pretreatment of the sections

1% potassium permanganate: 1 min. Rinse in cold running tap water: 2 min. 2% potassium disulphite cryst: 1 min. Rinse in cold running tap water: 2 min. Sensitize in 2% ammonium iron (III) sulphate: 3 min. Rinse in cold running tap water (rinse very quickly to avoid precipitation): 2 min. Wash 2 or 3 times with distilled water: 2 min in each.

A.13   Impregnation

Silver solution: 1 min. Wash with distilled water (2 ×): 1 min in each. Reduce in formaldehyde solution: 1 min. Wash in distilled water (3 or 4 times): 1 min in each. Check the impregnation under the microscope and repeat it until the impregnation is satisfactory. (Repeat 2–3 times, depending on the amount of reticulin fibrils in the section). Dip into the gold chloride solution. Wash with distilled water: 1 min. 2% potassium disulphite: 1 min. 1% sodium thiosulphate: 1 min. Rinse in cold running tap water: 5 min. Wash with distilled water: 1 min. Dry the slides with filter paper, dip into xylol and cover with mounting medium and cover glass.

A.13.1   Solutions

Potassium permanganate: 1 g; distilled water: 100 ml.
Potassium disulphite cryst: 2 g; distilled water: 100 ml.
Ammonium iron (III) sulphate, dodecahydrate: 2 g; distilled water: 100 ml.
Sodium thiosulphate pentahydrate: 1 g; distilled water: 100 ml.

A.13.2   Gold chloride solution

7 ml of a 1% gold chloride solution to 100 ml distilled water.

A.13.3   Silver solution (prepare just before use)

Silver nitrate: 3 g; distilled water: 30 ml. Add 2 ml of 10% caustic potash to 10 ml of the 10% silver solution. Dissolve the brown precipitate with strong ammonia solution (75 ml of c 25% ammonia solution (e.g. Merck No. 5432, BDH) and 25 ml distilled water). Titrate this solution with 10% silver solution until it becomes opalescent. Add several drops of strong ammonia solution until clear. Put the solution into a glass measuring cylinder and add an equal amount of distilled water. Keep the solution in darkness until used.

A.13.4   Formaldehyde solution

35% Formaldehyde solution: 6 ml; tap water: 54 ml.

A.14   B-5 Fixative

Solution A: Mercuric chloride: 6 g; anhydrous sodium acetate 1.25 g; hot distilled water 90 ml. Store at 4°C. Solution B: 10% buffered formalin. Add 1 ml of solution B to 9 ml of solution A immediately prior to use; fix thin blocks for 2–4 h (not longer), rinse and transfer to 70% ethyl alcohol for storage prior to dehydration and impregnation. Mercury crystals must be removed prior to staining with the aid of iodine followed by sodium thiosulphate solution. Buffered formal–acetone is the preferred fixative for cytochemical methods, and is prepared as follows:

Dissolve 20 mg $Na_2 HPO_4$ and 100 mg KH_3PO_4 in a mixture of 45 ml acetone, 30 ml water and 25 ml formalin (40% formaldehyde). The final pH should be about 6.6. Store at 4–10°C.

References

Banks, P. M., Caron, B. and Morgan, T. W. (1983), Use of imprints for monoclonal antibody studies: suitability of air-dried preparations from lymphoid tissues with an immunohistochemical method. *Am. J. clin. Pathol.*, **79**, 438–42.

Bartl, R., Burkhardt, R., Vondracek, H., Sommerfeld, W. and Hagemeister, E. (1978), Rationelle Beckenkammbiopsie. Längsteilung der Proben zur Anwendung von mehreren Präparationsverfahren ohne Materialverlust. *Klin. Wschr.*, **56**, 545–50.

Bordier, F., Matrait, H., Miravet, L. and Hioco, D. (1964), Mesure histologique de la masse et de la resorption des travees osseuses. *Pathol. Biol.*, **12**, 1238–43.

Burkhardt, R. (1971), *Farbatlas der klinischen Histopathologie von Knochenmark und Knochen*, Springer-Verlag, Berlin.

Catovsky, D., Crockard, A. D., Matutes, E. and O'Brien, M. (1981), Cytochemistry of leukaemic cells. In: *Histochemistry. The Widening Horizons of its Applications in the Biomedical Sciences* (eds P. J. Stoward and J. M. Polak), John Wiley and Sons, Chichester, p. 67–87.

Falini, B. and Taylor, C. R. (1983), New developments in immunoperoxidase techniques and their application. *Arch. Pathol. Lab. Med.*, **107**, 105–17.

Frisch, B. and Bartl, R. (1948), Bone marrow biopsies updated. *Biblthca haemat.*, **50**.

Harris, N. L and Data, R. E. (1982), The distribution of neoplastic and normal B-lymphoid cells in nodular lymphomas: use of an immunoperoxidase technique on frozen sections. *Human Pathol.*, **13**, 610–17.

Islam, A. (1982), A new bone marrow biopsy needle with core securing device. *J. clin. Pathol.*, **35**, 359–64.

Jamshidi, K. and Swaim, W. R. (1971), Bone marrow biopsy with unaltered architecture—a new biopsy device. *J. Lab. clin. Med.*, **77**, 335–42.

Janossy, G., Ganeshaguru, K. and Hoffbrand, A. V. (1982), Leukaemia and lymphoma: recent immunological and biochemical developments. In *Recent Advances in Haematology, Vol. 3* (ed. A. V. Hoffbrand), Churchill Livingstone, Edinburgh.

Jasmin, G. (1981), Cell markers. Methods and achievements. In: *Experimental Pathology, Vol. 10*, Karger, Basel.

Leong, A.S.-Y., and Forbes, I. J. (1982), Immunological and histochemical techniques in the study of the malignant lymphomas: a review. *Pathology*, **14**, 247–54.

Pizzola, G., Chilosi, M., Cetto, G. L., Fiore-Donati, L. and Janossy, G. (1982), tive disorders. *Brit. J. Haematol.*, **50**, 95–100.

Polak, J. M. and van Norden, S. (1983), *Immunocytochemistry. Practical Applications in Pathology and Biology.* Wright, Bristol.

Robb-Smith, A. H. T. and Taylor, C. R. (1981), *Lymph Node Biopsy. A Diagnostic Atlas*, Miller Heyden, London.

Stass, S. A., Dean, L., Peiper, S. C. and Bollum, J. F. (1982), Determination of terminal deoxynucleotidyl transferase on bone marrow smears by immunoperoxidase. *Am. J. clin. Pathol.*, **77**, 174–6.

Index